Workbook for

Fordney's Medical Insurance and Billing

Workbook for

Fordney's Medical Insurance and Billing

Sixteenth Edition

Linda M. Smith, CPC, CPC-I, CEMC, CMBS
Training and Consulting
MedOffice Resources
Greene, New York

ELSEVIER

Elsevier
3251 Riverport Lane
St. Louis, Missouri 63043

WORKBOOK FOR FORDNEY'S MEDICAL INSURANCE AND BILLING,   ISBN: 978-0-323-79536-4
SIXTEENTH EDITION

Notice

Practitioners and researchers must always rely on their own experience and knowledge in evaluating and using any information, methods, compounds or experiments described herein. Because of rapid advances in the medical sciences, in particular, independent verification of diagnoses and drug dosages should be made. To the fullest extent of the law, no responsibility is assumed by Elsevier, authors, editors or contributors for any injury and/or damage to persons or property as a matter of products liability, negligence or otherwise, or from any use or operation of any methods, products, instructions, or ideas contained in the material herein.

Previous editions copyrighted 2020, 2016, and 2014.

ISBN: 978-0-323-79536-4

Publishing Director: Kristin Wilhelm
Director, Content Development: Laurie Gower
Senior Content Strategist: Linda Woodard
Content Development Specialist: Brooke Kannady
Publishing Services Manager: Deepthi Unni
Project Manager: Thoufiq Mohammed
Cover Design: Gopalakrishnan Venkatraman

Printed in the United States of America

Last digit is the print number: 9   8   7   6   5   4   3   2

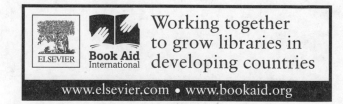

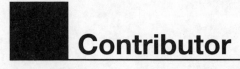

Contributor

Cheryl Fassett, CPC, CPMA, CRC, CDEO, CPB, CPPM, CPC-I
Educator
Practice Manager
Riverside Associates in Anesthesia, PC
Binghamton, New York

Contents

Instruction Guide to the Workbook

LEARNING OBJECTIVES

The student will be able to:

- Define and spell key terms and key abbreviations for each chapter.
- Answer review questions for each chapter of *Fordney's Medical Insurance*.
- Complete assignments to enhance and develop better critical thinking skills.
- Define abbreviations as they appear on a patient record.
- Abstract subjective and objective data from patient records.
- Review documentation on patient records.
- Code professional services properly, using the *Current Procedural Terminology* (CPT) Code Book.
- Select diagnostic code numbers, using the *International Classification of Diseases*, Tenth Revision, Clinical Modifications (ICD-10-CM).
- Locate errors on insurance claims before submission to insurance companies.
- Locate errors on returned insurance claims.
- Carry out collection procedures on delinquent accounts.
- Execute financial management procedures for tracing managed care plans.
- Extract information necessary to complete insurance claim forms from patient records and billing statements/ledger cards.
- Post payments, adjustments, and balances to patients' statements/ledger cards when submitting insurance claims.
- Compute mathematic calculations for Medicare and TRICARE cases.
- Analyze insurance claims for errors in both hospital inpatient and outpatient settings.
- Answer questions about the insurance verification process using patients' health insurance cards.
- Study case scenarios and explain how these violate security and confidentiality and give solutions to prevent the breaches.
- List important activities in each stage of the life cycle of an insurance claim.
- Prepare a cover letter, résumé, job application, and follow-up letter to search for employment.
- Access the Internet and visit websites to research and/or obtain data.

INSTRUCTIONS TO THE STUDENT

The 16th edition of *Workbook for Fordney's Medical Insurance and Billing* has been prepared for those who use the textbook, *Fordney's Medical Insurance and Billing*. It is designed to assist the learner in a practical approach to doing insurance billing and coding.

The key terms and key abbreviations are repeated for quick reference when studying. Each chapter's outline serves as a lecture guide to use for note taking. The review questions in the form of short answer, true/false, multiple choice, and matching are presented to reinforce learning of key concepts for each topic.

Some assignments give students hands-on experience in completing claim forms using National Uniform Claim Committee (NUCC) guidelines. Insurance claim forms and other sample documents that are easily removable are included for practice.

Current procedural and diagnostic code exercises are used throughout to facilitate and enhance coding skills for submitting a claim or making an itemized billing statement.

Critical thinking assignments require skills that help prepare you for real-world scenarios encountered in insurance billing.

KEY TERMS AND KEY ABBREVIATIONS

Key terms and key abbreviations are presented for each chapter, and definitions may be located in the glossary at the end of *Fordney's Medical Insurance and Billing*. It is suggested that you make up 3- by 5-inch index cards for each term or abbreviation and write in the definitions as you encounter them while reading each chapter in the *Fordney's Medical Insurance and Billing*. Doing this will reinforce your knowledge and help you learn the words and abbreviations. Your instructor may wish to select certain words for you to study for pop quizzes.

NOTE TAKING

Taking notes is an important key to success in studying and learning. Note taking helps an individual pay attention during class and retain information. Each chapter has a study outline for organizational purposes, and the outline may be used as a guide for writing down key points during lectures or when studying or reviewing from *Fordney's Medical Insurance and Billing* for tests. Use file cards, notepads, notebooks, computers, or tablets for taking notes. Underline or highlight important words or phrases. To improve the usefulness of notes, try the following format:

1. Using a tablet note-taking app, notepad sheet, or file card, draw a margin 3 inches from the left.
2. Use the left side for topic headings and the right side for notes.
3. Skip a few lines when the topic changes.

4. Write numbers or letters to indicate sub-ideas under a heading.
5. Be brief; do not write down every word except when emphasizing a quotation, rule, or law. Write notes in your own words because that is what you will understand.
6. Use abbreviations that you know how to translate.
7. Listen carefully to the lecture.
8. After the lecture, reread your notes. Highlight the word(s) on the left side of the page to identify the topic of the notes on the right.
9. For study purposes, cover the right side and see if you can explain to yourself or someone else the topic or word.
10. Remember: learning is by doing, and doing is up to you. So take notes for better understanding.

REVIEW QUESTION ASSIGNMENTS

Review questions have been designed to encompass important points for each chapter to assist you in studying insurance billing and coding theory.

SIMULATION ASSIGNMENTS

Assume that you have been hired as an insurance billing specialist and that you are working in a clinic setting for an incorporated group of medical doctors, other allied health specialists, and a podiatrist. You will be asked to complete various assignments. These doctors will be on the staff of a nearby hospital. Appendix A details this clinic's policies and procedures, which you must read completely before beginning the competency-based assignments. Within each chapter, the simulation assignments progress from easy to more complex. Some assignments are given with critical thinking problems, which the instructor may use for class discussion.

Always read the assignment entirely before starting.

MEDICAL TERMINOLOGY AND ABBREVIATIONS

A list of abbreviations is provided in Appendix A to help you learn how to abstract and read physicians' notes. Decode any abbreviations that you do not understand or that are unfamiliar to you. To reinforce learning these abbreviations, write their meanings on the assignment pages. If you do not have a background in medical terminology, it may be wise to use a good medical dictionary as a reference or, better yet, enroll in a terminology course to master that skill.

PATIENT RECORDS

Patient records, financial accounting records (ledgers), and encounter forms are presented, so the learner may have the tools needed to extract information to complete claim forms. Patient records have been abbreviated because of space and page constraints. The records contain pertinent data for each type of case, but it has been necessary to omit a lengthy physical examination. Because detailed documentation is encouraged in medical practices, the records all appear typewritten rather than in handwritten notes. The physician's signature appears after each dated entry on the record.

All the materials included in the assignments have been altered to prevent identification of the cases or parties involved. The names and addresses are fictitious, and no reference to any person living or dead is intended. No evaluation of medical practice or medical advice is to be inferred from the patient records, nor is any recommendation made toward alternative treatment methods or prescribed medications.

FINANCIAL RECORDS

Financial accounting record statements (ledgers) are included for practice in posting, totaling fees, and properly recording appropriate information when an insurance claim is submitted. Refer to Appendix A to obtain information about the Mock Fee Schedule and the physicians' fees for posting to the statements.

CMS-1500 CLAIM FORM

If you have access to a computer, use the practice management software that accompanies the *Workbook* to complete each assignment and print it out for evaluation. To complete the CMS-1500 claim form properly for each type of program, refer to the section in Chapter 14 of *Fordney's Medical Insurance and Billing* that describes in detail the correct information to be put in each block.

Do's and don'ts for claim completion and NUCC guidelines are mentioned in Chapter 14. If you do not have access to a computer, type or neatly write in the information on the insurance form as you abstract it from the patient record.

PERFORMANCE EVALUATION CHECKLIST

The 16th edition features a competency-based format for each assignment indicating performance objectives to let you know what is to be accomplished. The task (job assignment), conditions (elements needed to perform and complete the task), and standards (time management), as well as directions for the specific task, are included.

A two-part performance evaluation checklist used when completing a CMS-1500 claim form is depicted in Figures I.1 and I.2. Reproduce these sheets only for the assignments that involve completing the CMS-1500 claim form. Your instructor will give you the number of points to be assigned for each step.

STUDENT REFERENCE NOTEBOOK

A student reference notebook is recommended so that you can access information quickly to help you complete the *Workbook* assignments. Before beginning the assignments, tear out Appendix A and place it in a three-ring binder with the chapter indexes. Appendix A includes the clinic policies and guidelines, data about the clinic staff, medical and laboratory abbreviations, and the Mock Fee Schedule used while working as an insurance billing specialist for the College Clinic.

Besides these suggestions, you may wish to either tear out or make photocopies of other sections of *Fordney's Medical Insurance and Billing* for your personal use. In addition, your instructor may give you handouts from time to time, pertaining to regional insurance program policies and procedures, to place in your notebook.

TESTS

Tests appear at the end of the *Workbook* to provide a complete, competency-based educational program.

REFERENCE MATERIAL

To do the assignments in this *Workbook* and gain expertise in coding and insurance claims completion, an individual must have access to the books listed here. Addresses for obtaining these materials are given in parentheses. Additional books and booklets on these topics, as well as on Medicaid, Medicare, TRICARE, and more, can be found at bookstores or online retailers.

Dictionary

Dorland's Illustrated Medical Dictionary, 33rd edition, Elsevier, 2020 (6277 Sea Harbor Drive, Orlando, FL 32821-9989; 1-800-545-2522).

Code Books

Current Procedural Terminology, American Medical Association, published annually (515 North State Street, Chicago, IL 60610; 1-800-621-8335).

International Classification of Diseases, Tenth Revision, Clinical Modification, Elsevier, published annually (6277 Sea Harbor Drive, Orlando, FL 32821-9989; 1-800-545-2522).

Word Book

Sloane's Medical Word Book, 5th edition, by Ellen Drake, CMT, FAAMT, Elsevier (6277 Sea Harbor Drive, Orlando, FL 32821-9989; 1-800-545-2522).

Pharmaceutical Book

Optional publications for drug names and descriptions might be either drug books used by nurses (e.g., *Mosby's Gen RX*, Elsevier, published annually [3251 Riverport Lane, St. Louis, MO 63043; 1-800-325-4177; www.elsevier.com]) or ones used by physicians (e.g., *Physician's Desk Reference* [PDR], Medical Economics Company, published annually [5 Paragon Drive, Montvale, NJ, 07645; 1-800-432-4570]).

PERFORMANCE EVALUATION CHECKLIST

Assignment No. _____

Name:_____ Date:_____

Performance Objective

Task: Given access to all necessary equipment and information, the student will complete a CMS-1500 health insurance claim form.

Standards: Claim Productivity Management
Time _____ minutes
Note: Time element may be given by instructor.

Directions: See assignment.

NOTE TIME BEGAN _____ NOTE TIME COMPLETED _____

PROCEDURE STEPS	ASSIGNED POINTS	STEP PERFORMED SATISFACTORY	COMMENTS
1. Assembled CMS-1500 claim form, patient record, E/M code slip, ledger card, computer, pen or pencil, and code books.	_____	_____	_____
2. Posted ledger card correctly.	_____	_____	_____
3. Proofread form for spelling and typographical errors while form remained on computer screen.	_____	_____	_____
4. Points earned for correct completion of CMS-1500 block-by-block data.	_____	_____	_____

Figure I.1

Instruction Guide to the Workbook

PERFORMANCE EVALUATION CHECKLIST

BLOCK	INCORRECT	MISSING	NOT NEEDED	REMARKS	BLOCK	INCORRECT	MISSING	NOT NEEDED	REMARKS
					10				
1A					19				
2					20				
3					21				
4									
5					22				
6					23				
7					24A				
8					24B				
					24C				
9					24D				
9A									
9B									
9C					24E				
9D									
					24F				
10A					24G				
10B					24H, 24I				
10C					24J				
10D									
11					25, 26				
11A					27				
11B					28				
11C					29				
11D									
12					30				
13									
14					31				
15									
16					32				
17									
17A					33				
					Reference Initials				

TOTAL POINTS EARNED: _____

TOTAL POINTS POSSIBLE: _____

Evaluator's signature _____

NEED TO REPEAT: _____

Figure I.2

EMPLOYEE INSURANCE PROCEDURAL MANUAL

If you currently work in a health care office, you may custom design an insurance manual for your organization's practice as you complete insurance claims in this *Workbook*. Obtain a three-ring binder with indexes and label them "Group Plans," "Private Plans," "Medicaid," "Medicare," "Managed Care Plans," "State Disability," "TRICARE," and "Workers' Compensation." If many of your patients have group plans, complete an insurance data or fact sheet for each plan and organize them alphabetically by group plan (Figure I.3).

An insurance manual with fact sheets listing benefits can keep you up to date on policy changes and ensure maximum reimbursement. Fact sheets can be prepared from information obtained when patients bring in their benefit booklets. Obtain and insert a list of the procedures that must be performed as an outpatient and those that must have second opinions for each of the insurance plans.

As you complete the assignments in this *Workbook*, place them in the insurance manual as examples of completed claims for each particular program.

INSURANCE DATA

1. Employer's name _____

2. Address _____Telephone Number _____

3. Insurance Company Contact Person _____

4. Insurance Carrier _____

5. Address _____Telephone Number to Call for Benefits _____

6. Group Policy Number_____

7. Group Account Manager _____Telephone Number _____

8. **Insurance Coverage:**

   Annual Deductible_____ Patient Copayment Percentage _____

   Noncovered Procedures _____

   Maximum Benefits _____

9. **Diagnostic Coverage:**

   Limited Benefits _____

   Maximum Benefits _____

   Noncovered Procedures _____

10. **Major Medical:**

    Annual Deductible_____ Patient Copayment Percentage _____

    Limited Benefits_____

    Maximum Benefits_____

    Noncovered Procedures _____

Mandatory Outpatient Surgeries_____

Second Surgical Opinions _____

Preadmission Certification   Yes _____ No _____   Authorized Labs_____

Payment Plan:

UCR_____ Schedule of Benefits _____ CPT_____RVS_____

Send claims to: _____

_____

Date Entered_____ Date Updated _____

Figure I.3

Role of an Insurance Billing Specialist

Linda M. Smith

KEY TERMS

Your instructor may wish to select some specific words pertinent to this chapter for a test. For definitions of the terms, further study, and/or reference, the words, phrases, and abbreviations may be found in the glossary at the end of the Textbook. Key terms for this chapter follow.

accounts receivable
American Medical Association
cash flow
claims assistance professionals
claims examiner
cycle
dress code
electronic mail
emoticons
errors and omissions insurance
ethics
etiquette
facility billing
health record
independent contractor
insurance billing specialist

management service organizations
medical billing representative
medical record
non-physician practitioners
personal health record
physician extender
professional billing
professional liability insurance
reimbursement specialist
respondeat superior
revenue
self-pay patient
senior billing representative
text speak

KEY ABBREVIATIONS

See how many abbreviations and acronyms you can translate and then use this as a handy reference list. Definitions for the key abbreviations are located near the back of the Textbook in the glossary.

AMA _____

_____

_____

ASHD _____

CAPs _____

e-mail _____

_____

MSOs _____

NPPs _____

PERFORMANCE OBJECTIVES

The student will be able to:

- Define and spell the key terms and key abbreviations for this chapter, given the information from the *Textbook* glossary, within a reasonable time period and with enough accuracy to obtain a satisfactory evaluation.
- Answer the fill-in-the-blank, multiple choice, and true/false review questions after reading the chapter, with enough accuracy to obtain a satisfactory evaluation.

- Use critical thinking to write one or two grammatically correct paragraphs with sufficient information to obtain a satisfactory evaluation.
- Visit websites and site-search information via the Evolve website at http://evolve.elsevier.com/Smith/Fordneys/, with sufficient information to obtain a satisfactory evaluation.

1

STUDY OUTLINE

ASSIGNMENT 1.1 REVIEW QUESTIONS

Part I Fill in the Blank
Review the objectives, key terms, and chapter information before completing the following review questions.

1. Name some of the settings where facility billing is used.

   a. _____

   b. _____

   c. _____

   d. _____

   e. _____

2. Name some of the various types of providers who use professional billing.

   a. _____

   b. _____

   c. _____

   d. _____

   c. _____

3. Name examples of non-physician practitioners (NPPs).

   a. _____

   b. _____

   c. _____

   d. _____

   e. _____

   f. _____

   g. _____

   h. _____

4. Name several job titles associated with medical billing personnel in both small and large health care organizations.

   a. _____

   b. _____

   c. _____

5. List some of the responsibilities and duties an insurance billing specialist might perform generally, as well as when acting as a collection manager. Refer to the section on "Job Responsibilities" in Figs. 1.2 and 1.3 of the text.

   a. _____

   b. _____

   c. _____

   d. _____

   e. _____

   f. _____

   g. _____

6. List the duties of the claims assistance professionals (CAPs).

   a. _____

   b. _____

   c. _____

7. Insurance claims must be promptly submitted within _____ business days to ensure continuous cash flow.

8. Define *cash flow*.

   _____

9. An individual who takes a patient to a private area before their visit with the provider to discuss the practice's financial policies and review the patient's insurance coverage.

   _____

10. Reasons for a medical practice's large accounts receivable are:

    a. _____

    b. _____

    c. _____

    d. _____

11. Skills required for an insurance billing specialist are:

    a. _____

    b. _____

    c. _____

    d. _____

e. _____

f. _____

g. _____

h. _____

i. _____

j. _____

12. Standards of conduct by which an insurance billing specialist determines the propriety of his or her behavior in a relationship are known as _____.

13. Complete these statements with either the word *illegal* or *unethical*.

    a. To make critical remarks about another health care organization or physician is _____.

    b. To report incorrect information to a Medicare fiscal intermediary is _____.

14. When a physician is legally responsible for an employee's conduct during employment, it is known as _____.

15. A claims assistance professional (CAP) neglects to submit an insurance claim to a Medicare supplemental insurance carrier within the proper time limit. What type of insurance is needed for protection against this loss for the client?

    _____

Part II Multiple Choice

Choose the best answer.

16. Two billing components are facility billing and professional billing. Professional billing is done for:
    a. hospitals.
    b. skilled nursing facilities.
    c. ambulatory surgical centers.
    d. physicians.

17. *Physician extenders* are health care personnel trained to provide medical care under the direct or indirect supervision of a physician are also referred to as:
    a. independent contractors.
    b. claims assistance professionals (CAPs).
    c. non-physician practitioners (NPPs).
    d. insurance billing specialists.

18. The individual responsible for documenting the patient's clinical notes for assignment of a diagnosis code and procedure code for medical services rendered is a/an:
    a. physician.
    b. insurance biller.
    c. office manager.
    d. financial accounting clerk.

19. Insurance payers that require the provider to submit insurance claims for the patient are:
    a. federal and state programs.
    b. private insurance plans.
    c. managed care programs.
    d. health care insurance plans.

20. Facility billing is charging for services done by:
    a. hospitals.
    b. physicians.
    c. ambulatory surgical centers.
    d. both a and c.

Part III True/False

Write "T" or "F" in the blank to indicate whether you think the statement is true or false.

_____ 21. Insurance billing specialists have a well-defined scope of practice.

_____ 22. If you knowingly submit a false claim or allow such a claim to be submitted, you can be liable for a civil violation.

_____ 23. It is the coder's responsibility to inform the administration or his or her immediate supervisor if unethical or illegal coding practices are occurring.

_____ 24. Claims assistant professionals (CAPs) can interpret insurance policies for patients.

_____ 25. Independent contractors are covered under the health care organization's professional liability insurance whom they provide services to.

CRITICAL THINKING

To enhance your critical thinking skills, problems will be interspersed throughout the *Workbook*. Thinking is the goal of instruction and a student's responsibility. When trying to solve a problem by critical thinking, it is desirable to have more than one solution and to take time to think out answers. Remember that an answer may be changed when additional information is provided in a classroom setting.

ASSIGNMENT 1.2 CRITICAL THINKING

Performance Objective

Task: Describe why you are training to become an insurance billing specialist.

Conditions: Use one or two sheets of white typing paper and a pen or pencil.

Standards: Time: _____ minutes

             Accuracy: _____

             (Note: The time element and accuracy criteria may be given by your instructor.)

Directions: Write one or two paragraphs describing why you are training to become an insurance billing specialist. Or, if enrolled in a class that is part of a medical assisting course, explain why you are motivated to seek a career as a medical assistant. Make sure grammar, punctuation, and spelling are correct.

Performance Objective

Task: Access the Internet and visit several websites.

Conditions: Use a computer with a printer and/or a pen or pencil to make notes.

Standards: Time: _____ minutes

                       Accuracy: _____

                       (Note: The time element and accuracy criteria may be given by your instructor.)

Directions: Use a computer and use a browser to access the Internet. Go to some search engines to locate job opportunities.

1. Access the Internet and find one of the web search engines (Yahoo, Google, Bing). Begin a web search (e.g., key in "insurance billers") to search for information about insurance billers. List three to five websites found. Go to one or more of those resources and list the benefits that those sites might have for a student in locating job opportunities or networking with others for professional growth and knowledge. Bring the website addresses to share with the class.

2. Site-search information on standards of ethical coding by visiting the website of the American Health Information Management Association (AHIMA). Download and print a hard copy of this code of ethics developed by the AHIMA.

3. Site-search information on the standards of ethical coding by visiting the website of the American Academy of Professional Coders (AAPC). Download and print a hard copy of this code of ethics developed by the AAPC.

4. Site-search information to determine the median salary for a Certified Professional Biller (CPB) by visiting the website of the American Academy of Professional Coders AAPC).

ASSIGNMENT 1.4 COMPOSE EMAIL MESSAGES

Performance Objective

Task: Compose brief messages for electronic mail transmission after reading each scenario.

Conditions: List of scenarios, one sheet of 8½- × 11-inch plain typing paper, and a computer or a pen.

Standards: Time: _____ minutes

        Accuracy: _____

        (Note: The time element and accuracy criteria may be given by your instructor.)

Directions: Read each scenario. Compose polite, effective, and brief messages that, on the job, would be transmitted via e-mail. Be sure to list a descriptive subject line as the first item in each composition. Single-space the message. Insert a short signature at the end of the message to include your name and affiliation, and create an e-mail address for yourself if you do not have one. Print hard copies of e-mail messages for Scenarios 1 through 5 to give to your instructor. After the instructor has returned your work, either make the necessary corrections and place your work in a three-ring notebook for future reference or, if you received a high score, place it in your portfolio for use when applying for a job.

Scenario 1:

Ask an insurance biller, Mary Davis, in a satellite office to locate and fax you a copy of the billing done on account number 43500 for services rendered to Margarita Sylva on March 2, 20xx. Explain that you must telephone the patient about her account. Mary Davis' e-mail address is mdavis@aal.com.

Scenario 2:

Patient Ellen Worth was recently hospitalized; her hospital number is 20–9870-11. Compose an e-mail message to the medical record department at College Hospital (collegehospmedrecords@rrv.net) for her final diagnosis and the assigned diagnostic code needed to complete the insurance claim form.

Scenario 3:

You are working for a billing service and receive an encounter form that is missing the information about the patient's professional service received on August 2, 20xx. The patient's account number is 45098. You have the diagnosis data. Compose an e-mail message to Dr. Mason (pmason@email.mc.com) explaining what you must obtain to complete the billing portion of the insurance claim form.

Scenario 4:

A new patient, John Phillips, has e-mailed your office to ask what the outstanding balance is on his account. The account number is 42990. You look up the financial record and note the service was for an office visit on June 14, 20xx. The charge was $106.11. Compose an e-mail response to Mr. Phillips, whose e-mail address is jphillips@hotmail.com.

Chapter **1** **Role of an Insurance Billing Specialist**

2 Privacy, Security, and HIPAA

Cheryl Fassett

KEY TERMS

Your instructor may wish to select some specific words pertinent to this chapter for a test. For definitions of the terms, further study, and/or reference, the words, phrases, and abbreviations may be found in the glossary at the end of the Textbook. Key terms for this chapter follow.

Administrative safeguards
American Recovery and Reinvestment Act
authorization
authorization form
breach
business associate
clearinghouse
confidential communication
confidentiality
consent
covered entity
designated record sets
disclosure
electronic protected health information
health care organization
health care provider
Health Information Technology for Economic and Clinical Health Act
Health Insurance Portability and Accountability Act
HIPAA Omnibus Rule
Incidental use and disclosure

individually identifiable health information
Minimum Necessary Rule
mitigation
National Provider Identifier
nonprivileged information
Notice of Privacy Practices
Patient Protection and Affordable Care Act of 2010
portability
preexisting condition
privacy
privacy officer, privacy official
privacy rule
privileged information
protected health information
psychotherapy notes
security officer
Security Rule
State preemption
transaction
use

KEY ABBREVIATIONS

See how many abbreviations and acronyms you can translate, and then use this as a handy reference list. Definitions for the key abbreviations are located near the back of the Textbook *in the glossary.*

ARRA _____

CMS _____

DHHS _____

EIN _____

ePHI _____

FBI _____

FTP _____

HHS _____

HIPAA _____

HITECH _____

IIHI _____

NPI _____

NPP _____

OCR _____

OIG _____

P&P _____

PHI _____

PO _____

PPACA _____

TPO _____

The student will be able to:

- Define and spell the key terms and key abbreviations for this chapter, given the information from the Textbook glossary, within a reasonable time period and with enough accuracy to obtain a satisfactory evaluation.
- Answer the fill in the blank, multiple choice, and true/false review questions after reading the chapter, with enough accuracy to obtain a satisfactory evaluation.

- Decide when a situation is an incidental disclosure, HIPAA violation, or neither, with sufficient information to obtain a satisfactory evaluation.
- Research HIPAA and HIPAA violations on the internet.

STUDY OUTLINE

Health Information Portability and Accountability
Title I: Health Insurance Reform
Title II: Administrative Simplification
Transaction and Code Set Regulations
National Identifiers
The Privacy Rule: Confidentiality and Protected Health Information
Privacy, Confidentiality, Use and Disclosure
Covered Entities
Business Associates
Protected Health Information
Individually Identifiable Health Information
Privileged and Nonprivileged Information
Designated Record Set
Psychotherapy Notes
Consent and Authorization
Verification of Identity and Authority
Minimum Necessary Rule
Incidental Uses and Disclosures
State Preemption
Exceptions to HIPAA
    Patient Right's Under HIPAA
    1. Required Notice of Privacy Practices
    2. Restrictions on Certain Uses and Disclosures of PHI
    3. Confidential Communications
    4. Access to PHI

5. Amendment of PHI
6. Accounting of Disclosure of PHI
The Security Rule: Administrative, Technical, and Physical Safeguards
Administrative Safeguards
Technical Safeguards
Physical Safeguards
Health Information Technology for Economic and Clinical Health Act
Business Associates
Notification of Breach
HIPAA Omnibus Rule
HIPAA Compliance Audits
Consequences of Noncompliance with HIPAA and the HITECH Act
Penalties for Noncompliance with the Provisions of HIPAA
Refraining from Intimidating or Retaliatory Acts
Examples of Recent HIPAA Violations
Organization and Staff Responsibilities in Protecting Patient Rights
Obligations of the Health Care Organization
HIPAA and Social Media
Best Practices to Avoid Common HIPAA Violations

ASSIGNMENT 2.1 REVIEW QUESTIONS

Part I Fill in the Blank

Review the objectives, key terms, and chapter information before completing the following review questions.

1. What is the primary purpose of HIPAA Title I: Insurance Reform?

   _____

   _____

2. The focus on the health care practice setting and reduction of administrative costs and burdens are the goals of which part of HIPAA?

   _____

3. An independent organization that receives insurance claims from the physician's office, performs edits, and transmits claims to insurance carriers is known as a/an

   _____.

4. Name the standard code sets used for the following:

   a. Drugs and supplies _____

   b. Inpatient procedures _____

   c. Diagnosis coding _____

5. Under HIPAA guidelines, a health care coverage carrier, such as Blue Cross/Blue Shield, that transmits health information in electronic form in connection with a transaction is called a/an _____

   _____.

6. Dr. John Doe contracts with an outside billing company to manage claims and accounts receivable. Under HIPAA guidelines, the billing company is considered a/an _____ of the provider.

7. An individual designated to assist the provider by putting compliance policies and procedures regarding privacy and confidentiality in place and training office staff is known as a/an _____ under HIPAA guidelines.

8. If you give, release, or transfer information to another entity, it is known as

   _____

9. Define *protected health information* (PHI).

   _____

   _____

   _____

10. Unauthorized release of a patient's health information is called _____.

11. A confidential communication related to the patient's treatment and progress that may be disclosed only with the patient's permission is known as

_____

12. Under HIPAA, exceptions to the right of privacy are those records involving

a. _____

b. _____

c. _____

d. _____

e. _____

f. _____

g. _____

h. _____

13. At a patient's first visit, under HIPAA guidelines, the document that must be given so the patient acknowledges the provider's confidentiality of their PHI is the

_____.

14. If a breach of privacy is discovered, the health care provider is required to take affirmative action to respond to the breach and alleviate the severity of it. This is known as

_____

15. Name the three main sections of the HIPAA Security Rule for protecting electronic health information.

a. _____

b. _____

c. _____

16. Name the three specific areas of significant change that resulted from the Health Information Technology for Economic and Clinical Health (HITECH) Act.

a. _____

b. _____

c. _____

Part II Multiple Choice

Choose the best answer.

17. HIPAA transaction standards apply to the following, which are called *covered entities*:
    a. health care third-party payers.
    b. health care providers.
    c. health care clearinghouses.
    d. all of the above.

18. Oversight of the privacy standards of HIPAA is the responsibility of the:
    a. Health Care Fraud and Abuse Control Program (HCFAP).
    b. National Committee on Vital and Health Statistics (NCVHS).
    c. Office for Civil Rights (OCR).
    d. Federal Bureau of Investigation (FBI).

19. Verbal or written agreement that gives approval to some action, situation, or statement is called:
    a. authorization.
    b. consent.
    c. disclosure.
    d. release.

20. An individual's formal written permission to use or disclose his or her personally identifiable health information for purposes other than treatment, payment, or health care operations is called:
    a. authorization.
    b. disclosure.
    c. release.
    d. consent.

21. The Notice of Privacy Practices (NPP) document is given to patients:
    a. at the first visit to the practice.
    b. at every visit to the practice.
    c. on an annual basis.
    d. only on request of the patient.

22. Privacy regulations allow patients the right to obtain a copy of psychotherapy notes:
    a. under all circumstances.
    b. if they have a court order.
    c. only if the mental health provider has determined that it would be appropriate and it is allowed under state law.
    d. only if the patient can pay the associated fee for the copies.

23. Under HIPAA, patient sign-in sheets:
    a. are never permissible.
    b. are permissible.
    c. are permissible but limit the information that is requested.
    d. are permissible but require the practice to give the patient a number to be used when calling the patient.

24. Which section of the HIPAA Security Rule recommends unique usernames and passwords to log on to any computer with access to PHI?
    a. Administrative safeguards
    b. Technical safeguards
    c. Physical safeguards

25. Which section of the HIPAA Security Rule recommends use of screensavers that will activate after 1 to 60 minutes of inactivity?
    a. Administrative safeguards
    b. Technical safeguards
    c. Physical safeguards

26. Under HITECH, if a breach occurs, the covered entity:
    a. does not have to notify the affected party.
    b. only has to notify the affected party if they feel it is reasonable.
    c. must notify the affected party no later than 30 calendar days after the discovery of the breach.
    d. must notify the affected party no later than 60 calendar days after the discovery of the breach.

27. The HIPAA Omnibus Rule enhanced:
    a. patients' privacy rights and protections.
    b. patients' rights to restrict immunization records to schools.
    c. health care providers' rights limiting access to patient records.
    d. business associates' rights to use and disclose patient records.

28. Measurable solutions that have been taken, based on accepted standards, and are periodically monitored to demonstrate that an office is in compliance with HIPAA privacy rules are referred to as:
    a. reasonable safeguards.
    b. privacy safeguards.
    c. security safeguards.
    d. standards.

29. A person or organization that performs a function for a covered entity but is not employed by them is a/an:
    a. business associate.
    b. clearinghouse.
    c. provider.
    d. employee.

30. Health information that does not identify the patient is called:
    a. confidential communication.
    b. nonprivileged information.
    c. de-identified health information.
    d. protected health information.

Part III True/False

Write "T" or "F" in the blank to indicate whether you think the statement is true or false.

_____ 31. Individually identifiable health information (IIHI) is any part of a person's health data (e.g., demographic information, address, date of birth) obtained from the patient that is created or received by a covered entity.

_____ 32. HIPAA requirements protect disclosure of PHI outside of the organization but do not protect against internal use of health information.

_____ 33. Under HIPAA, patients may request confidential communications and may restrict certain disclosures of PHI.

_____ 34. It is not necessary to turn documents over or lock them in a secure drawer if you are only leaving your desk for a few moments.

_____ 35. Texting on cellphones is a secure method for discussing patient care.

_____ 36. Under HIPAA privacy regulations, patients do not have the right to access psychotherapy notes.

_____ 37. The HITECH Act requires that business associates comply with the HIPAA Security Rule in the same manner that a covered entity would.

_____ 38. A billing specialist does not need to be concerned about HIPAA violations because only providers may face penalties and imprisonment.

_____ 39. An allowable incidental disclosure occurs when someone hears you discussing a patient over dinner.

_____ 40. The penalty for violating HIPAA and HITECH can be $100 to $50,000 or more per violation.

ASSIGNMENT 2.2 CRITICAL THINKING: INCIDENTAL DISCLOSURE VERSUS HIPAA VIOLATION

Performance Objective

Task: Make a decision using your best judgment after reading each case study regarding whether it should be considered an incidental disclosure, a HIPAA violation, or neither.

Conditions: Use a pen or pencil.

Standards: Time: _____ minutes

Accuracy: _____

(Note: The time element and accuracy criteria may be given by your instructor.)

Directions: Read through each case study. Use your best judgment and circle whether you think it is an incidental disclosure (ID), a HIPAA violation (V), or neither (N). Briefly explain the answer that you selected.

Scenarios

1. Dr. Practon's office sign-in sheets ask patients to fill in their names, appointment times, and physicians' names.

   ID   V   N

   Explain:

   _____

   _____

2. It is Monday morning and you are inundated with work that needs to be done. You receive a telephone call and give patient information without confirming who is on the line.

   ID   V   N

   Explain:

   _____

   _____

3. You send a fax, but accidentally you switch the last two digits of the fax number and the patient's billing information is received in the wrong location.

   ID   V   N

   Explain:

   _____

   _____

4. You are in a high-traffic area where patients might overhear PHI, and you are careful to keep your voice down.

   ID   V   N

   Explain:

   _____

   _____

5. It is 10:30 am, and you go on a coffee break, leaving two patients' charts on the checkout counter.

    ID   V   N

    Explain:

    _____

    _____

6. In the reception room, a patient overhears your telephone conversation, even though you spoke quietly and shut the glass window.

    ID   V   N

    Explain:

    _____

    _____

7. You telephone a patient, Alex Massey, to remind him of tomorrow's appointment and leave a voicemail message on his answering machine.

    ID   V   N

    Explain:

    _____

    _____

8. Three patients near the reception area of the office overhear you telling another staff member that Daisy Dotson is scheduled for a Pap smear tomorrow at 4:00 pm.

    ID   V   N

    Explain:

    _____

    _____

9. You telephone a patient. She is not home, so you leave a message on her answering machine that her breast cancer biopsy results came back negative.

    ID   V   N

    Explain:

    _____

    _____

10. You call out Fran O'Donnell's complete name in the waiting room where other patients are sitting.

    ID   V   N

    Explain:

    _____

    _____

11. You do not close the glass window to the reception room when talking on the telephone with your sister.

ID   V   N

Explain:

_____

_____

12. The office nurse tells a patient, Hugo Wells, his test results in front of his relatives in a treatment area.

ID   V   N

Explain:

_____

_____

13. You leave Katy Zontag's medical chart open at the receptionist's counter.

ID   V   N

Explain:

_____

_____

14. You telephone a patient, José Ramirez, and leave your name, the physician's name, and your telephone number on his answering machine.

ID   V   N

Explain:

_____

_____

15. A patient, Kim Lee, is in the examination room and overhears a conversation concerning blood test results of another patient in an adjoining room. The doors to both examination rooms had been left ajar.

ID   V   N

Explain:

_____

_____

16. While waiting in the reception room, a patient, Xavier Gomez, overhears a receptionist talking with another patient on the telephone about a colonoscopy appointment. There was a closed window between the waiting area and the receptionist.

ID   V   N

Explain:

_____

_____

17. Betty Burton, a patient who is being weighed on the office scale by the medical assistant, overhears a conversation between an insurance billing specialist and an insurance company representative in which the billing specialist is trying to obtain preauthorization for another patient's medical procedure.

    ID   V   N

    Explain:

    _____

    _____

18. In a restaurant, a waitress overhears an insurance biller talking to a friend and telling her about a famous actress who visited her physician's office yesterday.

    ID   V   N

    Explain:

    _____

    _____

    _____

    _____

Performance Objective

Task:	Access the Internet and visit several websites.
Conditions:	Use a computer with printer and/or a pen or pencil to make notes.
Standards:	Time: _____ minutes
	Accuracy: _____
	(Note: The time element and accuracy criteria may be given by your instructor.)

Directions: Use a computer and use a browser to access the Internet. Go to some search engines to locate information.

1. Find information on patient confidentiality by visiting the website of the American Medical Association (www. ama-assn.org). At top left, click menu, click on Patient Care and then click on Ethics. Find information on patient confidentiality in health care by clicking on Ethics of Privacy, Confidentiality and Medical Records. Locate an article and print a hard copy to share and discuss with the class.

2. Search for information of settled HIPAA investigations by visiting the website for the Department of Human Services/ Office for Civil Rights (https://www.hhs.gov/hipaa/for-professionals/index.html) and click "Newsroom" at the top right. Print out a press release to share and discuss with the class.

Compliance, Fraud, and Abuse

Cheryl Fassett

KEY TERMS

Your instructor may wish to select some specific words pertinent to this chapter for a test. For definitions of the terms, further study, and/or reference, the words, phrases, and abbreviations may be found in the glossary at the end of the Textbook. Key terms for this chapter follow.

Abuse
Anti-Kickback Law
assumption coding
auditing
Civil False Claims Act
Civil Monetary Penalty
Clinical Laboratory Improvement Amendments
clustering
compliance
compliance plan
Comprehensive Error Rate Testing
corrective action plan
cost reports
Criminal False Claims Act
DRG upcoding/DRG creep
embezzlement
Emergency Medical Treatment and Labor Act
Exclusion Statute
Federal Deposit Insurance Corporation
fraud
Fraud Enforcement and Recovery Act
Health Care Fraud and Abuse Control

Health Care Fraud Prevention and Enforcement Action Team
kickback
medical necessity
Medicare Administrative Contractor
Medicare Integrity Program
monitoring
Occupational Safety and Health Administration
Office of the Inspector General
OIG Work Plan
Operation Restore Trust
patient dumping
phantom bills
Physician Self-Referral Law
qui tam
Recovery Audit Contractor
safe harbor
Self-Disclosure Protocol
Stark Law
undercoding
upcoding
Zone Program Integrity Contractor

KEY ABBREVIATIONS

See how many abbreviations and acronyms you can translate and then use this as a handy reference list. Definitions for the key abbreviations are located near the back of the Textbook *in the glossary.*

CERT _____

CLIA _____

CMP _____

CMS _____

DHHS _____

DOJ _____

EMTALA _____

FCA _____

FDIC _____

FERA _____

HCFAC _____

HEAT _____

MAC _____

MIP _____

OIG _____

ORT _____

OSHA _____

P&P _____

PPACA _____

RAC _____

SDP _____

ZPIC _____

23

PERFORMANCE OBJECTIVES

The student will be able to:

- Define and spell the key terms and key abbreviations for this chapter, given the information from the *Textbook* glossary, within a reasonable time period and with enough accuracy to obtain a satisfactory evaluation.
- Answer the fill-in-the-blank, multiple choice, and true/false review questions after reading the chapter, with enough accuracy to obtain a satisfactory evaluation.
- Make decisions after reading scenarios regarding whether the situations are considered fraud, abuse, or neither, with sufficient information to obtain a satisfactory evaluation.

STUDY OUTLINE

Compliance Defined
Fraud and Abuse Laws
    False Claims Act (1863)
    Exclusion Statute (42 US Code §1320a-7)
    Stark Laws (42 US Code §1395nn)
    Anti-Kickback Statute (42 US Code §1320a-7b[b])
    Civil Monetary Penalties Law (41 US Code §1320a-7a)
    Operation Restore Trust
    Additional Laws and Compliance
    Examples of Recent Fraud and Abuse Cases
Compliance Audits and Oversight
    Recovery Audit Program
    Medicare and Medicaid Integrity Programs
    Zone Program Integrity Contractors

    Comprehensive Error Rate Testing
    Health Care Fraud Prevention and Enforcement Action Team
    Special Alerts, Bulletins and Guidance Documents
Compliance Programs
    Purpose of a Compliance Plan
    Basic Components of a Compliance Plan
OIG Compliance Program Guidelines
    Individual and Small Group Practices
    Third-Party Medical Billing Companies
    Hospitals
What to Expect From Your Health Care Organization

Part I Fill in the Blank

Review the objectives, key terms, and chapter information before completing the following review questions.

1. *Compliance* is the process of

   _____

   _____

2. What is the first step health insurance specialists should take toward achieving compliance so they do not violate laws that could result in penalties or fines?

   _____

3. Indicate whether each of the following situations is one of fraud or abuse.

   a. Under the FCA, billing a claim for services not medically necessary _____

   b. Changing a figure on an insurance claim form to get increased payment _____

   c. Dismissing the copayment owed by a Medicare patient _____

   d. Neglecting to refund an overpayment to the patient _____

   e. Billing for a complex fracture when the patient suffered a simple break _____

4. The OIG publication that lists guidelines for compliance programs is the

   _____

5. CLIA certifies _____.

6. The law that prohibits self-referrals is the _____.

7. The term for providing appropriate care for the diagnosis is _____.

8. Accepting a gift for referring a patient to a specific physical therapy group is a

   _____

9. According to the Affordable Care Act, the seven steps required for an effective compliance program are:

   a. _____

   b. _____

   c. _____

   d. _____

   e. _____

   f. _____

   g. _____

10. The statute that requires the OIG to exclude individuals, providers, and health care organizations from participating in federal health care programs if they are found guilty of fraud or abuse is the _____.

Part II Multiple Choice

Choose the best answer.

11. One of the agencies charged with enforcing laws that regulate the health care industry is the:
    a. Drug Enforcement Agency (DEA).
    b. Office of the Inspector General (OIG).
    c. Committee on Vital and Health Statistics (NCVHS).
    d. Department of Internal Affairs (DIA).

12. Stealing money that has been entrusted in one's care is referred to as:
    a. fraud.
    b. abuse
    c. embezzlement.
    d. obstruction.

13. Under the Criminal False Claims Act, fines and imprisonment penalties for making a false claim in connection with payment for health care benefits can be imposed on:
    a. the physician who provided the services.
    b. the health care billing specialist who prepared the claim.
    c. the health care administrator who oversees the practice or organization.
    d. anyone who knowingly and willfully participated in the scheme.

14. The FCA provision that allows a private citizen to bring civil action for a violation on behalf of the federal government and share in any money recovered is referred to as:
    a. minimum necessary.
    b. qui tam.
    c. privileged information.
    d. exclusion statute.

15. The initiative that allowed the public to report issues that might indicate fraud, abuse, or waste is:
    a. Operation Restore Trust (ORT).
    b. Civil Monetary Penalty (CMP).
    c. Health Care Fraud Prevention and Enforcement Action Team (HEAT).
    d. Recovery Audit Contractor (RAC).

16. Health care providers who determine that they have submitted false claims should resolve the issue by seeking the Department of Health and Human Services (DHHS) and OIG guidance established in 2006 and referred to as:
    a. Operation Restore Trust.
    b. Stark I and II.
    c. Self-Disclosure Protocol.
    d. Safe Harbor.

17. The OIG recommends that health care staff should attend trainings in "general" compliance:
    a. as part of their initial orientation.
    b. at least annually.

    c. every 6 months.
    d. every 6 years.

18. When faced with a compliance offense or an error, health care organizations may receive reduced damages if:
    a. they submit a formal written apology to the OIG.
    b. they self-disclose the violation within 30 days of discovery.
    c. they conduct a thorough investigation and take corrective action.
    d. B and C.

19. Compliance is the responsibility of:
    a. physicians.
    b. coders.
    c. anyone working in health care.
    d. the compliance officer.

20. The following are parts of a well-rounded compliance program recommended by the OIG except:
    a. policies and procedures.
    b. staff education.
    c. open lines of communication.
    d. practice management software.

21. The OIG has published compliance guidelines for all of the following except:
    a. hospitals.
    b. private physician groups.
    c. patients.
    d. billing companies.

22. The law that states that emergency rooms must evaluate and stabilize patients regardless of ability to pay is called:
    a. EMTALA.
    b. The Stark Law.
    c. Anti-Kickback Statute.
    d. False Claims Act.

23. Fraudulent claims may include:
    a. multiple modifiers.
    b. unbundled codes.
    c. more than one diagnosis code.
    d. place of service codes.

24. Penalties for submitting false claims include:
    a. jail time.
    b. monetary penalties.
    c. termination.
    d. all of the above.

25. The purpose of an RAC audit is to:
    a. recoup overpayments.
    b. determine if a provider is clinically sound.
    c. investigate discrimination.
    d. all of the above.

Part III True/False

Write "T" or "F" in the blank to indicate whether you think the statement is true or false.

_____ 26. Every compliance program should include a method for employees to report issues anonymously.

_____ 27. To submit an insurance claim for medical services that were not medically necessary is a violation of the FCA.

_____ 28. Organizations that hire or contract with individuals who have been convicted of a misdemeanor or criminal offense and are on the OIG's list of excluded individuals may be subject to civil monetary penalties.

_____ 29. In the federal health care program, accepting discounts, rebates, or other types of reductions in price is encouraged.

_____ 30. Recovery audit contractors are highly motivated to find claim errors, as they are paid a percentage of the money they recover.

_____ 31. If fraud and abuse are detected, Zone Program Integrity Contractors (ZPICs) report to the Department of Justice (DOJ) for further investigation.

_____ 32. In the event of an OIG audit, the presence of an OIG compliance program will prevent any penalties and fines from being imposed.

_____ 33. Disciplinary standards for situations involving misconduct may result in termination of employment.

_____ 34. Hospitals are allowed to give free office space to physicians who use their radiology and laboratory departments.

_____ 35. In a qui tam lawsuit, the whistleblower shares in penalty money.

_____ 36. Reporting a higher level of service than the patient received is called up-coding.

_____ 37. A coding or billing specialist cannot be found guilty of fraud.

_____ 38. It is fraudulent to always adjust off deductibles and coinsurance.

_____ 39. If a health care organization receives an overpayment from a third-party payer, it is compliant to apply the amount to another patient's balance.

_____ 40. When a patient is transferred from one hospital to another, it is fraudulent for the first hospital to bill for a discharge.

Performance Objective

Task:　　　　Make a decision after reading each case study regarding whether it is considered fraud, abuse, or neither.

Conditions:　Use a pen or pencil.

Standards:　Time: _____ minutes

　　　　　　Accuracy: _____

　　　　　　(Note: The time element and accuracy criteria may be given by your instructor.)

Directions: Read through each scenario and circle whether it is a fraud (F) issue, practice of abuse (A), or neither (N). To distinguish the difference between fraud and abuse situations, remember that under the Medicare program, abuse relates to incidents or practices that are inconsistent with accepted sound business practices, whereas fraud is intentional deception that an individual knows, or should know, to be false, and the individual knows the deception could result in some unauthorized benefit to himself or herself or to some other person(s). Briefly explain the answer you selected.

Scenarios

1. Dr. Pedro Atrics has a friend whose child needs elective surgery. He agrees to perform the surgery and bill as an "insurance only" case.

　F　　A　　N

　Explain:

　_____

　_____

2. A patient, Carl Skinner, calls the office repeatedly about his prescriptions. When seen in the office the next time, Dr. Input bills a higher level of evaluation and management service to allow for the additional time.

　F　　A　　N

　Explain:

　_____

　_____

3. Dr. Skeleton sets a simple fracture and puts a cast on Mr. Davis. He bills for a complex fracture.

　F　　A　　N

　Explain:

　_____

　_____

4. A patient, Maria Gomez, asks a friendly staff member to change the dates on the insurance claim form. The medical assistant complies with the request.

　F　　A　　N

　Explain:

　_____

　_____

5. A patient, Roberto Loren, asks the physician to restate a diagnosis so the insurance company will pay because payment would be denied based on the present statement. The physician complies with the request.

   F   A   N

   Explain:

   _____

   _____

6. Dr. Rumsey sees a patient twice on the same day but bills as though the patient was seen on two different dates.

   F   A   N

   Explain:

   _____

   _____

7. A Medicare patient, Joan O'Connor, is seen by Dr. Practon, and the insurance claim shows a charge to the Medicare fiscal intermediary at a fee schedule rate higher than and different from that of non-Medicare patients.

   F   A   N

   Explain:

   _____

   _____

8. A patient, Hazel Plunkett, receives a service that is not medically necessary to the extent rendered, and an insurance claim is submitted.

   F   A   N

   Explain:

   _____

   _____

9. A patient, Sun Cho, paid for services that were subsequently declared not medically necessary, and Dr. Cardi failed to refund the payment to the patient.

   F   A   N

   Explain:

   _____

   _____

10. Dr. Ulibarri tells the insurance biller not to collect the deductible and copayments from Mrs. Gerry Coleman.

    F   A   N

    Explain:

    _____

    _____

Performance Objective

Task: Access the Internet and visit several websites.

Conditions: Use a computer with a printer and/or a pen or pencil to make notes.

Standards: Time: _____ minutes

                   Accuracy: _____

                   (Note: The time element and accuracy criteria may be given by your instructor.)

Directions: Use a computer and use a browser to access the Internet. Go to some search engines to locate information.

1. Search for information on fraud and abuse by visiting one or more of the federal websites. See what you can discover and either print out or take notes and bring back information to share with the class for discussion.

2. Search the AAPC site (http://www.aapc.com) for their Code of Ethics. How will this support your health care organization's compliance goals?

Basics of Health Insurance

Cheryl Fassett

KEY TERMS

Your instructor may wish to select some words pertinent to this chapter for a test. For definitions of the terms, further study, and/or reference, the words, phrases, and abbreviations may be found in the glossary at the end of the Textbook. Key terms for this chapter follow.

accounts receivable management
Affordable Care Act
Assignment
birthday rule
blanket contract
cancelable
capitation
claim
coinsurance
conditionally renewable
consumer directed health plan
contract
conversion privilege
coordination of benefits
copayment
cost share/cost sharing
daysheet
deductible
dependent
disability income insurance
electronic signature
emancipated minor
encounter form
exclusions
exclusive provider organization
expressed contract
fee-for-service
flexible spending account
group health insurance plan
guaranteed renewable
guarantor
Health Benefit Exchanges
Health Care and Education Reconciliation Act
Health insurance
health maintenance organization
health reimbursement account
health savings account
implied contract

indemnity health insurance
independent or individual practice association
institutional provider
insured
Life Cycle of a Claim
major medical
mandated benefits
Maternal and Child Health Program
Medicaid
Medical savings account
medically necessary
Medicare
Medicare/Medicaid
noncancelable policy
noncovered services
nonparticipating provider
optionally renewable
participating physician or provider
Patient Protection and Affordable Care Act
physician's representative
point-of-service plan
preauthorization
precertification
predetermination
preexisting conditions
preferred provider organization
premium
revenue cycle
self-funded health plans
self-pay
State Children's Health Insurance Program
State Disability Insurance
third-party payers
TRICARE
Unemployment Compensation Disability
Veterans Health Administration (CHAMPVA)
workers' compensation insurance

31

KEY ABBREVIATIONS

See how many abbreviations and acronyms you can translate and then use this as a handy reference list. Definitions for the key abbreviations are located near the back of the Textbook *in the glossary.*

ACA _____

A/R _____

CDHP _____

CHAMPVA _____

COB _____

COBRA _____

Copay _____

DOS _____

EPO _____

FSA _____

HCERA _____

HDHP _____

HMO _____

HRA _____

HSA _____

IPA _____

MCHP _____

Medi-Medi _____

MSA _____

nonpar _____

NPP _____

par _____

PMS _____

POS plan _____

PPACA _____

PPO _____

ROA _____

SCHIP _____

SDHP _____

SDI _____

SHOP _____

SOF _____

UCD _____

VA _____

WC _____

PERFORMANCE OBJECTIVES

The student will be able to:

- Define and spell the key terms and key abbreviations for this chapter, given the information from the *Textbook* glossary, within a reasonable time period and with enough accuracy to obtain a satisfactory evaluation.
- Answer the fill in the blank, multiple choice, and true/false review questions after reading the chapter, with enough accuracy to obtain a satisfactory evaluation.
- Arrange 18 administrative processing steps of an insurance claim in proper sequence, given data from the textbook, within a reasonable time period and with enough accuracy to obtain a satisfactory evaluation.

- Use critical thinking to explain some of the differences in insurance key terms, given data from the textbook, within a reasonable time period and with enough accuracy to obtain a satisfactory evaluation.
- Abstract data from some insurance identification cards, given data from the textbook, within a reasonable time period and with enough accuracy to obtain a satisfactory evaluation.

STUDY OUTLINE

History of Health Insurance in the United States
    Health Care Reform
Legal Principles of Insurance
    Insurance Contracts
    Implied or Expressed Contracts
    Self-pay Patients
    Guarantor
    Emancipated Minor
    Employment and Disability Examinations
    Workers' Compensation Patients
The Insurance Policy
    Policy Application
    Policy Renewal Provisions
    Policy Terms
    Coordination of Benefits
    General Policy Limitations
    Case Management Requirements
Choice of Health Insurance
    Conversion Privilege
    COBRA
    Medical Savings Accounts
    Health Savings Accounts
    Health Reimbursement Arrangements
    Flexible Spending Accounts
Types of Health Insurance Coverage
    Private Insurance
    Managed Care Plans
    Medicare

    Medicaid
    Military Plans
    Workers' Compensation Insurance
    Examples of Insurance Billing Exception
Handling and Processing Insurance Claims
Life Cycle of an Insurance Claim
    Step 1: Preregistration
    Step 2: Verification of Insurance
    Step 3: Notice of Privacy Practices
    Step 4: Insurance Identification Card
    Step 5: Patient's Signature Requirements
    Step 6: Assignment of Benefits
    Step 7: Patient's Financial Account
    Step 8: Encounter Form
    Step 9: Financial Accounting Record and Accounts
        Receivable Management
    Step 10: Insurance Claim
    Step 11: Submitting the Paper Claim
    Step 12: Transmitting the Electronic Claim
    Step 13: Provider's Signature
    Step 14: Track Pending Insurance Claims
    Step 15: Insurance Payments
    Step 16: Bank Deposit
    Step 17: Monthly Statement
    Step 18: Financial Records Retained
Keeping Up to Date

Part I Fill in the Blank

Review the objectives, key terms, glossary definitions to key terms, chapter information, and figures before completing the following review questions.

1. A/an _____ is a legally enforceable agreement between two or more parties.

2. An individual promising to pay for medical services rendered is known as a/an

   _____.

3. List five health insurance policy renewal provisions.

   a. _____

   b. _____

   c. _____

   d. _____

   e. _____

4. Traditional or fee-for-service health plans are also called _____.

5. Name two examples of services that are typically excluded in general health insurance policies.

   a. _____

   b. _____

6. Under PPACA, health plans must allow employees to keep their children on their plans until the children are _____ years old.

7. The act of determining whether treatment is covered under an individual's health insurance policy is called _____

   _____.

8. The procedure to obtain permission for a procedure before it is done, to determine whether the insurance program agrees it is medically necessary, is termed _____

   _____.

9. Determining the maximum dollar amount the insurance company will pay for a procedure before it is done is known as _____.

10. Name two ways an individual may obtain health insurance.

    a. _____

    b. _____

11. List four methods a health care organization may use to submit insurance claims to insurance companies.

    a. _____

    b. _____

    c. _____

    d. _____

12. A document signed by the insured directing the insurance company to pay benefits directly to the health care organization is known as a/an _____.

13. A patient service slip personalized to the health care organization and used as a communications/billing tool during routing of the patient can also be referred to as the following terms.

    a. _____

    b. _____

    c. _____

    d. _____

    e. _____

    f. _____

14. Digital data attached to a computerized document as verification of the provider's intent to sign the document is known as a/an _____.

15. A method of making an automatic deposit of funds from the payer into the provider's bank account and used in place of a mailed paper check is referred to as _____.

Part II Mix and Match

16. Match the following insurance terms in the right column with their descriptions, and fill in the blank with the appropriate letter.

_____ An insurance company considering benefits payable by another carrier in determining its own liability

_____ Transfer of one's right to collect an amount payable under an insurance contract

_____ Acts for insurance company or insured in settlement of claims

_____ Periodic payment to keep insurance policy in force

_____ Amount insured person must pay before policy will pay

_____ Time period in which a claim must be filed

_____ Certain illnesses or injuries listed in a policy that the insurance company will not cover

_____ Individual responsible for payment of health care services

_____ the policyholder, or insured of an insurance plan

a. Adjuster

b. Assignment

c. Guarantor

d. Coordination of benefits (COB)

e. Deductible

f. Exclusions

g. Premium

h. Subscriber

i. Time limit

Part III Multiple Choice

Choose the best answer.

17. When a patient goes to a health care organization seeking medical services, the health care organization accepts the patient and agrees to render treatment, and both parties agree. This contract is known as a/an:
    a. expressed contract.
    b. agreed contract.
    c. implied contract.
    d. written contract.

18. The process of checking and confirming that a patient is covered under an insurance plan is known as:
    a. precertification.
    b. eligibility verification.
    c. COB.
    d. predetermination.

19. A provision that allows the policyholder the right to refuse to renew the insurance policy on a premium due date is called:
    a. conditionally renewable.
    b. guaranteed renewable.
    c. optionally renewable.
    d. noncancelable.

20. A provision in a health insurance policy in which two insurance carriers work together for payment so that there is no duplication of benefits paid between the primary insurance carrier and the secondary insurance carrier is called:
    a. copayment.
    b. coinsurance.
    c. COB.
    d. cost-share rider.

21. A type of tax-free savings account that allows individuals and their employers to set aside money to pay for health care expenses is known as:
    a. a health savings account.
    b. a medical savings account.
    c. a flexible spending account.
    d. all of the above.

22. Time limits for filing insurance claims to a commercial carrier may have a range of:
    a. 10 days from the date medical service is received to 1 year.
    b. 30 days from the date of service to 1½ years.
    c. 60 days from the date of service.
    d. no time limit.

Part IV True/False

Write "T" or "F" in the blank to indicate whether you think the statement is true or false.

_____ 23. A preferred provider organization (PPO) occurs when a large employer or organization contracts with a hospital to offer medical care at a reduced rate.

_____ 24. The birthday rule is a change in the order of determination of COB regarding primary and secondary insurance carriers for dependent children.

_____ 25. The Consolidated Omnibus Budget Reconciliation Act of 1985 (COBRA) mandates that when an employee is laid off from a company, the group health insurance coverage must continue at group rates for up to 18 months.

_____ 26. A group policy usually provides better benefits; however, the premiums are generally higher than an individual contract would be.

_____ 27. A signature stamp is acceptable by all insurances as proof of the provider's signature on a CMS-1500 claim form.

ASSIGNMENT 4.2 CRITICAL THINKING: ADMINISTRATIVE SEQUENCE OF PROCESSING AN INSURANCE CLAIM

Performance Objective

Task: Number from 1 to 18 the proper sequence of processing an insurance claim.

Conditions: Use given data and a pen or pencil.

Standards: Time: _____ minutes

                  Accuracy: _____

                  (Note: The time element and accuracy criteria may be given by your instructor.)

Directions: Arrange the listed steps 1 through 18 in proper sequence by placing the correct number to the left of the statement. (Note: Each medical practice has its own order of the way office procedures are carried out; thus, these steps may vary slightly from practice to practice.)

_____ Bank deposit made and unpaid claims followed up

_____ Patient's financial account is pulled

_____ Insurance information (obtained and verified)

_____ Payer processing/payment received with explanation of benefits (EOB) document

_____ Patient's financial data posted and patient checkout

_____ Patient appointment and preregistration

_____ CMS-1500 paper claim forms submitted

_____ Provider's signature is obtained

_____ Electronic (Health Insurance Portability and Accountability Act [HIPAA] X12 837) claims transmitted

_____ Insurance claims preparation

_____ HIPAA Notice of Privacy is reviewed and signed

_____ Balance due statement mailed to patient

_____ Track pending insurance claims

_____ All required patient's signatures are obtained

_____ Assignment of benefits

_____ Medical services performed and encounter form completed

_____ Insurance identification card photocopied

_____ Full payment received and financial records retained

ASSIGNMENT 4.3 CRITICAL THINKING: DIFFERENCES IN INSURANCE KEYTERMS

Performance Objective

Task: Describe and/or explain your response to five questions.

Conditions: Use one or two sheets of white paper and a pen or pencil.

Standards: Time: _____ minutes

                    Accuracy: _____

                    (Note: The time element and accuracy criteria may be given by your instructor.)

Directions: Respond verbally or in writing to these questions or statements.

1. Explain the difference between the following:

Blanket contract _____

Individual contract _____

2. Explain the difference between a participating health care organization and a nonparticipating health care organization for the following:

Commercial insurance company or managed care plan participating health care organization:

_____

Commercial insurance company or managed care plan nonparticipating health care organization:

_____

Medicare participating health care organization:

_____

Medicare nonparticipating health care organization:

_____

3. State the difference between the following:

Implied contract: _____

Expressed contract: _____

4. Explain the birthday law (rule) and when it is used.

_____

ASSIGNMENT 4.4 ABSTRACT DATA FROM AN INSURANCE IDENTIFICATION CARD

Performance Objective

Task: Answer questions in reference to an insurance identification card for Case A.

Conditions: Use an insurance identification card (Fig. 4.1), the questions presented, and a pen or pencil.

Standards: Time: _____ minutes

                   Accuracy: _____

                   (Note: The time element and accuracy criteria may be given by your instructor.)

Directions: An identification card provides much of the information needed to establish a patient's insurance coverage. You have photocopied the front and back sides of three patients' cards and placed copies in their patient records, returning the originals to the patients. Answer the questions by abstracting or obtaining the data from the cards.

Case A

1. Name of patient covered by the policy. _____

2. Provide the insurance policy's effective date. _____

3. List the telephone number for preauthorization. _____

4. State name and address of insurance company. _____

5. List the telephone number to call for provider access. _____

6. Name the type of insurance plan. _____

7. List the insurance identification number (e.g., subscriber, certificate, or member numbers) _____
   _____

8. Furnish the group number. _____ Plan or coverage code. _____

9. State the copay requirements. _____

10. Does the card indicate the patient has pharmacy coverage?
    _____

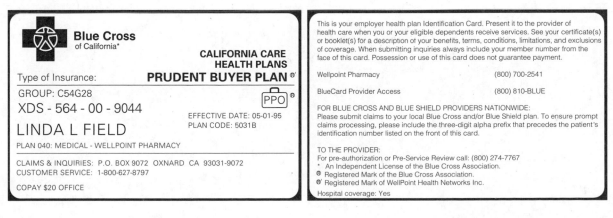

Fig. 4.1

Chapter **4 Basics of Health Insurance**

Performance Objective

Task: Answer questions in reference to the insurance identification card for Case B.

Conditions: Use an insurance identification card (Fig. 4.2), the questions presented, and a pen or pencil.

Standards: Time: _____ minutes

                   Accuracy: _____

                   (Note: The time element and accuracy criteria may be given by your instructor.)

Case B

1. Name of patient covered by the policy. _____

2. Provide the insurance policy's effective date. _____

3. List the telephone number for preauthorization. _____

4. State name of insurance company. _____

5. List the telephone number to call for patient benefits and eligibility. _____

6. Name the type of insurance plan. _____

7. List the insurance identification number (e.g., subscriber, certificate, or member numbers). _____

8. Furnish the group number. _____ Plan or coverage code. _____

9. State the copay requirements, if any. _____

10. List the Blue Shield website. _____

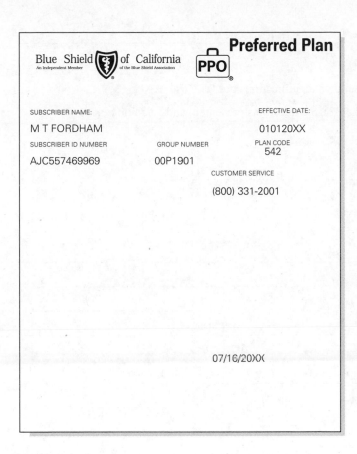

Fig. 4.2

The image shows a Blue Shield of California Preferred Plan PPO insurance card (front and back).

Front of card:

Blue Shield of California
An Independent Member of the Blue Shield Association

Preferred Plan
PPO

SUBSCRIBER NAME:
M T FORDHAM

EFFECTIVE DATE:
010120XX

SUBSCRIBER ID NUMBER
AJC557469969

GROUP NUMBER
00P1901

PLAN CODE
542

CUSTOMER SERVICE
(800) 331-2001

07/16/20XX

Back of card:

Use Blue Shield of California Preferred Physicians and Hospitals to receive maximum benefits.

Carry the Blue Shield Identification Card with you at all times and present it whenever you or one of your covered dependents receives medical services. Read your employee booklet/Health Services Agreement which summarizes the benefits, provisions, limitations and exclusions of your plan. Your health plan may require prior notification of any hospitalization and notification, within one business day, of an emergency admission. Review of selected procedures may be required before some services are performed. To receive hospital pre-admission and pre-service reviews, call 1-800-343-1691. Your failure to call may result in a reduction of benefits.

For questions, including those related to benefits, and eligibility, call the customer service number listed on the front of this card.

The PPO logo on the front of this ID Card identifies you to preferred providers outside the state of California as a member of the Blue Card PPO Program.

When you are outside of California call 1-800-810-2583 to locate the nearest PPO Provider. Remember, any services you receive are subject to the policies and provisions of your group plan.

ID-23200-PPO REVERSE   www.blueshieldca.com

Performance Objective

Task: Answer questions in reference to the insurance identification card for Case C.

Conditions: Use an insurance identification card (Fig. 4.3), the questions presented, and a pen or pencil.

Standards: Time: _____ minutes

               Accuracy: _____

               (Note: The time element and accuracy criteria may be given by your instructor.)

Case C

1. Name of patient covered by the policy. _____

2. Provide the insurance policy's effective date, if there is one. _____

3. List the number to call for out-of-network preauthorization. _____

4. State name and address of insurance company. _____

5. List the telephone number to call for member inquiries. _____

6. Name the type of insurance plan. _____

7. List the insurance identification number (e.g., subscriber, certificate, or member numbers). _____

8. Furnish the group number. _____

9. State the copay requirements, if any. _____

10. Who is the patient's primary care physician? _____

UNITEDhealthcare

LINDA L. FLORES
Member # 52170-5172

CALMAT

Group #   176422
COPAY: Office Visit $10 ER $50
   Urgent $35

Electronic Claims Payor ID 87726

Call 800-842-5751 for Member Inquiries

POS PCP Plan
WITH RX D - UHC
and MH/CD
PCP: G. LOMAN
805-643-9973

MTH

This identification card is not proof of membership nor does it guarantee coverage. Persons with coverage that remains in force are entitled to benefits under the terms and conditions of this group health benefit plan as detailed in your benefit description.

IMPORTANT MEMBER INFORMATION
In non-emergencies, call your Primary Care Physician to receive the highest level of benefits. If you have an emergency and are admitted to a hospital, you are required to call your Primary Care Physician within two working days.
For out of network services that require authorization, call the Member Inquiries 800 number on the front of this card.

Claim Address: P.O. Box 30990, Salt Lake City, UT 84130-0990

Fig. 4.3

5 The Blue Plans, Private Insurance, and Managed Care Plans

Linda M. Smith

KEY TERMS

Your instructor may wish to select some words pertinent to this chapter for a test. For definitions of the terms, further study, and/or reference, the words, phrases, and abbreviations may be found in the glossary at the end of the Textbook. Key terms for this chapter follow.

ancillary services
Blue Cross/Blue Shield Association
capitation
carve-out plans
Chapter 11
coinsurance
collection rate
concurrent review
consumer directed health plan
copayment
deductible
direct contract model HMO
direct referral
disenrollment
exclusive provider organization
fee-for-service
formal referral
gatekeeper
group model HMO
health maintenance organization
indemnity insurance plan
Individual Practice Association (IPA) HMO
managed care
managed care organization

National Committee for Quality Assurance
network model HMO
out-of-pocket
per capita
per member per month
point-of-service plan
preferred provider organization
prepaid group practice model
primary care physician
private health insurance
provider networks
provider sponsored organization
retrospective reviews
self-referral
staff model HMO
stop-loss
tertiary care
traditional insurance plan
triple option health plan
usual, customary, and reasonable
utilization review
utilization management
verbal referral
withhold

KEY ABBREVIATIONS

See how many abbreviations and acronyms you can translate and then use this as a handy reference list. Definitions for the key abbreviations are located near the back of the Textbook *in the glossary.*

BCBSA _____

CDHP _____

copay _____

_____

EPO _____

FFS _____

HMO _____

IPA _____

MCO _____

NCQA _____

PCP _____

PMPM _____

POS _____

PPO _____

UCR _____

UR _____

PERFORMANCE OBJECTIVES

The student will be able to:

- Define and spell the key terms and key abbreviations for this chapter, given the information from the *Textbook* glossary, within a reasonable time period and with enough accuracy to obtain a satisfactory evaluation.

- After reading the chapter, answer the fill in the blank, multiple choice, and true/false review questions with enough accuracy to obtain a satisfactory evaluation.

- Complete treatment authorization forms of managed care plans, given completed new patient information forms, within a reasonable time period and with enough accuracy to obtain a satisfactory evaluation.

STUDY OUTLINE

Private Health Insurance
    Blue Cross and Blue Shield Plans
    Fee-for-Service Plans
Managed Care
    Health Maintenance Organization Act of 1973
    Accreditation
    Participating Providers
    Primary Care Provider
    Identification Card
Managed Care Systems
    Health Maintenance Organizations
    Preferred Provider Organizations
    Exclusive Provider Organizations
    Point-of-Service Plans
    Triple-Option Health Plans
    Provider-Sponsored Organization
    Consumer Directed Health Plans
    Claim Forms
Utilization Management
    Preauthorization
    Concurrent Reviews
    Retrospective Reviews

Management of Insurance Plans
    Contracts
    Patient Information Letter
    Scheduling Appointments
    Verification of Benefits
    Referrals and Prior Approval
    Diagnostic Tests
    Insurance Plan Guide
Revenue Cycle Management
    Deductibles
    Copayments
    Payment Models and Mechanisms
    Contract Payment Time Limits
    Monitoring Payment
    Statement of Remittance
    Accounting
    Withhold
    Analysis of Insurance Plans
    Bankruptcy

Part I Fill in the Blank

Review the objectives, key terms, glossary definitions of key terms, figures, and chapter information before completing the following review questions.

1. An insurance plan requires the insured to pay a fixed monthly premium. The insurance that will pay the health care organization for services each time the service is rendered is referred to as

   _____.

2. A group of techniques used by insurance companies to reduce the cost of providing health care while improving access to care and the quality of care is referred to as _____

   _____.

3. What type of medical insurance provides coverage of health services for a prepaid fixed annual fee and requires enrollees to seek services through a panel of providers contracted with the insurance company? _____

   _____.

4. A not-for-profit organization that has built a set of standards to which health plans attest that they have met key elements required by state and federal laws allowing them to participate in managed care programs is called _____

   _____.

5. In a managed care setting, a primary care physician who controls patient access to specialists and diagnostic testing services is known as a/an _____.

6. Name four types of health maintenance organization (HMO) models.

   a. _____

   b. _____

   c. _____

   d. _____

7. If a physician or hospital in a managed care plan is paid a fixed, per capita amount for each patient enrolled, regardless of the type and number of services rendered, this is a payment system known as

   _____.

8. A health benefit program in which enrollees may choose any physician or hospital for services but obtain a higher level of benefits if preferred providers are used is known as a/an _____

   _____.

9. HMOs and preferred provider organizations (PPOs) consisting of a network of physicians and hospitals that provide an insurance company or employer with discounts on their services are referred to collectively as a/an _____

   _____.

10. To control health care costs, the process of reviewing and establishing medical necessity for services and providers' use of medical care resources is termed _____

   _____.

11. Explain the meaning of a "stop-loss" provision that might appear in a managed care contract.

_____

_____

12. When a certain percentage of the monthly capitation payment or a percentage of the allowable charges to physicians is set aside to operate a managed care plan, it is known as a/an

_____.

Part II Multiple Choice

Choose the best answer.

13. A specified dollar amount that the patient must pay annually before an insurance plan begins covering health care costs is called:
    a. coinsurance.
    b. copayment.
    c. deductible.
    d. withhold.

14. A type of managed care plan regulated under insurance statutes that combines features of HMOs and PPOs and requires that employers agree not to contract with any other plan is known as a/an:
    a. independent practice association (IPA).
    b. exclusive provider organization (EPO).
    c. physician provider group (PPG).
    d. point-of-service (POS) plan.

15. A utilization review technique used to look at services that were already provided and compare them with treatment guidelines to ensure care is adequate and medically current, for the condition.
    a. concurrent review
    b. retrospective review
    c. medical necessity review
    d. preauthorization

16. Medical services that are not included in a managed care contract's capitation rate but that may be contracted for separately are referred to as:
    a. carve outs.
    b. stop-loss limits.
    c. payment mechanisms.
    d. copayments.

17. When the primary care physician informs the patient and telephones the referring physician that the patient is being referred for an appointment, it is called a:
    a. direct referral.
    b. formal referral.
    c. self-referral.
    d. verbal referral.

18. Plan-specified facilities listed in managed care plan contracts where patients are required to have laboratory and radiology tests performed are called:
    a. hospital facilities.
    b. medical facilities.
    c. network facilities.
    d. outside facilities.

19. A type of payment model in which the patient pays a monthly or annual retainer fee to the physician is known as:
    a. capitation.
    b. cash only practice.
    c. concierge medicine.
    d. copayment.

20. A value-based reimbursement model in which providers receive performance-based incentives to share cost savings combined with disincentives to share the excess costs of health care delivery is called:
    a. shared risk.
    b. shared savings.
    c. one-sided risk.
    d. full risk.

Part III True/False

Write "T" or "F" in the blank to indicate whether you think the statement is true or false.

_____ 21. Private health insurances are government-sponsored programs.

_____ 22. Blue Cross plans provide health care coverage for hospital expenses.

_____ 23. All managed care plans are alike.

_____ 24. A provider-sponsored organization is a managed care plan that can be owned and operated by a hospital rather than an insurance company.

_____ 25. Consumer-driven health plans (CDHP) are referred to as low deductible plans.

_____ 26. Utilization management techniques should help patients get the best care, at the best price, in the best setting.

_____ 27. Obtaining preapproval for services always ensures payment of a claim by the insurance company.

_____ 28. Value-based reimbursement programs reward health care providers with incentive payments for the quality of care they provide.

_____ 29. When a health care organization agrees to accept a single negotiated fee to deliver all medical services related to a patient's hip replacement surgery, it is referred to as pay for performance.

_____ 30. State laws dictate the time limit within which a private insurance or managed care plan must pay a bill once it is submitted.

Performance Objective

Task: Complete a treatment authorization form to obtain permission for an office consultation for a patient covered by a managed care plan.

Conditions: Use a treatment authorization form (Fig. 5.1), a new patient information form (Fig. 5.2), a computer, and a printer.

Standards: Time: _____ minutes

                      Accuracy: _____

                      (Note: The time element and accuracy criteria may be given by your instructor.)

Directions: Complete a treatment authorization form (see Fig. 5.1) for Mrs. Cohn's managed care plan to obtain permission for the office consultation and date it August 2 of the current year. To obtain information, refer to the New Patient Information form completed by Mrs. Cohn when she came into the office for her visit with Dr. Practon (see Fig. 5.2). Dr. Practon's Family Health Plan provider number is FHP C01402X.

Scenario: Meriweather B. Cohn's primary care physician, Dr. Gerald Practon, took her clinical history. Physical examination revealed a normal blood pressure (120/80); however, abnormal heart sounds were heard, and a diagnosis of a heart murmur (ICD-10-CM code R01.1) was made. Dr. Practon decided to make a semiurgent request to refer Mrs. Cohn for a cardiac consultation (other service) to Dr. Victor M. Salazar, whose office is located at 20 Excalibur Street, Woodland Hills, XY 12345, and whose office telephone number is 555-625-7344. Dr. Salazar will take a detailed history, perform a detailed examination, and make low-complexity medical decisions (CPT-4 Code 99243) to evaluate Mrs. Cohn's heart murmur.

    After the instructor has returned your work to you, either make the necessary corrections and place your work in a three-ring notebook for future reference or, if you receive a high score, place it in your portfolio for reference when applying for a job.

IPA TREATMENT AUTHORIZATION FORM

FHP®
HEALTH CARE

_____ Referral
_____ Participating
_____ Nonparticipating
_____ Commercial
_____ Senior

For Billing Instructions, Patient and Nonaffiliated Providers, and Consultants please see reverse side for instructions

THIS PORTION COMPLETED BY PHYSICIAN

Patient Name _____ Date _____ / _____ / _____

M _____ F _____ Age _____ FHP # _____ Home Phone _____

Address _____

Primary Care MD_____ Primary Care MD's FHP # _____

Referring MD _____ Referring MD's FHP # _____

Referred To _____ Address _____

_____ Office Phone _____

Type of Service: ☐ In-Patient ☐ Out-Patient Services ☐ Initial Visit ☐ Return Visit ☐ Other

Clinical History and Findings _____

_____

Diagnosis _____

ICD-10-CM CODE

Evaluation and Treatment to Date _____

_____

Procedure _____

RVS CPT-4 CODE

Reason for Referral/Consultation/Procedure _____

_____

Accident: ☐ Yes ☐ No   Where Occurred: ☐ Home ☐ Work ☐ Auto ☐ Other
☐ Urgent ☐ Semi-Urgent ☐ Elective

Facility to be Used: _____ Estimated Length of Stay _____

☐ Office ☐ Out-Patient ☐ In-Patient

THIS PORTION COMPLETED BY FHP UR
THIS AUTHORIZATION GOOD FOR 60 DAYS ONLY

Type of Contract: ☐ Capitation ☐ Fee For Service ☐ Per Diem

Projected Cost of Procedure _____ Projected Cost of Facility _____

HMO Verification: Effective _____ Group # _____

Benefits: Co-Pay Per Visit _____ Hospital _____

Limitations: _____

_____ Authorized   Date _____ Initials _____ Reason _____ Authorization #_____

_____ Deferred   Date _____ Initials _____ Reason _____

_____ Denied   Date _____ Initials _____ Reason _____

_____ Modified   Date _____ Initials _____ Reason _____

WHITE – UR Copy   CANARY – Hospital Copy   PINK – Physician Copy   GOLDENROD – Claims Copy

Fig. 5.1

49

Welcome To Our Office

NEW PATIENT INFORMATION

DATE _____ 8-2-20xx _____

PATIENT'S NAME (PLEASE PRINT) Meriweather B. Cohn	S.S. # 430-XX-0261	MARITAL STATUS S [X] W D SEP	SEX M [X]	BIRTH DATE 11-14-65	AGE	RELIGION (optional)

STREET ADDRESS PERMANENT TEMPORARY 267 Blake Street	CITY AND STATE Woodland Hills XY	ZIP CODE 12345	HOME PHONE # 555-263-0911

PATIENT'S OR PARENT'S EMPLOYER Sun Corporation	OCCUPATION (INDICATE IF STUDENT) sales representative	HOW LONG EMPLOYED 5 yrs	BUS. PHONE # EXT # 555-263-0099

EMPLOYER'S STREET ADDRESS 74 Rain Street	CITY AND STATE Woodland Hills XY	ZIP CODE 12345

DRUG ALLERGIES, IF ANY
Penicillin

SPOUSE OR PARENT'S NAME Starkweather L. Cohn	S.S. # 273-XX-9961	BIRTH DATE 7-9-63

SPOUSE OR PARENT'S EMPLOYER B & L Stormdrain Co.	OCCUPATION (INDICATE IF STUDENT) accountant	HOW LONG EMPLOYED 10 yrs	BUS. PHONE # 555-421-0091

EMPLOYER'S STREET ADDRESS 20 South Wind Road	CITY AND STATE Woodland Hills XY	ZIP CODE 12345

*SPOUSE'S STREET ADDRESS, IF DIVORCED OR SEPARATED	CITY AND STATE	ZIP CODE	HOME PHONE #

PLEASE READ: ALL CHARGES ARE DUE AT THE TIME OF SERVICES. IF HOSPITALIZATION IS INDICATED, THE PATIENT IS RESPONSIBLE FOR FURNISHING INSURANCE CLAIM FORMS TO THE OFFICE PRIOR TO HOSPITALIZATION.

PERSON RESPONSIBLE FOR PAYMENT, IF NOT ABOVE	STREET ADDRESS, CITY, STATE	ZIP CODE	HOME PHONE #

BLUE SHIELD (GIVE NAME OF POLICYHOLDER) [ ]	EFFECTIVE DATE	CERTIFICATE #	GROUP #	COVERAGE CODE

OTHER (WRITE IN NAME OF INSURANCE COMPANY) [ ] FHP Healthcare	EFFECTIVE DATE 1-1-8X	POLICY # FHP # A4932

OTHER (WRITE IN NAME OF INSURANCE COMPANY) [ ]	EFFECTIVE DATE	POLICY #

MEDICARE (PLEASE GIVE NUMBER) [ ]	RAILROAD RETIREMENT (PLEASE GIVE NUMBER) [ ]

MEDICAID [ ]	EFFECTIVE DATE	PROGRAM #	COUNTY #	CASE #	ACCOUNT #

INDUSTRIAL [ ]	WERE YOU INJURED ON THE JOB? [ ] YES [X] NO	DATE OF INJURY	INDUSTRIAL CLAIM #

ACCIDENT [ ]	WAS AN AUTOMOBILE INVOLVED? [ ] YES [X] NO	DATE OF ACCIDENT	NAME OF ATTORNEY

WERE X-RAYS TAKEN OF THIS INJURY OR PROBLEM? [ ] YES [X] NO	IF YES, WHERE WERE X-RAYS TAKEN? (HOSPITAL, ETC)	DATE X-RAYS TAKEN

HAS ANY MEMBER OF YOUR IMMEDIATE FAMILY BEEN TREATED BY OUR PHYSICIAN(S) BEFORE? INCLUDE NAME OF PHYSICIAN AND FAMILY MEMBER
No

REFERRED BY BREEZIE N. CLOUD	STREET ADDRESS, CITY, STATE 521 N. Wind Rd., Woodland Hills XY	ZIP CODE 12345	PHONE # 555-721-9641

ALL PROFESSIONAL SERVICES RENDERED ARE CHARGED TO THE PATIENT. NECESSARY FORMS WILL BE COMPLETED TO HELP EXPEDITE INSURANCE CARRIER PAYMENTS. HOWEVER, THE PATIENT IS RESPONSIBLE FOR ALL FEES, REGARDLESS OF INSURANCE COVERAGE. IT IS ALSO CUSTOMARY TO PAY FOR SERVICES WHEN RENDERED UNLESS OTHER ARRANGEMENTS HAVE BEEN MADE IN ADVANCE WITH OUR OFFICE BOOKKEEPER.

INSURANCE AUTHORIZATION AND ASSIGNMENT

Name of Policy Holder _____ Meriweather B. Cohn _____ HC Number _____

I request that payment of authorized Medicare/Other Insurance company benefits be made either to me or on my behalf to _____ College Clinic _____
for any services furnished me by that party who accepts assignment/physician. Regulations pertaining to Medicare assignment of benefits apply.

I authorize any holder of medical or other information about me to release to the Social Security Administration and Health Care Financing Administration or its intermediaries or carrier or any other insurance company any information needed for this or a related Medicare/Other Insurance company claim.

I understand my signature requests that payment be made and authorizes release of medical information necessary to pay the claim. If item 9 of the HCFA-1500 claim form is completed, my signature authorizes releasing of the information to the insurer or agency shown. In Medicare/Other Insurance company assigned cases, the physician or supplier agrees to accept the charge determination of the Medicare/Other Insurance company as the full charge, and the patient is responsible only for the deductible, coinsurance, and noncovered services. Coinsurance and the deductible are based upon the charge determination of the Medicare/Other Insurance company.

Signature _____ Meriweather B. Cohn _____ Date _____ 8-2-20XX _____

NEW PATIENT INFORMATION

Fig. 5.2

50

ASSIGNMENT 5.3 OBTAIN AUTHORIZATION FOR PHYSICAL THERAPY FROM A MANAGED CARE PLAN

Performance Objective

Task: Complete a treatment authorization form to obtain permission for physical therapy for a patient covered by a managed care plan.

Conditions: Use a treatment authorization form (Fig. 5.3), computer, and printer.

Standards: Time: _____ minutes

Accuracy: _____

(Note: The time element and accuracy criteria may be given by your instructor.)

Directions: Complete the treatment authorization form for this patient (see Fig. 5.3), date it July 7 of the current year, and submit it to the managed care plan.

Scenario: Mrs. Rosario Jimenez comes into Dr. Gerald Practon's office complaining of neck pain. Mrs. Jimenez is a member of the managed care program HealthNet, and Dr. Practon is her primary care physician. Mrs. Jimenez lives at 350 South Carib Street, Woodland Hills, XY 12345-0003. Her telephone number is 555-450-9987, and she was born April 6, 1960. Her plan identification number is JIM40896, and the effective date is January 1, 20xx. After taking a history, completing a physical examination, and taking and reviewing radiographs, Dr. Practon makes a diagnosis of cervical radiculitis (diagnosis code M54.12). He gives Mrs. Jimenez a prescription for some medication and says it is necessary to order outpatient physical therapy; one area, for 15 minutes; therapeutic exercises to develop strength, motion, and flexibility (Procedure code 97110) twice a week for 6 weeks at College Hospital; 4500 Broad Avenue, Woodland Hills, XY 13245-0001 (telephone # 555-487-6789). Authorization must be obtained for this treatment. Dr. Practon's NPI number is 46278897XX; College Hospital's NPI number is 95073167.

After the instructor has returned your work to you, either make the necessary corrections and place your work in a three-ring notebook for future reference or, if you receive a high score, place it in your portfolio for reference when applying for a job.

College Clinic
4567 Broad Avenue
Woodland Hills, XY 12345-0001
Telephone No. (555) 487-8976
Fax No. (555) 487-8976

MANAGED CARE PLAN AUTHORIZATION REQUEST

❑ Health Net	❑ Met Life
❑ Pacificare	❑ Travelers
❑ Secure Horizons	❑ Pru Care
❑ Other	

Member/Group No.

TO BE COMPLETED BY PRIMARY CARE PHYSICIAN OR OUTSIDE PROVIDER

Patient Name_____ Date_____

❑ Male ❑ Female Birthdate_____ Home Telephone Number _____

Address _____

Primary Care Physician_____ NPI_____

Referring Physician _____ NPI_____

Referred to _____ NPI_____

Address _____ Telephone No. _____

Diagnosis Code_____ Diagnosis_____

Diagnosis Code_____ Diagnosis_____

Treatment Plan _____

Authorization Requested for: ❑ Consult Only   ❑ Treatment Only   ❑ Consult/Treatment
                              ❑ Consult/Procedure/Surgery   ❑ Diagnostic Tests

Procedure Code: _____ Description: _____

Procedure Code: _____ Description: _____

Place of Service ❑ Office ❑ Outpatient ❑ Inpatient ❑ Other   Number of Visits: _____

Facility: _____ Length of Stay: _____

Physician's Signature: _____

TO BE COMPLETED BY PRIMARY CARE PHYSICIAN

PCP Recommendations: _____ PCP Initials: _____

Date Eligibility Checked: _____

TO BE COMPLETED BY UTILIZATION MANAGEMENT

Authorized: _____ Auth. No:_____ Not Authorized _____

Deferred: _____ Modified: _____

Effective Date: _____ Expiration Date: _____ No. of Visits: _____

Fig. 5.3

ASSIGNMENT 5.4 OBTAIN AUTHORIZATION FOR DIAGNOSTIC ARTHROSCOPY FROM A MANAGED CARE PLAN

Performance Objective

Task: Complete a treatment authorization form to obtain permission for diagnostic arthroscopy with debridement for a patient covered by a managed care plan.

Conditions: Use a treatment authorization form (Fig. 5.4), computer, and printer.

Standards: Time: _____ minutes

                     Accuracy: _____

                     (Note: The time element and accuracy criteria may be given by your instructor.)

Directions: Complete the treatment authorization form for this patient (see Fig. 5.4), date it August 12 of the current year, and submit it to the managed care plan.

Scenario: Daniel Chan has been referred by his primary care physician, Dr. Gerald Practon, to an orthopedic surgeon, Dr. Raymond Skeleton. Both physicians are members of his managed care plan, Metropolitan Life. The patient comes into Dr. Skeleton's office complaining of pain, swelling (diagnosis code M79.89), and crepitus of the right knee (diagnosis code M23.91). The patient is having difficulty walking (diagnosis code R26.2) but indicates no recent injury to the knee.

   Mr. Chan lives at 226 West Olive Avenue, Woodland Hills, XY 12345-0001, and his telephone number is 555-540-6700. His plan identification number is FTW90876, effective February 1, 20xx, and he was born February 23, 1971.

   After taking a history, completing a physical examination, and taking and reviewing radiographs, Dr. Skeleton suspects the patient has a tear of the medial meniscus and may require debridement of articular cartilage. This procedure will be performed on an outpatient basis at College Hospital; 4500 Broad Avenue, Woodland Hills, XY 12345-0001; telephone number 555-486-3322. Authorization must be obtained for the surgical arthroscopy with debridement of articular cartilage (procedure code 29877). Dr. Practon's NPI number is 46278897XX; Dr. Skeleton's NPI number is 12678547XX; College Hospital's NPI number is 95073167.

   After the instructor has returned your work to you, either make the necessary corrections and place your work in a three ring notebook for future reference or, if you received a high score, place it in your portfolio for reference when applying for a job.

College Clinic
4567 Broad Avenue
Woodland Hills, XY 12345-0001
Telephone No. (555) 487-8976
Fax No. (555) 487-8976

MANAGED CARE PLAN AUTHORIZATION REQUEST

❏ Health Net   ❏ Met Life
❏ Pacificare   ❏ Travelers
❏ Secure Horizons   ❏ Pru Care
❏ Other

Member/Group No.

TO BE COMPLETED BY PRIMARY CARE PHYSICIAN OR OUTSIDE PROVIDER

Patient Name_____ Date_____

❏ Male ❏ Female Birthdate_____ Home Telephone Number _____

Address _____

Primary Care Physician_____ NPI_____

Referring Physician _____ NPI_____

Referred to _____ NPI_____

Address _____ Telephone No. _____

Diagnosis Code _____ Diagnosis_____

Diagnosis Code _____ Diagnosis_____

Treatment Plan _____

Authorization Requested for: ❏ Consult Only   ❏ Treatment Only   ❏ Consult/Treatment
           ❏ Consult/Procedure/Surgery   ❏ Diagnostic Tests

Procedure Code: _____ Description: _____

Procedure Code: _____ Description: _____

Place of Service ❏ Office ❏ Outpatient ❏ Inpatient ❏ Other   Number of Visits: _____

Facility: _____ Length of Stay: _____

Physician's Signature: _____

TO BE COMPLETED BY PRIMARY CARE PHYSICIAN

PCP Recommendations: _____ PCP Initials: _____

Date Eligibility Checked: _____

TO BE COMPLETED BY UTILIZATION MANAGEMENT

Authorized: _____ Auth. No:_____ Not Authorized _____

Deferred: _____ Modified: _____

Effective Date: _____ Expiration Date: _____ No. of Visits: _____

Fig. 5.4

ASSIGNMENT 5.5 OBTAIN AUTHORIZATION FOR CONSULTATION FROM A MANAGED CARE PLAN

Performance Objective

Task: Complete a treatment authorization form to obtain permission for consultation for a patient from a managed care plan.

Conditions: Use a treatment authorization form (Fig. 5.5), computer, and printer.

Standards: Time: _____ minutes

                Accuracy: _____

                (Note: The time element and accuracy criteria may be given by your instructor.)

Directions: Complete the treatment authorization form for this patient (see Fig. 5.5), date it September 3 of the current year, and submit it to the managed care plan.

Scenario: Frederico Fellini, with a history of getting up four times during the night with a slow urinary stream, was seen by his primary care physician, Dr. Gerald Practon (NPI 46278897XX). An intravenous pyelogram yielded negative results except for distention of the urinary bladder. Physical examination of the prostate showed an enlargement. The preliminary diagnosis is benign prostatic hypertrophy (BPH) (diagnosis code N40.0).

    The patient will be referred to Dr. Douglas Lee, a urologist, for a level 4 office consultation (procedure code 99244) and cystoscopy (procedure code 52000). Transurethral resection of the prostate is possible at a future date. Dr. Lee's address is 4300 Cyber Street, Woodland Hills, XY 12345, and his office telephone number is 555-675-3322. His National Provider Identifier (NPI) is 55026717XX.

    The patient is enrolled in a managed care plan through PruCare; Dr. Practon is a contracted provider in the plan.

    Mr. Fellini lives at 476 Miner Street, Woodland Hills, XY 12345, and his telephone number is 555-679-0098. His PruCare plan identification number is VRG87655, effective January 1, 20xx. His birth date is May 24, 1944.

    After the instructor has returned your work to you, either make the necessary corrections and place your work in a three-ring notebook for future reference or, if you received a high score, place it in your portfolio for reference when applying for a job.

College Clinic
4567 Broad Avenue
Woodland Hills, XY 12345-0001
Telephone No. (555) 487-8976
Fax No. (555) 487-8976

MANAGED CARE PLAN AUTHORIZATION REQUEST

❏ Health Net   ❏ Met Life
❏ Pacificare   ❏ Travelers
❏ Secure Horizons   ❏ Pru Care
❏ Other

Member/Group No.

TO BE COMPLETED BY PRIMARY CARE PHYSICIAN OR OUTSIDE PROVIDER

Patient Name_____ Date_____

❏ Male ❏ Female Birthdate_____ Home Telephone Number _____

Address _____

Primary Care Physician _____ NPI_____

Referring Physician _____ NPI_____

Referred to _____ NPI_____

Address _____ Telephone No. _____

Diagnosis Code_____ Diagnosis_____

Diagnosis Code_____ Diagnosis_____

Treatment Plan _____

Authorization Requested for: ❏ Consult Only   ❏ Treatment Only   ❏ Consult/Treatment
                              ❏ Consult/Procedure/Surgery   ❏ Diagnostic Tests

Procedure Code: _____ Description: _____

Procedure Code: _____ Description: _____

Place of Service ❏ Office ❏ Outpatient ❏ Inpatient ❏ Other   Number of Visits: _____

Facility: _____ Length of Stay: _____

Physician's Signature: _____

TO BE COMPLETED BY PRIMARY CARE PHYSICIAN

PCP Recommendations: _____ PCP Initials: _____

Date Eligibility Checked: _____

TO BE COMPLETED BY UTILIZATION MANAGEMENT

Authorized: _____ Auth. No:_____ Not Authorized _____

Deferred: _____ Modified: _____

Effective Date: _____ Expiration Date: _____ No. of Visits: _____

Fig. 5.5

ASSIGNMENT 5.6 OBTAIN AUTHORIZATION FOR DIAGNOSTIC BODY SCAN FROM A MANAGED CARE PLAN

Performance Objective

Task: Complete a treatment authorization form to obtain permission for diagnostic complete body bone scan and mammogram for a patient covered by a managed care plan.

Conditions: Use a treatment authorization form (Fig. 5.6), computer, and printer.

Standards: Time: _____ minutes

             Accuracy: _____

             (Note: The time element and accuracy criteria may be given by your instructor.)

Directions: Complete the treatment authorization form for this patient (see Fig. 5.6), date it October 23 of the current year, and submit it to the managed care plan.

Scenario: A patient, Debbie Dye, sees her primary care physician, Dr. Gerald Practon (NPI 46278897XX), for complaint of midback pain. She underwent a lumpectomy 2 years ago for a malignant neoplasm of the lower left breast; thus she has a history of breast cancer (diagnosis code Z85.3). She has been referred by Dr. Practon (PacifiCare identification number PC C01402X) to Dr. Donald Patos, an oncologist, for a complete workup. He finds that her complaint of midback pain (diagnosis code M54.6) warrants the need to refer her to XYZ Radiology for bilateral diagnostic mammography (procedure code 77066) and a complete body bone scan (procedure code 78306).

Dr. Patos' address is 4466 East Canter Drive, Woodland Hills, XY 12345, and his office telephone number is 555-980-5566. His NPI is 6520101678XX.

Ms. Dye lives at 6700 Flora Road, Woodland Hills, XY 12345-0002, and her telephone number is 555-433-6755. Her PacifiCare plan identification number is SR45380, effective January 1, 20xx. Her birth date is August 6, 1952.

XYZ Radiology's address is 4767 Broad Avenue, Woodland Hills, XY 12345-0001, and the office telephone number is 555-486-9162. NPI is 77542134XX.

After the instructor has returned your work to you, either make the necessary corrections and place your work in a three-ring notebook for future reference or, if you received a high score, place it in your portfolio for reference when applying for a job.

57

College Clinic
4567 Broad Avenue
Woodland Hills, XY 12345-0001
Telephone No. (555) 487-8976
Fax No. (555) 487-8976

MANAGED CARE PLAN AUTHORIZATION REQUEST

❑ Health Net	❑ Met Life
❑ Pacificare	❑ Travelers
❑ Secure Horizons	❑ Pru Care
❑ Other	

Member/Group No.

TO BE COMPLETED BY PRIMARY CARE PHYSICIAN OR OUTSIDE PROVIDER

Patient Name_____ Date_____

❑ Male ❑ Female Birthdate_____ Home Telephone Number _____

Address _____

Primary Care Physician_____ NPI_____

Referring Physician _____ NPI_____

Referred to _____ NPI_____

Address _____ Telephone No. _____

Diagnosis Code _____ Diagnosis_____

Diagnosis Code _____ Diagnosis_____

Treatment Plan _____

Authorization Requested for: ❑ Consult Only   ❑ Treatment Only   ❑ Consult/Treatment
                              ❑ Consult/Procedure/Surgery   ❑ Diagnostic Tests

Procedure Code: _____ Description: _____

Procedure Code: _____ Description: _____

Place of Service ❑ Office ❑ Outpatient ❑ Inpatient ❑ Other   Number of Visits: _____

Facility: _____   Length of Stay: _____

Physician's Signature: _____

TO BE COMPLETED BY PRIMARY CARE PHYSICIAN

PCP Recommendations: _____ PCP Initials: _____

Date Eligibility Checked: _____

TO BE COMPLETED BY UTILIZATION MANAGEMENT

Authorized: _____ Auth. No:_____ Not Authorized _____

Deferred:_____ Modified: _____

Effective Date: _____ Expiration Date: _____ No. of Visits: _____

Fig. 5.6

6 Medicare

Linda M. Smith

KEY TERMS

Your instructor may wish to select some words pertinent to this chapter for a test. For definitions of the terms, further study, and/or reference, the words, phrases, and abbreviations may be found in the glossary at the end of the Textbook. *Key terms for this chapter follow.*

adjudication
adjustment
Advance Beneficiary Notice of Noncoverage
Advanced Alternative Payment Model
approved charges
assignment
beneficiaries
benefit period
Centers for Medicare and Medicaid Services
Correct Coding Initiative
crossover claim
custodial services
disability
donut hole
dual eligible
durable medical equipment
end-stage renal disease
formulary
generic drugs
hospice
hospital insurance
jurisdiction
limiting charge
Local Coverage Determination
medical necessity
Medicaid
Medicare
Medicare administrative contractor
Medicare Access and CHIP Reauthorization Act of 2015
Medicare Advantage Plan
Medicare Beneficiary Identifier

Medicare Claims Processing Manual—Internet Only Manual
Medicare fee schedule
Medicare Improvements for Patients and Providers Act
Medicare Learning Network
Medicare/Medicaid
Medicare Part A
Medicare Part B
Medicare Part C
Medicare Part D
Medicare secondary payer
Medicare Select
Medicare Summary Notice
Medigap
Merit-based Incentive Payment System
National Coverage Determination
national health insurance
national provider identifier
nonparticipating provider
nursing facility
participating provider
premium
prepayment screen
preventive services
prospective payment system
Quality Improvement Organization
Recovery Audit Contractor Initiative
remittance advice
resource-based relative value scale
respite care
United States Preventive Services Task Force (USPSTF_
value-based programs

KEY ABBREVIATIONS

See how many abbreviations and acronyms you can translate and then use this as a handy reference list. Definitions for the key abbreviations are located near the back of the Textbook *in the glossary.*

ABN _____

APM _____

CCI _____

CMS _____

DHHS _____

DME _____

ERA _____

ESRD _____

GPCIs _____

ICU _____

LCDs _____

LGHP _____

59

MA Plan _____

MAC _____

MACRA _____

MBI _____

Medi-Medi _____

MFS _____

MIPAA _____

MIPS _____

MG _____

MLN _____

MMA _____

MSA _____

MSN _____

MSP _____

NCDs _____

NF _____

nonpar _____

NPI _____

par _____

PFFS plan _____

PPS _____

PSO _____

QIO _____

RA _____

RAC Initiative _____

RBRVS _____

USPSTF _____

PERFORMANCE OBJECTIVES

The student will be able to:

- Define and spell the key terms and key abbreviations for this chapter, given the information from the *Textbook* glossary, within a reasonable time period and with enough accuracy to obtain a satisfactory evaluation.

- After reading the chapter, answer the fill in the blank, multiple choice, and true/false review questions, with enough accuracy to obtain a satisfactory evaluation.

- Compute mathematical calculations, given Medicare problem situations, within a reasonable time period and with enough accuracy to obtain a satisfactory evaluation.

- Complete an ABN form.

STUDY OUTLINE

Background
Policies and Regulations
 The Parts of Medicare
 Eligibility Requirements
 Medicare Enrollment
 Non U.S. Citizens
 Health Insurance Card
 Benefits
Additional Insurance Programs
 Medicare/Medicaid
 Medicare/Medigap
 Medicare Secondary Payer
 Managed Care and Medicare
 Automobile or Liability Insurance Coverage
Utilization and Quality Control
 Quality Improvement Organizations
 Medicare Billing Compliance Issues
Program Fundamentals
 Provider
 Prior Authorization

 National and Local Coverage Determinations
 Prepayment Screens
Medicare Reimbursement
 Medicare Fee Schedule
 Prospective Payment System
 Value-Based Programs
Claim Submission
 Medicare Administrative Contractors
 Provider Identification Numbers
 Time Limit for Claims Submission
 Instructions for Claims Submission
After Claim Submission
 Remittance Advice
 Medicare Summary Notice
 Posting Payments
 Medicare Overpayments

ASSIGNMENT 6.1 REVIEW QUESTIONS

Part I Fill in the Blank

Review the objectives, key terms, glossary definitions of key terms, chapter information, and figures before completing the following review questions.

1. Medicare is administered by the federal agency _____.

2. Medicare Part A is _____ coverage, and Medicare Part B is _____ _____ coverage.

3. A program designed to provide pain relief, symptom management, and supportive services to terminally ill individuals and their families is known as _____

    _____.

4. An individual becomes eligible for Medicare Parts A and B at age _____.

5. Individuals who are unable to engage in any substantial employment due to physical or mental impairment which can be expected to last for 12 continuous months or result in death are defined by The Social Security Administration as: _____

6. To be eligible for Medicare, an individual must have lived in the United States as a permanent resident for ____ consecutive years.

7. Patients who are entitled to received Medicare benefits are referred to as _____ _____.

8. The 11 character number that replaced social security numbers on Medicare insurance cards is referred to as the ___ _____.

9. Define a Medicare Part A hospital benefit period.

    _____

    _____

    _____

10. Short-term inpatient medical care for terminally ill individuals to give temporary relief to the caregiver is known as _____.

11. The independent panel of national experts in disease prevention who recommends which preventive service benefits will be offered to Medicare beneficiaries is: _____

12. Medicare coverage plans offered by private insurance companies to Medicare beneficiaries are known as _____ _____.

13. _____ is a temporary limit on what a Medicare drug plan will cover.

14. A list of covered drugs kept by each Medicare drug plan is called a/an _____ _____.

15. A document by Medicare explaining the decision made on a claim for services that were paid is called a/an _____.

16. Private insurance policies that helps to pay copayments, coinsurance and deductibles that traditional Medicare plans do no cover are known as: _____ insurance policies.

17. The performance of services and procedures that are consistent with the diagnosis in accordance with standards of good medical practice, performed at the proper level and provided in the most appropriate setting is referred to by CMS as: _____.

18. The amount that a nonparticipating provider can charge the Medicare beneficiary above the Medicare allowed amounts is referred to as:_____.

Choose the best answer.

19. The fee that Medicare decides a medical service is worth, is referred to as the:
    a. reasonable charge for services.
    b. assigned amount.
    c. approved amount.
    d. paid amount.

20. Physicians who are nonparticipating with the Medicare program are only allowed to bill the limiting charge to the patient, which is:
    a. the provider's usual fee.
    b. 80% of the provider's fee schedule.
    c. 20% of the Medicare fee schedule allowed amount.
    d. 115% of the Medicare fee schedule allowed amount.

21. National Coverage Determinations are coverage guidelines that are mandated:
    a. at the federal level.
    b. at the Medicare contractor level.
    c. at the Medicare Advantage Plan level.
    d. by Recovery Audit Contractors Initiative.

22. A decision by a Medicare administrative contractor (MAC) whether to cover (pay) a particular medical service on a contractor-wide basis in accordance with whether it is reasonable and necessary is known as a/an:
    a. Local Coverage Determination.
    b. Correct Coding Initiative edit.
    c. prepayment screen.
    d. redetermination process.

23. A Medicare prepayment screen which would suspend a claim for the excision of an appendix performed by an audiologist would be referred to as:
    a. diagnosis to procedure edits.
    b. procedure to procedure edits.
    c. procedure to specialty code edits.
    d. procedure to place of service edits.

24. The resource-based relative value scale establishes fees, taking into account:
    a. physician's specialty, work value, and overhead expense.
    b. work value, overhead expense, and malpractice expense.
    c. work value, physician's specialty, and malpractice expense.
    d. physician's specialty, overhead expense, and malpractice expense.

25. The prospective payment system is a method of reimbursement to:
    a. physicians.
    b. ambulance services.
    c. hospitals.
    d. pharmacies.

26. The number of Medicare administrative contractors that currently process claims for DME suppliers is:
    a. 1
    b. 4
    c. 12
    d. 50

27. The 10-digit identification number required on a claim form to identify a service provider is the:
    a. SSN
    b. MBI
    c. NPI
    d. PIP

28. According to regulations, a Medicare patient must be billed for a copayment:
    a. at least once before a balance is adjusted off as uncollectible.
    b. at least two times before a balance is adjusted off as uncollectible.
    c. at least three times before a balance is adjusted off as uncollectible.
    d. no more than four times before a balance is adjusted off as uncollectible.

29. How many days does a health care organization have to report and return any Medicare overpayment that the organization identifies?
    a. None; they can keep it until they are asked to return it.
    b. 30 days
    c. 60 days
    d. 180 days

30. How many days does a health care organization have to repay an overpayment identified by a Medicare Administrative Contractor before interest will be charged?
    a. None, interest will never be charged.
    b. 30 days
    c. 60 days
    d. 180 days

Part III True/False

Write "T" or "F" in the blank to indicate whether you think the statement is true or false.

_____ 31. All patients who have a Medicare health insurance card have Part A hospital and Part B medical coverage.

_____ 32. Prescription drug plans refer to the drugs in their formularies by tier numbers.

_____ 33. Nonparticipating physicians may decide on a case-by-case basis whether to accept assignment when providing medical services to Medicare patients.

_____ 34. Medicare's Correct Coding Initiative was implemented by the Centers for Medicare and Medicaid Services to identify procedures that are usually described by a single code or are inherent to another procedure.

_____ 35. When patients have both Medicare and Medicaid coverage, Medicare is always considered to be the payer of last resort.

_____ 36. A Medicare preventive health benefit is a screening mammogram.

_____ 37. Medicare patients must pay for diabetes screening.

_____ 38. Intensive behavioral therapy for obesity is a Medicare preventive health benefits.

_____ 39. The Pneumococcal vaccine may be administered to Medicare patients, but the patient is required to pay a 20% coinsurance.

_____ 40. Glaucoma screening is a covered benefit for Medicare patients if the patient has met their annual deductible.

Performance Objective

Task: Calculate and insert the correct amounts for the following Medicare scenarios.

               Conditions: Use a pen or pencil and the description of the problem.

Standards: Time: _____ minutes

               Accuracy: _____

               (Note: The time element and accuracy criteria may be given by your instructor.)

Directions: Submitting insurance claims, particularly Medicare claims, involves a bit of math. Several problems are given here so that you will gain experience with situations encountered daily in your work. The Medicare deductible is always subtracted from the allowed amount first before mathematical computations continue.

Problem 1: Mr. Doolittle has Medicare Parts A and B coverage. He was well during the entire past year. On January 1, Mr. Doolittle is rushed to the hospital, where Dr. Input performs an emergency gastric resection. The hospital bills Medicare under the Part A coverage, and under the Part B coverage, the physician bills $450 for surgical services. The doctor participates in the Medicare program and agrees to accept assignment. The patient has not met any of his deductible for 2020 which is $198. Complete the following statements by putting in the correct amounts.

Original Bill

    a. Medicare allows $400. Medicare payment: _____

    b. Patient owes Dr. Input: _____

    c. Dr. Input's contractual adjustment: _____

    Mathematical computations:

Problem 2: Mrs. James has Medicare Parts A and B coverage. She met her deductible when she was ill in March of this year. On November 1, Dr. Caesar performs a bilateral salpingo-oophorectomy. The hospital bills Medicare under the Part A coverage, and under Part B coverage, the physician bills $300 for surgical services. The doctor participates in the Medicare program and agrees to accept a Medicare assignment.

Original Bill

    a. Medicare allows $275. Medicare payment: _____

    b. Patient owes Dr. Caesar: _____

    c. Dr. Caesar's contractual adjustment: _____

    Mathematical computations for surgeon:

The assistant surgeon in Mrs. James case, does not participate with Medicare and does not accept assignment. The assistant surgeon charged Mrs. James $60 (the Medicare limiting charge. After receiving her check from Medicare, Mrs. James sends the surgeon his $60. Medicare has allowed $55 for the fee.

a. How much of the money was from Mrs. James' private funds? $ _____

b. How much did Medicare pay? _____

Mathematical computations:

Problem 3: You work for Dr. Coccidioides. He does not participate in the Medicare program and does not accept assignments. He is treating Mr. Robinson in his office for allergies. Mr. Robinson has Medicare Part A, but he does not have Medicare Part B. What portion of the $135 bill for the office visit will Medicare pay? _____

Problem 4: In June, Mr. Fay has an illness that incurs $89 in medical bills. He asks you to bill Medicare, and the physician does not participate in the Medicare program and does not accept assignments. He has paid the deductible at another physician's office.

a. If Medicare allows the entire amount of your fees, the Medicare check to the patient is $_____.

b. The patient's part of the bill to you is_____.

Mathematical computations:

Problem 5: Mr. Iba, a Medicare patient with a Medigap insurance policy, is seen for an office visit, and the fee is $80. The Medicare-approved amount is $54.44. The patient has met his deductible for the year.

a. The Medicare payment check is $ _____.

b. After the claim is submitted to the Medigap insurance, the Medigap payment check is $ _____.

c. To zero out the balance, the Medicare contractual adjustment is _____.

Mathematical computations:

Problem 6: Mrs. Smith, a Medicare patient, had surgery, and the participating physician's fee is $1250. This patient is working part-time, and her employer group health plan (primary insurance) allowed $1100, applied $500 to the deductible, and paid 80% of $600.

a. Amount paid by this plan: $_____

b. The spouse's employer group health plan (secondary insurance) is billed for the balance, which is $ _____. This program also has a $500 deductible. This plan pays 100% of the fee billed, minus the deductible.

c. The spouse's employer group plan makes a payment of _____.

You send copies of the remittance advice from the two group health plans and submit a claim to Medicare (the third insurance) for $1250. The balance at this point is $ _____.

Mathematical computations:

Problem 7: Beverly James has Medicare Part B coverage. She has $242 in medical bills and has met $100 of the $198 (2020 deductible). Dr. Practon participates with Medicare and agrees to accept assignment.

Original Bill

a. Medicare allows $200. Medicare payment: _____

b. Beverly James owes Dr. Practon: _____

c. Dr. Practon's contractual adjustment: _____

Mathematical computations:

Problem 8: Oliver Mills has Medicare Part B coverage. He fell at home and suffered a sprain and Dr. Skeleton treated him. His medical bill totaled $370, and he has met $60 of the $198 (2020 deductible). Dr. Skeleton participates in the Medicare program and agrees to accept assignment.

Original Bill

    a. Medicare allows $280. Medicare payment: _____

    b. Oliver Mills owes Dr. Skeleton: _____

    c. Dr. Skeleton's contractual adjustment: _____

    Mathematical computations:

Problem 9: Maria Sanchez has Medicare Part B coverage. She has $565 in medical bills at Dr. Cardi's office and met $45 of the $198 (2020 deductible) at another physician's office. Dr. Cardi participates in the Medicare program and agrees to accept assignment.

Original Bill

    a. Medicare allows $480. Medicare payment: _____

    b. Maria Sanchez owes Dr. Cardi: _____

    c. Dr. Cardi's contractual adjustment: _____

    Mathematical computations:

ASSIGNMENT 6.3 COMPLETE A MEDICARE ADVANCE BENEFICIARY NOTICE OF NONCOVERAGE

Performance Objective

Task: Complete Medicare ABN.

Conditions: Use the ABN form (Fig. 6.1)

Standards: ABN Completion Productivity Measurement

                    Time: _____ minutes

                    Accuracy: _____

                    (Note: The time element and accuracy criteria may be given by your instructor.)

Directions:

1. Complete an ABN form using the information provided below.

2. Patient: Raymond Fay (Medicare ID # A887661235A)
   a. Procedure performed: nystagmus test (CPT 92531) is a noncovered service and requires that an ABN be on file.
   b. The estimated cost of the nystagmus test is $30.00 .
   c. After review of the ABN with the patient, the patient would like to proceed with the test and understands that they may be responsible for payment of the service.
   d. Provider of Services: Concha Antrum, MD; College Clinic; 4567 Broad Ave., Woodland Hills, XY 12345

A. Notifier:

B. Patient Name: **C. Identification Number:**

Advance Beneficiary Notice of Non-coverage (ABN)

<u>**NOTE:**</u> If Medicare doesn't pay for **D.**_____below, you may have to pay.

Medicare does not pay for everything, even some care that you or your health care provider have good reason to think you need. We expect Medicare may not pay for the **D.**_____below.

D.	E. Reason Medicare May Not Pay:	F. Estimated Cost

WHAT YOU NEED TO DO NOW:

- Read this notice, so you can make an informed decision about your care.
- Ask us any questions that you may have after you finish reading.
- Choose an option below about whether to receive the **D.**_____listed above.
  Note: If you choose Option 1 or 2, we may help you to use any other insurance that you might have, but Medicare cannot require us to do this.

G. OPTIONS: Check only one box. We cannot choose a box for you.
☐ **OPTION 1.** I want the **D.**_____listed above. You may ask to be paid now, but I also want Medicare billed for an official decision on payment, which is sent to me on a Medicare Summary Notice (MSN). I understand that if Medicare doesn't pay, I am responsible for payment, but I can appeal to Medicare by following the directions on the MSN. If Medicare does pay, you will refund any payments I made to you, less co-pays or deductibles.
☐ **OPTION 2.** I want the **D.**_____listed above, but do not bill Medicare. You may ask to be paid now as I am responsible for payment. I cannot appeal if Medicare is not billed.
☐ **OPTION 3.** I don't want the **D.**_____listed above. I understand with this choice I am **not** responsible for payment, and I cannot appeal to see if Medicare would pay.

H. Additional Information:

This notice gives our opinion, not an official Medicare decision. If you have other questions on this notice or Medicare billing, call **1-800-MEDICARE** (1-800-633-4227/**TTY:** 1-877-486-2048).
Signing below means that you have received and understand this notice. You also receive a copy.

I. Signature:	**J. Date:**

CMS does not discriminate in its programs and activities. To request this publication in an alternative format, please call: 1-800-MEDICARE or email: AltFormatRequest@cms.hhs.gov.

According to the Paperwork Reduction Act of 1995, no persons are required to respond to a collection of information unless it displays a valid OMB control number. The valid OMB control number for this information collection is 0938-0566. The time required to complete this information collection is estimated to average 7 minutes per response, including the time to review instructions, search existing data resources, gather the data needed, and complete and review the information collection. If you have comments concerning the accuracy of the time estimate or suggestions for improving this form, please write to: CMS, 7500 Security Boulevard, Attn: PRA Reports Clearance Officer, Baltimore, Maryland 21244-1850.

Form CMS-R-131 (Exp. 06/30/2023)   Form Approved OMB No. 0938-0566

Fig. 6.1

7 Medicaid and Other State Programs

Linda M. Smith

KEY TERMS

Your instructor may wish to select some words pertinent to this chapter for a test. For definitions of the terms, further study, and/or reference, the words, phrases, and abbreviations may be found in the glossary at the end of the Textbook. *Key terms for this chapter follow.*

categorically needy
Children's Health Insurance Program
coinsurance
copayment
covered services
Early and Periodic Screening, Diagnosis, and Treatment
federal poverty level
fiscal agent
Medicaid
Medi-Cal

medically needy
Medicare Savings Programs
payer of last resort
prior approval
recipient
share of cost
spousal impoverishment
Supplemental Security Income
Temporary Assistance for Needy Families

KEY ABBREVIATIONS

See how many abbreviations and acronyms you can translate and then use this as a handy reference list. Definitions for the key abbreviations are located near the back of the Textbook *in the glossary.*

CHIP _____

DEFRA _____

EPSDT _____

FPL _____

MN _____

MSP _____

OBRA _____

OOY claims _____

POS machine _____

QI program _____

QMB _____

RA _____

SLMB _____

SSI _____

TANF _____

PERFORMANCE OBJECTIVES

The student will be able to:

- Define and spell the key terms and key abbreviations for this chapter, given the information from the *Textbook* glossary, within a reasonable time period and with enough accuracy to obtain a satisfactory evaluation.

- After reading the chapter, answer the fill in the blank, multiple choice, and true/false review questions with enough accuracy to obtain a satisfactory evaluation.
- Determine if prior authorization is required for a specific scenario.

STUDY OUTLINE

Medicaid
   History
Medicaid Programs
   Children's Health Insurance Program
   Medicare Savings Programs
Medicaid Eligibility
   Categorically Needy
   Medically Needy
   Spousal Impoverishment Protection Law
   Verifying Eligibility
Medicaid Benefits
   Covered Services
   Non-Covered Services

Medicaid Managed Care
Accepting Medicaid Patients
   Program Participation
Claims Procedures
   Copayment
   Prior Approval
   Hospital-Acquired Condition
   Time Limit
   Reciprocity
   Claim Form
After Claim Submission
   Remittance Advice
   Appeals

Part I Fill in the Blank

Review the objectives, key terms, glossary definitions of key terms, chapter information, and figures before completing the following review questions.

1. Medicaid is not considered an insurance program. It is a/an _____ program.

2. The Medicaid program is jointly funded by the _____ and _____ governments.

3. Because the federal government sets minimum requirements, states are free to enhance the Medicaid program. Name two ways in which Medicaid programs vary from state to state.

   a. _____

   b. _____

4. Title XIX of the Social Security Act became federal law and created Medicaid in the year _____.

5. Health care reform legislation passed in 2010, known as _____affected the Medicaid program by expanding access for childless adults and nonelderly and nonpregnant individuals.

6. To help compensate for budget cuts, many Medicaid programs instituted required specific dollar amounts, known as _____, to be collected at each office visit from the individual seeking medical services.

7. The measure of income issued every year by HHS and used to determine Medicaid eligibility is known as _____.

8. In most states, the medical assistance program is known as *Medicaid*, however, some states may have different names for the program. In California the program is called _____ _____.

9. Name the four Medicare Savings Programs for low-income Medicare patients.

   a. _____

   b. _____

   c. _____

   d. _____

10. Medicare beneficiaries who are disabled but have annual incomes below the federal poverty level may be eligible for the _____ program.

11. _____ is the portion the patient pays of the Medicare allowed amount.

12. States have the option to cover nonimmigrant and unauthorized aliens who are pregnant or who are children and can meet the definition of _____ in the U.S.

13. When health care services are rendered, the Medicaid identification card or electronic verification must show eligibility for the _____ that the service is rendered.

14. Name two broad classifications of people eligible for Medicaid assistance.

   a. _____

   b. _____

15. A _____ is an individual certified by the local welfare department to receive benefits of Medicaid.

16. The name of the program for the prevention, early detection, and treatment of conditions of children receiving welfare is known as _____. It is abbreviated as _____.

17. Items that must be abstracted from the patient's insurance card for claim submission are:

   a. _____

   b. _____

   c. _____

   d. _____

18. The time limit for submitting a Medicaid claim varies from _____ to _____.

19. The insurance claim form for submitting Medicaid claims in all states is

   _____.

20. Your Medicaid patient also has TRICARE. What billing procedure do you follow? Be exact in your steps for a dependant of an active military person.

   a. _____

   b. _____

21. Claim adjudication can be detailed on a Medicaid remittance advice as:

   a. _____

   b. _____

   c. _____

   d. _____

   e. _____

   f. _____

   g. _____

22. Name three levels of Medicaid appeals.

   a. _____

   b. _____

   c. _____

23. _____ is the processing of an insurance claim through a series of edits for final determination of coverage (benefits) for possible payment.

Part II Multiple Choice

Choose the best answer.

24. An organization under contract with the state to process claims for a state Medicaid program is a/the:
    a. Medicaid administrative contractor.
    b. Department of Social Services.
    c. Centers for Medicare and Medicaid Services.
    d. fiscal agent.

25. A patient's Medicaid eligibility may be verified by:
    a. real-time online access via the internet.
    b. verification by telephone with an automated voice response system.
    c. point-of-service machine.
    d. all of the above.

26. When a Medicaid patient requires a piece of durable medical equipment, the physician must:
    a. write a prescription.
    b. obtain prior authorization, preferably written.
    c. instruct the patient on how to use the equipment.
    d. give the name and address of where to purchase the equipment.

27. Which of the following services are mandated Medicaid basic benefits?
    a. Ambulance services
    b. Podiatric care
    c. Immunizations
    d. Dental care

28. If a patient is eligible for group health insurance coverage through an employer and they are also eligible for Medicaid benefits, Medicaid is referred to as the:
    a. payer of last resort.
    b. primary payer.
    c. co-insurance.
    d. fiscal agent.

29. If a patient is eligible for Medicare and Medicaid, Medicare is referred to as the:
    a. payer of last resort.
    b. primary payer.
    c. co-insurance.
    d. fiscal agent.

Part III True/False

Write "T" or "F" in the blank to indicate whether you think the statement is true or false.

_____ 30. Medicaid managed care plans require gatekeepers to approve all specialty care.

_____ 31. Providers must enroll for participation in the Medicaid program with the fiscal agent for their region.

_____ 32. Medicaid spend down eligibility is determined annually to find out the patient's copayment amount.

_____ 33. In some states, the phrase *prior approval* may be referred to as *prior authorization*.

_____ 34. There is only one type of copayment requirement in the Medicaid program.

_____ 35. Hospital-acquired conditions are payable by the Medicaid program.

_____ 36. All states have a Medicaid time limit of 12 months from the date of service for filing claims.

_____ 37. If a Medicaid patient requires medical care while out of state, the claim for services should be filed with the patient's home state Medicaid program.

_____ 38. If a Medicaid managed care patient requires medical care, the claim for services should be filed with the state Medicaid's fiscal agent.

_____ 39. A state agency that investigates complaints of mistreatment in long-term care facilities is the Medicaid Fraud Control Unit (MFCU).

_____ 40. The Office of the Inspector General oversees and assess the MFCU for performance and compliance with federal requirements.

ASSIGNMENT 7.2 CRITICAL THINKING

Performance Objective

Task: After reading the scenario, answer the following questions, using critical thinking skills.

Conditions: Use a pen or pencil.

Standards: Time: _____ minutes

               Accuracy: _____

               (Note: The time element and accuracy criteria may be given by your instructor.)

Directions: After reading the following scenarios, answer the question, using your critical thinking skills. Record your answers on the blank lines.

#1: Scenario: Mrs. Ho, a Medicaid recipient, suddenly experiences a pain in her right lower abdominal area and rushes to a local hospital for emergency care. Laboratory work verifies that she has a ruptured appendix, and immediate surgery is recommended. Is prior authorization required in a situation like this?

1. _____

    Reason: _____

#2: Scenario: Mary Decker, a 4-year-old who is covered under the CHIP program, presents to her pediatrician for her annual well-child check and immunizations. Is prior authorization required for the immunizations?

2. _____

    Reason:_____

#3: Scenario: Ethel Ramsey, a Medicaid recipient, has been diagnosed with chronic kidney disease and will require hemodialysis. Is prior authorization required for hemodialysis to begin?

3. _____

    Reason:_____

#4: Scenario: A cancer patient, covered by Medicaid, has acquired a Stage III pressure ulcer following her hospital admission. Is prior authorization required for treatment of the pressure ulcer?

4. _____

    Reason: _____

8 TRICARE and Veterans' Health Care

Linda M. Smith

KEY TERMS

Your instructor may wish to select some words pertinent to this chapter for a test. For definitions of the terms, further study, and/or reference, the words, phrases, and abbreviations may be found in the glossary at the end of the Textbook. *Key terms for this chapter follow.*

active duty service member
allowable charge
authorized provider
beneficiary
catastrophic cap
catchment area
Civilian Health and Medical Program of the Department of Veterans Affairs
Civilian Health and Medical Program of the Uniformed Services
cooperative care
coordination of benefits
cost share
Defense Enrollment Eligibility Reporting System
Department of Veterans Affairs
emergency
Explanation of benefits
Fiscal Intermediary
health benefits advisor
health care finder
medically (or psychologically) necessary
Military Health System
Military Treatment Facility
Network provider
nonparticipating provider

other health insurance
participating provider
partnership program
point-of-service option
preauthorization
Prime Service Area
primary care manager
regional contractor
service benefit program
service-connected injury
service retiree (military retiree)
sponsor
Supplemental Health Care Program
total, permanent, service-connected disability
Transitional Assistance Management Program (TAMP)
TRICARE
TRICARE for Life
TRICARE Prime
TRICARE service center
TRICARE Select
urgent care
veteran
Veterans Choice Act
Veterans Health Administration
Veterans Health Care

KEY ABBREVIATIONS

See how many abbreviations and acronyms you can translate and then use this as a handy reference list. Definitions for the key abbreviations are located near the back of the Textbook *in the glossary.*

ADSM _____

CHAMPUS _____

CHAMPVA _____

COB _____

DEERS _____

FI _____

HBA _____

HCF _____

MHS _____

MTF _____

nonpar _____

OHI _____

par _____

PCM _____

POS _____

PSA _____

SHCP _____

TAMP _____

TFL _____

TMA _____

TPR _____   VA _____

TSC _____

PERFORMANCE OBJECTIVES

The student will be able to:

- Define and spell the key terms and key abbreviations for this chapter, given the information from the *Textbook* glossary, within a reasonable time period and with enough accuracy to obtain a satisfactory evaluation.

- After reading the chapter, answer the fill in the blank, multiple choice, and true/false review questions with enough accuracy to obtain a satisfactory evaluation.

STUDY OUTLINE

TRICARE
    History of TRICARE
    TRICARE Eligibility
    TRICARE Authorized Providers
    TRICARE Health Plans
Veterans Health Administration Program
    Eligibility
    Enrollment
    Identification Card
    Benefits
    Provider
    Preauthorization

TRICARE and CHAMPVA Claims Procedure
    Regional Contractor
    TRICARE
    TRICARE and CHAMPVA Claim Offices
    TRICARE and CHAMPVA Time Limits for
       Claim Filing
After Claims Submission
    Explanation of Benefits
    Claim Inquiries and Appeals

Part I Fill in the Blank

Review the objectives, key terms, glossary definitions of key terms, chapter information, and figures before completing the following review questions.

1. CHAMPUS, the acronym for Civilian Health and Medical Program of the Uniformed Services, is now called _____ and was organized to control escalating medical costs and to standardize benefits for active duty families and military retirees.

2. The regional contractor for TRICARE East is _____.

3. An active duty service member is known as a/an _____; once retired, this former member is called a/an _____.

4. An individual who qualifies for TRICARE is known as a/an _____.

5. A system for verifying an individual's TRICARE eligibility is called _____.

6. Children of military sponsors are eligible for TRICARE benefits until the age of _____, unless they are enrolled in college. Children enrolled in college are eligible for benefits until the age of _____.

7. Active duty uniformed service personnel are issued a/an _____ to be used for standard identification.

8. Military family members and retirees are issued a/an _____ to access health care benefits.

9. The maximum dollar amount that a TRICARE member has to pay in any fiscal year for covered medical benefits is referred to as the _____, after which TRICARE pays 100% of the allowable charges for the rest of the year.

10. The two primary TRICARE programs are _____ and _____.

11. Programs that allow TRICARE Select beneficiaries to receive treatment, services, or supplies from civilian providers are called _____ and _____.

12. An individual who is located at TRICARE service centers who can help TRICARE beneficiaries and providers with preauthorization of medical services is a/an _____.

13. A TRICARE managed care plan option available to individuals on active duty which limits freedom of choice in providers but offers fewer out-of-pocket costs is known as:_____ _____.

14. A physician who is responsible for coordinating and managing all of the TRICARE Prime beneficiary's health care unless there is an emergency is a/an _____.

15. TRICARE Prime provides the same covered services as TRICARE Select beneficiaries, plus there are additional _____ and _____ services.

16. A _____ is an individual at military hospitals or clinics who is available to assist TRICARE beneficiaries to obtain medical care needed through the military and through TRICARE.

17. TRICARE Young Adult enrollees must be a dependant of an eligible uniformed service sponsor, unmarried, at least age _____, and not eligible to enroll in an employer-sponsored health plan.

18. TRICARE for Life is a program for TRICARE-eligible beneficiaries who are age _____.

19. The TRICARE _____ program is designed to provide care and comfort to patients who are terminally ill.

20. CHAMPVA is the acronym for _____ now known as the _____ _____.

21. Those individuals who serve in the United States Armed Forces, finish their service, and are honorably discharged are known as _____.

22. Veterans Health Administration (CHAMPVA) is not an insurance program but is considered as a/an _____ program.

23. Which individuals are entitled to Veterans Health Administration (CHAMPVA) medical benefits?

    a. _____

    b. _____

    _____

    c. _____

    _____

24. A specific region defined by zip codes that is within a 40-mile radius from the closest VA medical facility is known as a:_____

25. An organization that contracts with the government to process TRICARE and Veterans Health Administration (CHAMPVA) health insurance claims is known as a/an _____ _____.

26. The time limit for submitting a TRICARE Standard or CHAMPVA claim for outpatient service is _____ _____; for inpatient service, it is _____.

Part II Multiple Choice

Choose the best answer.

27. Effective January 1, 2018, the two primary TRICARE regions are designated as:
    a. Region West and Region South.
    b. Region North and Region South.
    c. Region East and Region West.
    d. Region South and Region East.

28. The catchment area for a specific geographic region is defined by zip code and is based on an area surrounding each Medical Treatment Facility in the U.S. of approximate radius:
    a. 30 miles.
    b. 40 miles.
    c. 50 miles.
    d. 100 miles.

29. An authorized civilian provider who has not signed a contract with a regional TRICARE contractor to give medical care to TRICARE beneficiaries but agrees to accept assignment on a case-by-case basis is known as a/an:
    a. authorized provider.
    b. network provider.
    c. non-network participating provider.
    d. non-network not-participating provider.

30. The 4 different types of military treatment facilities which provide different levels of service are:
    a. Primary care offices, medical centers, trauma centers and hospitals
    b. Primary care offices, specialty offices, trauma centers and clinics
    c. Multi-service markets, outpatient clinics, inpatient facilities, and ambulatory surgical centers.
    d. Multi-service markets, medical centers, hospitals, clinics

31. A health care professional who helps a patient who is under the TRICARE program obtain preauthorization for care is called a:
    a. primary care physician (PCP).
    b. health care finder (HCF).
    c. health benefits advisor (HBA).
    d. participating provider.

32. TRICARE Prime Remote is a managed plan that can only be used if the distance from both the sponsor's home and work addresses to a military hospital or clinic is more than:
    a. 30 miles.
    b. 40 miles.
    c. 50 miles.
    d. 100 miles.

33. TRICARE Prime Remote Overseas is a managed care plan available in the designated remote overseas locations of:
    a. Europe-Australia, and Canada.
    b. Africa, Canada, and the Pacific.
    c. Latin America, Australia, and Canada.
    d. Eurasia-Africa, Latin America, Canada, and the Pacific.

34. Under the U.S. Family Health Plan, the designated provider for Upstate New York is:
    a. Johns Hopkins Medicine.
    b. Martin's Point Health Care.
    c. US Family Health Plan of Southern New England
    d. St. Vincent Catholic Medical Centers.

35. To qualify for TRICARE for Life (TFL), a beneficiary must be:
    a. a TRICARE beneficiary.
    b. eligible for Medicare Part A.
    c. enrolled in Medicare Part B.
    d. all of the above.

Part III True/False

Write "T" or "F" in the blank to indicate whether you think the statement is true or false.

_____ 36. TRICARE is funded by both the state and federal governments.

_____ 37. Retired service members and their families are entitled to medical benefits under TRICARE.

_____ 38. TRICARE beneficiaries who use nonauthorized providers and receive medical services may be responsible for their entire bill.

_____ 39. The catastrophic cap does not apply to noncovered TRICARE services.

_____ 40. The TRICARE Select program became effective January 1, 2017.

_____ 41. Referrals are not required for the TRICARE Select program.

_____ 42. TRICARE Prime Remote (TPR) is a program designed for military retirees and their families.

_____ 43. Beneficiaries of the Veterans Health Administration (CHAMPVA) program have complete freedom of choice in selecting their civilian health care providers.

_____ 44. A patient enrolled in the Veterans Health Administration (CHAMPVA) program does not need preauthorization for hospice services.

_____ 45. By law, Veterans Health Administration is usually the second payer when a beneficiary is enrolled in other health insurance.

_____ 46. When transmitting a TRICARE claim for medical care received in the U.S. or U.S territories, always send it to the TRICARE claims office nearest to the residence of the military sponsor.

_____ 47. TRICARE is considered primary to Medicare for persons younger than age 65 who have Medicare Part A as a result of a disability and who have enrolled in Medicare Part B.

_____ 48. CHAMPVA is considered primary to Medicare for persons younger than age 65 who are enrolled in Medicare Parts A and B.

_____ 49. TRICARE is considered primary to Worker's Compensation if the beneficiary is injured on the job or becomes ill because of his or her work.

_____ 50. If a provider participates with TRICARE, accepts assignment, and receives payment directly from the regional contractor, the patient will have access to the EOB statement.

Chapter **8** **TRICARE and Veterans' Health Care**

Performance Objective

Task: After reading the scenarios, answer the following questions, using critical thinking skills.

Conditions:

Standards: Time: _____minutes

                     Accuracy: _____

                     (Note: The time element and accuracy criteria may be given by your instructor.)

Directions: After reading the scenarios, answer the following questions, using your critical thinking skills. Record your answers on the blank lines.

1. If Bertha Evans is seen for an office visit and has other insurance besides TRICARE, and she is the dependant of an active military person, whom do you bill first?

   _____

   Reason: _____

2. If Jason Williams, a TRICARE beneficiary who became disabled at age 10 years and who is also receiving Medicare Part A and Medicare Part B benefits, is seen for a consultation, whom do you bill first?

   _____

   Reason: _____

3. If Tanner Vine, a Veterans Health Administration (CHAMPVA) and Medicaid beneficiary, is seen on an emergency basis in the office, whom do you bill first?

   _____

   Reason: _____

9 Workers' Compensation

Linda M. Smith

KEY TERMS

Your instructor may wish to select some words pertinent to this chapter for a test. For definitions of the terms, further study, and/or reference, the words, phrases, and abbreviations may be found in the glossary at the end of the Textbook. Key terms for this chapter follow.

accident
adjudication
claims examiner
conversion factor
compromise and release
deposition
ergonomic
extraterritorial
Federal Employees' Compensation Act
injury
insurance adjuster
lien
medical service order
nondisability claim
occupational illness or disease
Occupational Safety and Health Administration
Office of Workers' Compensation Programs
permanent and stationary
permanent disability

petition
physician of record
reexamination report
relative value scale
second-injury fund
sequelae
self-insure
State Compensation Insurance Fund
state-run program
sub rosa films
subrogation
subsequent-injury fund
temporary disability
third-party liability
third-party subrogation
waiting period
work hardening
Workers' Compensation Board
workers' compensation insurance

KEY ABBREVIATIONS

See how many abbreviations and acronyms you can translate and then use this as a handy reference list. Definitions for the key abbreviations are located near the back of the Textbook in the glossary.

AME _____

C and R _____

ERISA _____

FECA _____

IME _____

LHWCA _____

ND _____

OSHA _____

OWCP _____

P and S _____

PD _____

POR _____

QME _____

ROM _____

SCIF _____

SIF _____

TD _____

WP _____

PERFORMANCE OBJECTIVES

The student will be able to:

- Define and spell the key terms and key abbreviations for this chapter, given the information from the *Textbook* glossary, within a reasonable time period and with enough accuracy to obtain a satisfactory evaluation.

- After reading the chapter, answer the fill in the blank, multiple choice, and true/false review questions with enough accuracy to obtain a satisfactory evaluation.

- Given a list of common medical abbreviations and symbols that appear in chart notes, fill in the correct meaning of each abbreviation within a reasonable time period and with enough accuracy to obtain a satisfactory evaluation. Students may use a medical dictionary or internet resource.

- Given the patients' medical chart notes and blank workers' compensation forms, complete each workers' compensation form related to billing within a reasonable time period and with enough accuracy to obtain a satisfactory evaluation.

STUDY OUTLINE

Workers' Compensation Defined

History
 Workers' Compensation Statutes
 Workers' Compensation Reform
 Purposes of Workers' Compensation Laws

Workers' Compensation Insurance Programs
 State Compensation Insurance Fund
 Private Insurance Workers Compensation Carriers
 Self-Insurance
 Second-Injury Fund (Subsequent-Injury Fund)

Eligibility
 Work-Related Accident
 Occupational Illness
 Volunteer Workers
 Agricultural Workers

Federal and State Laws
 Federal Laws
 State Laws

Types of State Compensation Benefits

Types of State Workers' Compensation Claims
 Nondisability Claim
 Temporary Disability Claim
 Permanent Disability Claim

Fraud and Abuse

Legal Situations
 Medical Evaluator
 Depositions
 Medical Testimony
 Liens
 Third-Party Subrogation

Medical Reports
 Health Information Record Keeping
 Terminology

Reporting Requirements
 Employer's Report of Injury
 Medical Service Order
 Health Care Provider's First Report of Injury
 Health Care Provider's Progress or Supplemental Report
 Final Report

Claim Submission
 Financial Responsibility
 Fee Schedules
 Helpful Billing Tips
 Out-of-State Claims
 Delinquent or Slow Pay Claims

ASSIGNMENT 9.1 REVIEW QUESTIONS

Part I Fill in the Blank

Review the objectives, key terms, glossary definitions of key terms, chapter information, and figures before completing the following review questions.

1. Individuals who are paid by someone in exchange for labor or services are referred to as _____ _____.

2. Name two kinds of statutes under workers' compensation.

    a. _____

    b. _____

3. List five reasons that workers' compensation laws were developed.

    a. _____

    b. _____

    c. _____

    d. _____

    e. _____

4. _____ pays the workers' compensation insurance premiums.

5. State three methods used for funding workers' compensation.

    a. _____

    b. _____

    c. _____

6. Self-insured employers are governed by _____, a federal law that sets minimum requirements for group health plans.

7. A form of self-insurance that is owned by its policyholders and serves smaller or mid-size companies is known as _____.

8. When an employee with a preexisting condition is injured at work and the injury produces a disability greater than what would have been caused by the second injury alone, the benefits are drawn from a/an _____.

9. An unexpected, unintended event that occurs at a particular time and place, causing injury to an individual not of his or her own making, is called a/an _____.

10. Maria Cardoza works in a plastics manufacturing company and inhales some fumes that cause bronchitis. Because this condition is associated with her employment, it is called a/an _____.

11. Name the federal workers' compensation acts that cover workers.

    a. _____

    b. _____

    c. _____

    d. _____

12. Federal law mandates that states set up laws to meet _____ requirements.

13. State compensation laws that require each employer to accept its provisions and to provide for specialized benefits for employees who are injured at work are called

    _____.

14. State compensation laws that may be accepted or rejected by the employer are known as _____

    _____

    _____.

15. When billing for an injury of a patient who lives out-of-state, the insurance billing specialist should follow the rules and fee schedule of the state in which the workers' compensation claim was _____ filed.

16. In most states, the waiting period for workers' compensation to pay for medical bills resulting from a workplace injury or illness begins: _____

17. List five types of workers' compensation benefits.

    a. _____

    b. _____

    c. _____

    d. _____

    e. _____

18. Who can provide medical treatment for an industrial injury?

    _____

    _____

19. What are three types of workers' compensation claims and the differences among them?

    a._____

    b._____

    c._____

20. Weekly temporary disability payments are based on

    _____.

21. After suffering an industrial injury, Mr. Fields is in a treatment program in which he is given real work tasks for building strength and endurance. This form of therapy is called _____
    _____.

22. When an industrial case reaches the time for rating the disability, this is accomplished by what state agency? _____
    _____

23. May an injured person appeal his or her case if he or she is not satisfied with the rating?_____
    If so, to whom does he or she appeal? _____ or _____
    _____

24. When fraud or abuse is suspected in a workers' compensation case, the physician should report the situation to ___
    _____.

25. Physicians who conduct medical–legal evaluations of injured workers must pass a complex medical examination to become certified by the _____ Council.

26. A proceeding that generally takes place in an attorney's office in which an attorney asks a witness questions about a case and the witness answers under oath is referred to as a/an _____.

27. In a workers' compensation case, when a claim is made against a separate person or company, but not the employer, it is referred to as a _____ liability.

28. Explain third-party subrogation.

    _____

    _____

29. When an individual suffers a work-related injury or illness, the employer must complete and send a form called a/an _____ to the insurance company and workers' compensation state offices, and if the employee is sent to a physician's office for medical care, the employer must complete a form called a/an _____ _____, which authorizes the physician to treat the employee.

30. Temporary disability ends when the patient is able to return to work or if the disability lasts longer than _____ months.

Part II Multiple Choice

Choose the best answer.

31. Employers are required to meet health and safety standards for their employees under federal and state statutes known as the:
    a. Occupational Safety and Health Administration (OSHA) Act of 1970.
    b. Health Insurance Portability and Accountability Act (HIPAA).
    c. Clinical Laboratory Improvement Amendment (CLIA).
    d. Employee Retirement Income Security Act (ERISA).

32. The process of carrying on a lawsuit is called:
    a. lien.
    b. litigation.
    c. deposition.
    d. adjudication.

33. A proceeding during which an attorney questions a witness who answers under oath but not in open court is called a:
    a. subpoena.
    b. subrogation.
    c. petition.
    d. deposition.

34. The legal claim on the property of another for payment of a debt is termed a:
    a. medical service order.
    b. subpoena.
    c. lien.
    d. promissory note.

35. The contract for treatment and the financial responsibility in a workers' compensation case is between:
    a. the health care organization and the patient.
    b. the health care organization and the employer.
    c. the health care organization and the workers' compensation insurance carrier.
    d. the employer and the workers' compensation insurance carrier.

36. Workers' compensation fee schedules that consider the time, skills, and extent of the service provided by the physician are:
    a. maximum fee schedules.
    b. relative value scale fee schedules.
    c. Medicare-based fee schedules.
    d. compulsory fee schedules.

Part III True/False

Write "T" or "F" in the blank to indicate whether you think the statement is true or false.

_____ 37. When working for the ABC Machining Company, an employee cuts his finger off while using a lathe. He is covered under workers' compensation.

_____ 38. A roofer takes his girlfriend to a roofing job and she is injured. She is covered under workers' compensation insurance.

_____ 39. A private duty nurse employed by the XYZ homecare service is injured while moving a patient. She is covered under workers' compensation insurance.

_____ 40. A Department of Energy employee diagnosed with a disease resulting from exposure to radiation is covered under workers' compensation.

_____ 41. A postal worker twists his ankle while delivering mail. He is covered under workers' compensation.

_____ 42. An employee who is at an official company retreat suffers from a concussion due to a fall. The injury would be covered under workers' compensation.

87

_____ 43. An independent contractor is injured while working for a local construction company. The construction company's workers' compensation would cover the related medical bills.

_____ 44. If an individual seeks medical care for a workers' compensation injury from another state, the state's regulations are followed in which the injured person's claim was originally filed.

_____ 45. When a patient arrives at a medical office and says he or she was hurt at work, you should verify insurance information with the benefits coordinator for the employer.

_____ 46. A stamped physician's signature is acceptable on the Doctor's First Report of Occupational Injury or Illness form.

ASSIGNMENT 9.2 COMPLETE A DOCTOR'S FIRST REPORT OF OCCUPATIONAL INJURY OR ILLNESS FORM FOR A WORKERS' COMPENSATION CASE

Performance Objective

Task: Complete a Doctor's First Report of Occupational Injury or Illness form and define patient record abbreviations.

Conditions: Use the patient's record (Fig. 9.1), a Doctor's First Report of Occupational Injury or Illness form (Fig. 9.2), and a computer.

Standards: Claim Productivity Measurement

   Time: _____ minutes

   Accuracy: _____

   (Note: The time element and accuracy criteria may be given by your instructor.)

***Directions*:**

1. Complete the Doctor's First Report of Occupational Injury or Illness form (see Fig. 9.2) for this nondisability type of claim. The patient was seen by Gerald Practon, MD; 4567 Broad Avenue, Woodland Hills, XY 12345. (Phone number: 555-486-9002) (License#: C01402X) (IRS Number: 70-34597XX).

2. Using a medical dictionary or an internet resource, define abbreviations found in the patient's medical record.

   After the instructor has returned your work to you, either make the necessary corrections and place your work in a three-ring notebook for future reference or, if you received a high score, place it in your portfolio for reference when applying for a job.

Abbreviations pertinent to this record:

apt _____	CT _____
lt _____	ncg _____
pt _____	DC _____
ED _____	FU _____
hosp _____	wks _____
ER _____	approx _____
c/o _____	RTW _____
L _____	WC _____

PATIENT RECORD NO. 15-2-3

Hiranuma	Glen	M.	12-24-55	M	555-467-3383
LAST NAME	FIRST NAME	MIDDLE NAME	BIRTH DATE	SEX	HOME PHONE

4372 Hanley Avenue	Woodland Hills	XY	12345
ADDRESS	CITY	STATE	ZIP CODE

555-908-3433		555-467-3383		hiranuma@wb.net
CELL PHONE	PAGER NO.	FAX NO.		E-MAIL ADDRESS

558-XX-9960	U3402189
PATIENT'S SOC. SEC. NO.	DRIVER'S LICENSE

house painter	Pittsburgh Paint Company (commercial painting company)
PATIENT'S OCCUPATION	NAME OF COMPANY

3725 Bonfeld Avenue, Woodland Hills, XY 12345	555-486-9070
ADDRESS OF EMPLOYER	PHONE

Esme M. Hiranuma	homemaker
SPOUSE OR PARENT	OCCUPATION

EMPLOYER	ADDRESS	PHONE

State Compensation Insurance Fund, 14156 Magnolia Boulevard, Torres, XY 12349
NAME OF INSURANCE

016-2432-211
POLICY/CERTIFICATE NO.   GROUP NO.

REFERRED BY: Pittsburgh Paint Company

DATE	PROGRESS NOTES
5-22-xx	At 9:30 a.m. this ♂ house painter was painting an apt ceiling (apt located at 3540 W. 87th Street, Woodland Hills, XY 12345, County of Woodland Hills) when he slipped and fell from a tall ladder landing on his head and lt side of body; brief unconsciousness for approximately 15 minutes. Employer was notified by coworker and pt was sent to College Hosp ED. I was called to the hosp at the request of the employer and saw pt in ER at 5 PM (performed a comprehensive history and exam. Pt c/o L shoulder pain and swelling; L leg and hip pain; neck and head pain. X-rays were taken of lt hip (complete), lt femur (2 views), and cervical spine (3 views) as well as CT of the brain (without contrast)—all neg. I admitted pt for overnight stay in hosp for concussion. Applied sling for L shoulder sprain. Cleaned and dressed L hip and leg abrasions (moderate complexity/medical decision making). Plan to DC 5/23/xx. No PD expected. Pt to FU in 2 wks. Approx. RTW 6/6 xx. Prepared WC report. GP/llf *Gerald Practon, MD*
5-23-xx	Pt's HA gone. Vital signs normal. Discharged home. RTO 1 wk. GP/llf *Gerald Practon, MD*

Fig. 9.1: Patient Record

DOCTOR'S FIRST REPORT OF OCCUPATIONAL INJURY OR ILLNESS

Within 5 days of your initial examination, for every occupational injury or illness, send two copies of this report to the employer's workers' compensation insurance carrier or the insured employer. Failure to file a timely doctor's report may result in assessment of a civil penalty. In the case of diagnosed or suspected pesticide poisoning, send a copy of the report to Division of Labor Statistics and Research, P.O. Box 420603, San Francisco, CA 94142-0603, and notify your local health officer by telephone within 24 hours.

	PLEASE DO NOT USE THIS COLUMN
1. INSURER NAME AND ADDRESS	
2. EMPLOYER NAME	Case No.
3. Address No. and Street City Zip	Industry
4. Nature of business (e.g., food manufacturing, building construction, retailer of women's clothes.)	County
5. PATIENT NAME (first name, middle initial, last name)	6. Sex □ Male □ Female	7. Date of Mo. Day Yr. Birth	Age
8. Address. No. and Street City Zip	9. Telephone number ( )	Hazard
10. Occupation (Specific job title)	11. Social Security Number	Disease
12. Injured at: No. and Street City County	Hospitalization
13. Date and hour of injury Mo. Day Yr. Hour _____ a.m. _____ p.m. or onset of illness	14. Date last worked Mo. Day Yr.	Occupation
15. Date and hour of first Mo. Day Yr. Hour _____ a.m. _____ p.m. examination or treatment	16. Have you (or your office) previously treated patient? □ Yes □ No	Return Date/Code

Patient please complete this portion, if able to do so. Otherwise, doctor please complete immediately, inability or failure of a patient to complete this portion shall not affect his/her rights to workers' compensation under the California Labor Code.

17. **DESCRIBE HOW THE ACCIDENT OR EXPOSURE HAPPENED.** (Give specific object, machinery or chemical Use reverse side if more space is required.)

18. SUBJECTIVE COMPLAINTS (Describe fully Use reverse side if more space is required.)

19. OBJECTIVE FINDINGS (Use reverse side if more space is required.)
   A. Physical examination

   B. X-ray and laboratory results (State if non or pending.)

20. **DIAGNOSIS** (if occupational illness specify etiologic agent and duration of exposure.) Chemical or toxic compounds involved?   □ Yes □ No
   ICD-9 Code ___ ___ ___ - ___ ___

21. Are your findings and diagnosis consistent with patient's account of injury or onset of illness? □ Yes   □ No   If "no", please explain.

22. Is there any other current condition that will impede or delay patient's recovery? □ Yes   □ No   If "yes", please explain.

23. TREATMENT RENDERED (Use reverse side if more space is required.)

24. If further treatment required, specify treatment plan/estimated duration.

25. If hospitalized as inpatient, give hospital name and location   Date   Mo. Day Yr.   Estimated stay admitted

26. WORK STATUS -- Is patient able to perform usual work?   □ Yes   □ No
   If "no", date when patient can return to: Regular work ____/____/____
                                              Modified work ____/____/____   Specify restrictions _____

Doctor's Signature _____   CA License Number _____

Doctor Name and Degree (please type) _____   IRS Number _____

Address _____   Telephone Number (____) _____

FORM 5021 (Rev. 4)
1992

Any person who makes or causes to be made any knowingly false or fraudulent material statement or material representation for the purpose of obtaining or denying workers' compensation benefits or payments is guilty of a felony.

Fig. 9.2: Doctor's First Report of Occupational Injury or Illness

ASSIGNMENT 9.3 COMPLETE A DOCTOR'S FIRST REPORT OF OCCUPATIONAL INJURY OR ILLNESS FORM FOR A WORKERS' COMPENSATION CASE

Performance Objective

Task: Complete a Doctor's First Report of Occupational Injury or Illness form and define patient record abbreviations.

Conditions: Use the patient's record (Fig. 9.3a and 9.3b), a Doctor's First Report of Occupational Injury or Illness form (Fig. 9.4), and a computer.

Standards: Claim Productivity Measurement

             Time: _____ minutes

             Accuracy: _____

             (Note: The time element and accuracy criteria may be given by your instructor.)

Directions:

1. Complete the Doctor's First Report of Occupational Injury or Illness form for this temporary disability type of claim. Refer to Carlos A. Giovanni's patient record for November 11 through November 15. The patient was seen by Astro Parkinson, MD; 4567 Broad Avenue, Woodland Hills, XY 12345. (Phone number: 555-486-9002) (License#: C02600X) (IRS Number: 75-44530XX).

2. Using a medical dictionary or an internet resource, define abbreviations found in the patient's medical record.

After the instructor has returned your work to you, either make the necessary corrections and place your work in a three-ring notebook for future reference or, if you received a high score, place it in your portfolio for reference when applying for a job.

Abbreviations pertinent to this record:

pt _____

ER _____

CT _____

R _____

tr _____

adm _____

DC _____

hosp _____

HA _____

BP _____

RTO _____

wks _____

TD _____

RTW _____

approx _____

PO _____

X _____

adv _____

trt _____

reg _____

W _____

Cons _____

PATIENT RECORD NO. 15-4-5

Giovanni	Carlos	A.	10-24-55	M	555-677-3485
LAST NAME	FIRST NAME	MIDDLE NAME	BIRTH DATE	SEX	HOME PHONE

89 Beaumont Court	Woodland Hills	XY	12345	
ADDRESS	CITY	STATE	ZIP CODE	

	555-230-7788	555-677-3485		giovannic@wb.net
CELL PHONE	PAGER NO.	FAX NO.		E-MAIL ADDRESS

556-XX-9699	Y0394876
PATIENT'S SOC. SEC. NO.	DRIVER'S LICENSE

TV repairman	Giant Television Co. (TV repair company)
PATIENT'S OCCUPATION	NAME OF COMPANY

8764 Ocean Avenue, Woodland Hills, XY 12345	555-647-8851
ADDRESS OF EMPLOYER	PHONE

Maria B. Giovanni	homemaker
SPOUSE OR PARENT	OCCUPATION

EMPLOYER	ADDRESS	PHONE

State Compensation Insurance Fund, 600 S. Lafayette Park Place, Ehrlich, XY 12350
NAME OF INSURANCE

57780	
POLICY/CERTIFICATE NO.	GROUP NO.

REFERRED BY: Giant Television Company

Fig. 9.3a: Patient Record

DATE	PROGRESS NOTES
	Patient: Giovanni, Carlos A. Patient Record No. 15-04-05
11-11-xx	Pt referred to College Hospital ER by employer for workers' compensation injury. I was called in as on-call neurosurgeon to evaluate the pt. Pt states that today at 2 PM he fell from the roof of a private home while installing an antenna at 2231 Duarte St., Woodland Hills, XY 12345 in Woodland Hills County. He describes the incident as follows: "When I was attaching the base of an antenna, the weight of the antenna shifted and knocked me off the roof." Pt complains of head pain and indicates brief loss of consciousness. I performed a comprehensive history and exam. Complete skull x-rays showed fractured skull. CT of head/brain (without contrast) indicates well-defined R. subdural hematoma. Pt suffering from cerebral concussion; no open wound. Tr plan: Adm pt to College Hospital (5 PM) and schedule R infratentorial craniotomy to evacuate hematoma. (high medical decision making). Obtained authorization and prepared Dr.'s First Report.
	AP/llf *Astro Parkinson, MD*
11-12-xx	Performed R infratentorial craniotomy and evacuated subdural hematoma. Pt stable and returned to room; will be seen daily. TD: Estimated RTW 1-15-xx. Possible cranial defect & head disfigurement resulting. Pt to be hospitalized for approx 2 weeks.
	AP/llf *Astro Parkinson, MD*
11-13-xx	Hospital Visit. (Expanded problem focused history exam/moderate medical decision making). Pt improving; recommend consult with Dr. Graff for cranial defect. Authorization obtained from adjuster (Steve Burroughs) at State Comp.
	AP/llf *Astro Parkinson, MD*
11-14-xx	Pt seen in cons by Dr. Cosmo Graff who stated he does not recommend correcting PO cranial defect. Both Dr. Graff and I explained how the defect resulted from the injury; there may be some improvement over time. Pt states he is grateful to be alive (Expanded problem focused history and exam/moderate medical decision making.)
	AP/llf *Astro Parkinson, MD*
11-15-xx	Daily hospital visit. (Expanded problem focused history and exam/moderate medical decision making). Pt progressing appropriately; no complications have occurred.
thru	
11-29-xx	AP/llf *Astro Parkinson, MD*
11-30-xx	DC from hosp. Permanent cranial defect resulting from fracture and surgery. RTO 1 wk.
	AP/llf *Astro Parkinson, MD*
12-7-xx	Office visit (Expanded problem focused history and exam/low complexity medical decision making). Pt doing very well. No HA or visual disturbances, BP 120/80, alert and oriented. He is anxious to return to work. Pt cautioned about maintaining low activity level until released. RTO 2 wks.
	AP/llf *Astro Parkinson, MD*
12-21-xx	Office visit (problem focused history and exam/straightforward medical decision making). Pt continues to improve. Suggested he start a walking program 3 x wk and monitor symptoms. May do light activity and lifting (10 lbs). Adv to call if any symptoms return. RTO 10 days.
	AP/llf *Astro Parkinson, MD*
12-29-xx	Office visit (problem focused history and exam/straightforward medical decision making). Pt did not experience any symptoms with increased activity. No further trt necessary. Pt will increase activity and call if any problems occur. Pt scheduled to resume reg W on 1-15-xx. Final report submitted to workers' compensation carrier.
	AP/llf *Astro Parkinson, MD*

Fig. 9.3b, cont'd: Patient Record – Progress note

94

STATE OF CALIFORNIA
DOCTOR'S FIRST REPORT OF OCCUPATIONAL INJURY OR ILLNESS

Within 5 days of your initial examination, for every occupational injury or illness, send two copies of this report to the employer's workers' compensation insurance carrier or the insured employer. Failure to file a timely doctor's report may result in assessment of a civil penalty. In the case of diagnosed or suspected pesticide poisoning, send a copy of the report to Division of Labor Statistics and Research, P.O. Box 420603, San Francisco, CA 94142-0603, and notify your local health officer by telephone within 24 hours.

	PLEASE DO NOT USE THIS COLUMN
1. INSURER NAME AND ADDRESS	
2. EMPLOYER NAME	Case No.
3. Address No. and Street City Zip	Industry
4. Nature of business (e.g., food manufacturing, building construction, retailer of women's clothes.)	County
5. PATIENT NAME (first name, middle initial, last name) 6. Sex ☐ Male ☐ Female 7. Date of Birth Mo. Day Yr.	Age
8. Address: No. and Street City Zip 9. Telephone number ( )	Hazard
10. Occupation (Specific job title) 11. Social Security Number - -	Disease
12. Injured at: No. and Street City County	Hospitalization
13. Date and hour of injury or onset of illness Mo. Day Yr. Hour _____ a.m. _____ p.m. 14. Date last worked Mo. Day Yr.	Occupation
15. Date and hour of first examination or treatment Mo. Day Yr. Hour _____ a.m. _____ p.m. 16. Have you (or your office) previously treated patient? ☐ Yes ☐ No	Return Date/Code

Patient please complete this portion, if able to do so. Otherwise, doctor please complete immediately, inability or failure of a patient to complete this portion shall not affect his/her rights to workers' compensation under the California Labor Code.

17. DESCRIBE HOW THE ACCIDENT OR EXPOSURE HAPPENED. (Give specific object, machinery or chemical. Use reverse side if more space is required.)

18. SUBJECTIVE COMPLAINTS (Describe fully. Use reverse side if more space is required.)

19. OBJECTIVE FINDINGS (Use reverse side if more space is required.)
    A. Physical examination

    B. X-ray and laboratory results (State if non or pending.)

20. DIAGNOSIS (if occupational illness specify etiologic agent and duration of exposure.) Chemical or toxic compounds involved?   ☐ Yes   ☐ No
    ICD-9 Code ___ ___ ___ - ___ ___

21. Are your findings and diagnosis consistent with patient's account of injury or onset of illness? ☐ Yes   ☐ No   If "no", please explain.

22. Is there any other current condition that will impede or delay patient's recovery? ☐ Yes   ☐ No   If "yes", please explain.

23. TREATMENT RENDERED (Use reverse side if more space is required.)

24. If further treatment required, specify treatment plan/estimated duration.

25. If hospitalized as inpatient, give hospital name and location   Date   Mo. Day Yr.   Estimated stay
admitted

26. WORK STATUS -- Is patient able to perform usual work?   ☐ Yes   ☐ No
    If "no", date when patient can return to: Regular work ___/___/___
                                                Modified work ___/___/___   Specify restrictions _____

Doctor's Signature _____   CA License Number _____

Doctor Name and Degree (please type) _____   IRS Number _____

Address _____   Telephone Number (____) _____

FORM 5021 (Rev. 4)
1992

Any person who makes or causes to be made any knowingly false or fraudulent material statement or material representation for the purpose of obtaining or denying workers' compensation benefits or payments is guilty of a felony.

Fig. 9.4: Doctor's First Report of Occupational Injury or Illness

10 Disability Income Insurance and Disability Benefits Programs

Linda M. Smith

KEY TERMS

Your instructor may wish to select some words pertinent to this chapter for a test. For definitions of the terms, further study, and/or reference, the words, phrases, and abbreviations may be found in the glossary at the end of the Textbook.

Some of the insurance terms presented in this chapter are shown marked with an asterisk (*) and may seem familiar from previous chapters. However, their meanings may or may not have a slightly different connotation when referring to disability income insurance. Key terms for this chapter follow.

accidental death and dismemberment
benefit period*
Civil Service Retirement System
consultative examiner
cost-of-living adjustment
Department of Defense Disability
disability
Disability Determination Services
disability income insurance
double indemnity
exclusions*
Family and Medical Leave Act Federal Employees
    Retirement System
future purchase option
guaranteed renewable*
hearing
indemnity benefits
long-term disability insurance
noncancelable clause*

Paid family and medical leave insurance
partial disability*
reconsideration
residual benefits*
residual disability
short-term disability insurance
Social Security Administration
Social Security Disability Insurance program
State Disability Insurance
supplemental benefits
Supplemental Security Income
temporary disability*
temporary disability insurance
total disability*
unemployment compensation disability
Veterans Affairs disability program
voluntary disability insurance
waiting period*
waiver of premium*

KEY ABBREVIATIONS

See how many abbreviations and acronyms you can translate and then use this as a handy reference list. Definitions for the key abbreviations are located near the back of the Textbook *in the glossary.*

CE _____

COLA _____

CSRS _____

DDS _____

DoD _____

FERS _____

FMLA _____

PFML _____

SDI _____

SSA _____

SSDI _____

SSI _____

TD _____

TDI _____

UCD _____

VA _____

WP _____

PERFORMANCE OBJECTIVES

The student will be able to:

- Define and spell the key terms and key abbreviations for this chapter, given the information from the *Textbook* glossary, within a reasonable time period, and with enough accuracy to obtain a satisfactory evaluation.
- After reading the chapter, answer the fill in the blank, multiple choice, and true/false review questions with enough accuracy to obtain a satisfactory evaluation.

- Fill in the correct meaning of each abbreviation, given a list of common medical abbreviations and symbols that appear in chart notes, within a reasonable time period and with enough accuracy to obtain a satisfactory evaluation.
- Complete each state disability form, given the patients' medical chart notes and blank state disability forms, within a reasonable time period and with enough accuracy to obtain a satisfactory evaluation.

STUDY OUTLINE

Disability Income Insurance Defined
  Types of Disability
  Waiting Period
  Benefit Period
History
Disability Income Insurance Policies
  Individual
  Group
Federal Disability Programs
  Work-Related Disability
  Disability Benefit Programs

State Disability Insurance
  Eligibility
  Benefits
  Time Limits
  Medical Examinations
  Restrictions
  Voluntary Disability Insurance
Disability Income Claims Submission Guidelines
  Federal Disability Claims
  State Disability Claims

Part I Fill in the Blank

Review the objectives, key terms, glossary definitions of key terms, chapter information, and figures before completing the following review questions.

1. Insurance that provides monthly or weekly income when an individual is unable to work because of a nonindustrial illness or injury is called

   _____.

2. A _____ is the maximum amount of time that benefits will be paid to the injured or ill person for the disability.

3. When an individual who is insured under a disability income insurance policy cannot perform one or more of his or her regular job duties, this is known as _____ or _____ _____ disability.

4. Compensation which is paid to an insured disable person is referred to as _____.

5. Some insurance contracts that pay twice the face amount of the policy if accidental death occurs may have a provision titled _____.

6. When an individual becomes permanently disabled and cannot pay the insurance premium, a desirable provision in an insurance contract is _____.

7. Give three examples of preexisting conditions that may be written into a disability contract as exclusions:

   a. _____

   b. _____

   c. _____

8. Two federal programs for individuals younger than 65 years of age who cannot work for at least 1 year because of a severe disability are

   a. _____

   b. _____

9. The strict definition of *Disability* given by Social Security is _____ _____.

10. When applying for SSDI benefits, there is a _____ waiting period during which time the individual will not receive SSA benefits.

11. The _____ program pays monthly income benefits to adults and children with limited income and resources who are disabled, blind, or age 65 or older.

12. The Social Security Administration may hire a physician to evaluate an applicant's disability. A physician's role may be any one of the following:

   a. _____

   b. _____

   c. _____

13. If Disability Determination Services determines that the claimant is not eligible for disability benefits, the first level of the appeals process is referred to as _____.

14. The two types of federal retirement systems which have provisions for those who become disabled are _____ and _____.

15. Jamie Woods, a Navy petty officer aboard the USS *Denebola*, suffered an accident at his home three weeks after his honorable discharge. To receive veteran's benefits for this injury, the time limit in which a claim must be filed is ___
_____.

16. Name the states and the territory that have nonindustrial state disability programs.

    a. _____

    b. _____

    c. _____

    d. _____

    e. _____

    f. _____

17. In the state of Hawaii, the waiting period for state disability benefits to begin is: _____ days.

18. How long can a person living in New York State continue to draw state disability insurance benefits?
_____

19. After a claim begins, when do basic state disability benefits become payable if the patient is confined to his or her home or hospitalized? _____

20. Nick Tyson has recovered since a previous illness ended and becomes ill again with the same ailment. Is he entitled to state disability benefits? _____

21. John S. Thatcher stubbed his toe as he was leaving work and going to his car parked on the street. Because the injury was only slightly uncomfortable, he thought no more about it. The next morning he found that his foot was too swollen to fit in his shoe, so he stayed home. When the swelling did not subside after three days, John went to the doctor. Radiographs showed a broken toe, which kept John home for two weeks. After one week he applied for temporary state disability benefits.

    Will he be paid? _____

    Why or why not? _____

22. Peggy Jonson has an ectopic pregnancy and is unable to work because of complications of this condition. Can she receive state temporary disability benefits?
_____

23. Five states that allow for maternity benefits in normal pregnancy are

    a. _____

    b. _____

    c. _____

    d. _____

    e. _____

24. Betty T. Kraft had to stay home from her job because her 10-year-old daughter had measles. She applied for temporary state disability benefits.

    Will she be paid? _____

    Why or why not? _____

25. Vincent P. Michael was ill with a bad cold for one week. Will he receive temporary state disability benefits? _____
_____

    Why or why not? _____

26. Betsy C. Palm works in Hawaii and had an emergency appendectomy. She was hospitalized for three days and is returning to work within 3 days from discharge. Will she receive state disability benefits?

_____

Why or why not? _____

27. Frank E. Thompson is a box boy at a supermarket on Saturdays and Sundays while a full-time student at college. He broke his leg while skiing and cannot work at the market, but he is able to attend classes with his leg in a cast. Can he collect state disability benefits for his part-time job? _____ Why or why not? _____

28. Jerry L. Slate is out of a job and is receiving unemployment insurance benefits. He is now suffering from severe intestinal flu. The employment office calls him to interview for a job, but he is too ill to go. Can he collect temporary state disability benefits for this illness when he might have been given a job?

_____

Why or why not? _____

29. While walking the picket line with other employees on strike, Gene J. Berry came down with pneumonia and was ill for two weeks. Can he collect temporary state disability benefits?

Why or why not? _____

Gene went back to work for three weeks and then developed a slight cold and cough, which again was diagnosed as pneumonia. The doctor told him to stay home from work. Would he be able to collect temporary disability benefits?

_____

Why or why not? _____

30. A month after he retired, Roger Reagan had a gallbladder operation. Can he receive temporary state disability benefits?

Why or why not? _____

31. Jane M. Lambert, a resident of New Jersey fell in the back yard of her home and fractured her left ankle. She had a nonunion fracture and could not work for 28 weeks. For how long will she collect temporary state disability benefits?

_____

32. Dr. Kay examines Ben Yates and completes a disability income claim form because of a prolonged illness. On receiving the information, the insurance adjuster notices some conflicting data. Name other documents that may be requested to justify payment of benefits.

a. _____

b. _____

c. _____

33. Trent Walters, a permanently disabled individual, applies for federal disability benefits. To establish eligibility for benefits under this program, data allowed must be _____ year/years old.

34. When following up on State Disability Claims, all correspondence should include the patient's name and _____

_____.

Part II Multiple Choice

Choose the best answer.

35. Compensation paid to the insured disabled person can be received:
    a. daily.
    b. weekly.
    c. monthly.
    d. varies, depending on the policy.

36. When the purchase of insurance is investigated, the words to look for in the insurance contract that mean the premium cannot be increased at renewal time are:
    a. guaranteed renewable.
    b. conditional provision.
    c. noncancelable clause.
    d. optional provision.

37. Provisions that limit the scope of insurance coverage are known as:
    a. clauses.
    b. deductibles.
    c. conditions.
    d. exclusions.

38. A Social Security Administration division that determines an individual's eligibility to be placed under the federal disability program is called:
    a. Disability Determination Services.
    b. Social Security Disability.
    c. Supplemental Security Income.
    d. none of the above.

39. The time period from the beginning of disability to receiving the first payment of benefits is called a/an
    a. exclusion period.
    b. waiting period.
    c. insurance period.
    d. elimination phase.

40. The second level of appeals for a determination of disability is:
    a. a reconsideration.
    b. a hearing.
    c. an Appeals Council review.
    d. and Administrative Law Judge review.

Part III True/False

Write "T" or "F" in the blank to indicate whether you think the statement is true or false.

_____ 41. When a person insured under a disability income insurance policy cannot, for a limited period of time, perform all functions of his or her regular job duties, it is known as permanent disability.

_____ 42. Disability income policies provide medical expense benefits.

_____ 43. There is no standard definition for total disability.

_____ 44. Eligibility for the SSI program is based strictly on financial need.

_____ 45. To be eligible to apply for disability benefits under Social Security, an individual must be unable to perform any type of work for a period of not less than 12 months.

_____ 46. Hospital benefits may be paid for nonoccupational illness or injury under state temporary disability benefits.

_____ 47. If a woman has an abnormal condition that arises from her pregnancy (e.g., diabetes or varicose veins) and is unable to work because of the condition, she may not receive state disability benefits.

_____ 48. When a claim form is submitted for a patient applying for state disability benefits, the most important item required on the form is the claimant's Social Security number.

_____ 49. To justify payment of disability benefits, an insurance company may request an employee's wage statements.

_____ 50. A person receiving state disability benefits must report any income received to the state disability insurance office because it can affect benefits.

ASSIGNMENT 10.2 COMPLETE A STATE DISABILITY INSURANCE FORM

Performance Objective

Task: Complete a state disability insurance form and define patient record abbreviations.

Conditions: Use the patient's record (Fig. 10.1), a New York State Notice and Proof of Claim for Disability Benefits (Fig. 10.2), and a computer.

Standards: Time: _____minutes

                Accuracy: _____

                (Note: The time element and accuracy criteria may be given by your instructor.)

Directions:

1. To familiarize you with what information the employee must furnish, this assignment will encompass completing the New York State Notice and Proof of Claim for Disability Benefits.

2. Mr. Broussard (see Fig. 10.1) is applying for state disability benefits, and he does not receive sick leave pay from his employer. The language he prefers is English. He does not want any disclosure of benefit payment information to his employer. During his disability, he was not in the custody of law enforcement authorities for any violation and he has no alcoholic tendencies.

3. Date the Claimant's Information November 5 of the current year, and date the Health Care Provider's Statement November 10 of the current year.

4. The patient was treated by Raymond Skeleton, MD, 4567 Broad Ave, Woodland Hills, XY 12345 (Phone 555-486-9002) (license # C04561X).

After the instructor has returned your work to you, either make the necessary corrections and place your work in a three-ring notebook for future reference or, if you received a high score, place it in your portfolio for reference when applying for a job.

Abbreviations pertinent to this record:

LBP _____   pt _____

lt _____   wk _____

reg _____   exam _____

SLR _____   rt _____

WNL _____   STAT _____

MRI _____   RTO _____

imp _____

PATIENT RECORD

Broussard	Jeff	L.	03-09-52	M	555-466-2490
LAST NAME	FIRST NAME	MIDDLE NAME	BIRTH DATE	SEX	HOME PHONE

3577 Plain Street	Woodland Hills	XY	12345
ADDRESS	CITY	STATE	ZIP CODE

555-667-7654	555-399-5903	555-466-2490	broussard@wb.net
CELL PHONE	PAGER NO.	FAX NO.	E-MAIL ADDRESS

566-XX-0090	F0394588
PATIENT'S SOC. SEC. NO.	DRIVER'S LICENSE

carpenter Payroll #2156	Ace Construction Company
PATIENT'S OCCUPATION	NAME OF COMPANY

4556 West Eighth Street, Dorland, XY 12347	555-447-8900
ADDRESS OF EMPLOYER	PHONE

Harriet M. Broussard	secretary
SPOUSE OR PARENT	OCCUPATION

Merit Accounting Company, 6743 Main Street, Woodland Hills, XY 12345	555-478-0980
EMPLOYER ADDRESS	PHONE

Blue Cross	Jeff L. Broussard
NAME OF INSURANCE	INSURED OR SUBSCRIBER

466-XX-9979	6131
POLICY/CERTIFICATE NO.	GROUP NO.

REFERRED BY: Harold B. Hartburn (friend)

DATE	PROGRESS NOTES
10-21-xx	8:30 a.m. New patient seen complaining of ongoing LBP. On 9-12-xx after swinging a golf club, pt had sudden
	onset of severe pain in low back with radiation to lt side. Pt unable to work 9-13 but resumed wk on 8-17 and
	has been working full time but doing no lifting while working. Pain is exacerbating affecting his work and reg
	duties. Exam showed SLR strongly positive on lt, on rt causes pain into lt side. Neurological exam WNL.
	Ordered STAT MRI. Off work. RTO.
	RS/mtf *Raymond Skeleton, MD*
10-23-xx	Pt returns for test results. MRI showed huge defect of L4-5. Imp: acute herniated disc L4-5 with spinal stenosis.
	Recommended laminotomy, foraminotomy, and diskectomy L4-5.
	RS/mtf *Raymond Skeleton, MD*
11-1-xx	Admit to College Hospital. Operation: Lumbar laminotomy with exploration and decompression of spinal
	cord with diskectomy L4-5; lumbar anterior arthrodesis.
	RS/mtf *Raymond Skeleton, MD*
11-5-xx	Pt seen daily in hosp. At 3 p.m. pt discharged to home. Will retn to wk 12-15-XX.
	RS/mtf *Raymond Skeleton, MD*

Fig. 10.1: Patient Record

DB-450 9-17

New York State
NOTICE AND PROOF OF CLAIM FOR DISABILITY BENEFITS

Use this form if you became disabled **while employed** or if you became disabled **within four (4) weeks after termination of employment** OR if you became **disabled after having been unemployed for more than four (4) weeks.** Please answer all questions in Part A and questions 1 through 3 in Part B. Read all instructions on this form carefully. Health care providers must complete Part B on page 2.

PART A - CLAIMANT'S INFORMATION (Please Print or Type)

1. Last Name: _____ First Name: _____ MI: ___

2. Mailing Address (Street & Apt. #): _____
   City: _____ State: _____ Zip: _____ Country: _____

3. Daytime Phone #: _____ 4. Email Address: _____

5. Social Security #: ____ - ___ - ____ 6. Date of Birth: ___ - ___ - ____ 7. Gender: ☐ Male ☐ Female

8. My disability is (if injury, also state <u>how</u>, <u>when</u> and <u>where</u> it occurred): _____
_____

9. I became disabled or became ineligible for Unemployment Insurance because of this disability on: ___ / ___ / _____
   I worked on that day: ☐ Yes ☐ No
   Have you recovered from this disability? ☐ Yes ☐ No   If Yes, what was the date you were able to work: ___ / ___ / _____
   Have you since worked for wages or profit? ☐ Yes ☐ No   If Yes, list dates: _____

10. Give name of last employer. If more than one employer during last eight (8) weeks, name all employers. Average Weekly Wage is based on all wages earned in last eight (8) weeks worked.

LAST EMPLOYER			PERIOD OF EMPLOYMENT		**Average Weekly Wage** (Include Bonuses, Tips, Commissions, Reasonable Value of Board, Rent, etc.)
Firm or Trade Name	Address	Phone Number	First Day	Last Day Worked	
			Mo. Day Yr.	Mo. Day Yr.	

OTHER EMPLOYER (during last eight (8) weeks)			PERIOD OF EMPLOYMENT		**Average Weekly Wage** (Include Bonuses, Tips, Commissions, Reasonable Value of Board, Rent, etc.)
Firm or Trade Name	Address	Phone Number	First Day	Last Day Worked	
			Mo. Day Yr	Mo. Day Yr.	
			Mo. Day Yr.	Mo. Day Yr.	

11. My job is or was: _____ 12. Union Member: ☐ Yes ☐ No If "Yes": _____
    <small>Occupation</small> Name of Union or Local Number

13. Were you claiming or receiving unemployment prior to this disability? ☐ Yes ☐ No
    If you did **not** claim or if you claimed but did **not** receive unemployment insurance benefits after LAST DAY WORKED, explain reasons fully: _____
    _____

14. For the period of disability covered by this claim:
    A. Are you <u>receiving</u> wages, salary or separation pay: ☐ Yes ☐ No
    B. Are you <u>receiving</u> or **claiming**:
       1. Workers' compensation for work-connected disability: ☐ Yes ☐ No
       2. Paid Family Leave: ☐ Yes ☐ No
       3. No-Fault motor vehicle accident (check box): ☐ Yes ☐ No or personal injury involving third party (check box): ☐ Yes ☐ No
       4. Long-term disability benefits under the Federal Social Security Act for this disability: ☐ Yes ☐ No

IF "YES" IS CHECKED IN ANY OF THE ITEMS IN 14, COMPLETE THE FOLLOWING:
I have: ☐ received ☐ claimed from: _____ for the period: ___ / ___ / _____ to: ___ / ___ / _____

15. In the year (52 weeks) **before** your disability began, have you received disability benefits for other periods of disability? ☐ Yes ☐ No
    If "Yes", fill in the following: Paid by: _____ from: ___ / ___ / _____ to: ___ / ___ / _____

16. In the year (52 weeks) **before** your disability began, have you received Paid Family Leave? ☐ Yes ☐ No
    If "Yes", fill in the following: Paid by: _____ from: ___ / ___ / _____ to: ___ / ___ / _____

I hereby claim Disability Benefits and certify that for the period covered by this claim I was disabled. If my disability began while I was unemployed, I certify that I had been unemployed for more than four (4) weeks. I have read the instructions on page 2 of this form and that the foregoing statements, including any accompanying statements are, to the best of my knowledge, true and complete.

_____ _____
        Claimant's Signature   **Date**
An individual may sign on behalf of the claimant only if he or she is legally authorized to do so and the claimant is a minor, mentally incompetent or incapacitated. If signed by other than claimant, print information below and complete and submit Form OC-110A, Claimant's Authorization to Disclose Workers' Compensation Records.

_____ _____ _____
        On behalf of Claimant   **Address**   **Relationship to Claimant**

DB-450 (9-17) Page 1 of 2

Fig. 10.2 (From New York State Workers' Compensation Board.)

Continued

Chapter **10** Disability Income Insurance and Disability Benefits Programs

PART B - HEALTH CARE PROVIDER'S STATEMENT (Please Print or Type)

THE HEALTH CARE PROVIDER'S STATEMENT MUST BE FILLED IN COMPLETELY. THE ATTENDING HEALTH CARE PROVIDER SHALL COMPLETE AND RETURN TO THE CLAIMANT WITHIN SEVEN (7) DAYS OF RECEIPT OF THIS FORM. For item 7-d, you must give estimated date. If disability is caused by or arising in connection with pregnancy, enter estimated delivery date in item 9. **INCOMPLETE ANSWERS MAY DELAY PAYMENT OF BENEFITS.**

1. Last Name: _____ First Name: _____ MI: ___

2. Gender: ☐ Male ☐ Female   3. Date of Birth: ___ / ___ / _____

4. Diagnosis/Analysis: _____ Diagnosis Code: _____

    a. Claimant's symptoms: _____

    b. Objective findings: _____

5. Claimant hospitalized?: ☐ Yes ☐ No   From: ___ / ___ / _____   To: ___ / ___ / _____

6. Operation indicated?: ☐ Yes ☐ No   a. Type _____ b. Date ___ / ___ / _____

7.	ENTER DATES FOR THE FOLLOWING	MONTH	DAY	YEAR
a	Date of your first treatment for this disability			
b.	Date of your most recent treatment for this disability			
c.	Date Claimant was unable to work because of this disability			
d.	Date Claimant will again be able to perform work (Even if considerable question exists, estimate date. Avoid use of terms such as unknown or undetermined.)			
e.	If pregnancy related, please check box and enter the date ☐ estimated delivery date OR ☐ actual delivery date			

8. In your opinion, is this disability the result of injury arising out of and in the course of employment or occupational disease?: ☐ Yes ☐ No   If "Yes", has Form C-4 been filed with the Board? ☐ Yes ☐ No

I certify that I am a:

_____   _____   _____
(Physician, Chiropractor, Dentist, Podiatrist, Psychologist, Nurse-Midwife)   Licensed or Certified in the State of   License Number

_____   _____   _____
Health Care Provider's Printed Name   Health Care Provider's Signature   Date

_____   _____
Health Care Provider's Address   Phone #

CLAIMANT: READ THESE INSTRUCTIONS CAREFULLY

PLEASE NOTE: Do not date and file this form prior to your first date of disability. In order for your claim to be processed, Parts A and B must be completed.

1. If you are using this form because you became disabled **while employed** or you became disabled **within four (4) weeks after termination of employment**, your completed claim should be mailed **within thirty (30) days to your employer or your last employer's insurance carrier.** You may find your employer's disability insurance carrier on the Workers' Compensation Board's website using Employer Coverage Search.

2. If you are using this form because you became **disabled after having been unemployed for more than four (4) weeks**, your completed claim should be mailed to: **Workers' Compensation Board, Disability Benefits Bureau, 328 State Street, Schenectady, NY 12305.** If you answered "Yes" to question 14.B.3, please complete and attach Form DB-450.1.

If you have any questions about claiming disability benefits, you may contact the Board's Disability Benefits Bureau at (800) 353-3092. Additional information may be obtained at the Board's website: www.wcb.ny.gov, or you may write to the Disability Benefits Bureau at the address listed above.

Notification Pursuant to the New York Personal Privacy Protection Law (Public Officers Law Article 6-A) and the Federal Privacy Act of 1974 (5 U.S.C. § 552a). The Workers' Compensation Board's (Board's) authority to request that claimants provide personal information, including their social security number, is derived from the Board's investigatory authority under Workers' Compensation Law (WCL) § 20, and its administrative authority under WCL § 142. This information is collected to assist the Board in investigating and administering claims in the most expedient manner possible and to help it maintain accurate claim records. Providing your social security number to the Board is voluntary. There is no penalty for failure to provide your social security number on this form; it will not result in a denial of your claim or a reduction in benefits. The Board will protect the confidentiality of all personal information in its possession, disclosing it only in furtherance of its official duties and in accordance with applicable state and federal law

HIPAA NOTICE - In order to adjudicate a workers' compensation claim or disability benefits claim, WCL 13-a(4)(a) and 12 NYCRR 325-1.3 require health care providers to regularly file medical reports of treatment with the Board and the insurance carrier or employer. Pursuant to 45 CFR 164.512 these legally required medical reports are exempt from HIPAA's restrictions on disclosure of health information.

Disclosure of Information: The Board will not disclose any information about your case to any unauthorized party without your consent. If you choose to have such information disclosed to an unauthorized party, you must file with the Board an original signed Form OC-110A, Claimant's Authorization to Disclose Workers' Compensation Records, or an original signed, notarized authorization letter. You may telephone your local WCB office to have Form OC-110A sent to you, or you may download it from our website, www.wcb.ny.gov. It can be found under Forms on the 'List of All Common Workers' Compensation Board Forms' web page. Mail the completed authorization form to the address listed above.

An employer or insurer, or any employee, agent, or person acting on behalf of an employer or insurer, who KNOWINGLY MAKES A FALSE STATEMENT OR REPRESENTATION as to a material fact in the course of reporting, investigation of, or adjusting a claim for any benefit or payment under this chapter for the purpose of avoiding provision of such payment or benefit SHALL BE GUILTY OF A CRIME AND SUBJECT TO SUBSTANTIAL FINES AND IMPRISONMENT.

DB-450 (9-17) Page 2 of 2

Fig. 10.2, cont'd

ASSIGNMENT 10.3 COMPLETE A STATE DISABILITY INSURANCE FORM

Performance Objective

Task: Complete a state disability insurance form and define patient record abbreviations.

Conditions: Use the patient's record (Fig. 10.3), a New York State Notice and Proof of Claim for Disability Benefits (Fig. 10.4), and a computer.

Standards: Time:_____minutes

               Accuracy: _____

               (Note: The time element and accuracy criteria may be given by your instructor.)

Directions:

1. Assume that the Claim Statement of Employee has been completed satisfactorily by Mr. Fred E. Thorndike (see Fig. 10.3). Complete the New York State Notice and Proof of Claim for Disability Benefits (Fig. 10.4) and date it December 2. In completing this portion of the assignment, look at the first entry made by Dr. Practon on November 25 only.

2. Mr. Thorndike returns to see Dr. Practon on December 7, at which time his disability leave needs to be extended. Complete the Health Care Provider's Statement (Fig. 10.4) by referring to the entry made during the second visit, and date the certificate December 7. Remember that this is not a claim for payment to the physician, so no ledger card has been furnished for this patient.

3. The patient was treated by Gerald Practon, MD, 4567 Broad Ave, Woodland Hills, XY 12345 (Phone 555-486-9002) (license # C01402X).

After the instructor has returned your work to you, either make the necessary corrections and place your work in a three-ring notebook for future reference or, if you received a high score, place it in your portfolio for reference when applying for a job.

Abbreviations pertinent to this record:

pt _____   SDI _____

PE _____   Wks _____

dx _____   wk _____

RTO _____   FU _____

reg _____   CXR _____

        Chapter **10** Disability Income Insurance and Disability Benefits Programs

PATIENT RECORD

Thorndike	Fred	E.	02-17-54	M	555-465-7820
LAST NAME	FIRST NAME	MIDDLE NAME	BIRTH DATE	SEX	HOME PHONE

5784 Helen Street	Woodland Hills	XY	12345
ADDRESS	CITY	STATE	ZIP CODE

555-432-7744	555-320-5500	555-466-7820	thorndike@wb.net
CELL PHONE	PAGER NO.	FAX NO.	E-MAIL ADDRESS

549-XX-8721	M00430548
PATIENT'S SOC. SEC. NO.	DRIVER'S LICENSE

salesman Payoll No. 6852	Easy on Paint Company
PATIENT'S OCCUPATION	NAME OF COMPANY

4586 West 20th Street, Woodland Hills, XY 12345	555-467-8898
ADDRESS OF EMPLOYER	PHONE

Jennifer B. Thorndike	homemaker
SPOUSE OR PARENT	OCCUPATION

EMPLOYER	ADDRESS	PHONE

Pacific Mutual Insurance Company,120 South Main Street, Merck, XY 12346
NAME OF INSURANCE

	6709	Fred E. Thorndike
POLICY/CERTIFICATE NO.	GROUP NO.	INSURED OR SUBSCRIBER

REFERRED BY: John Diehl (Friend)

DATE	PROGRESS NOTES
11-25-xx	On or about 11-3-xx, pt began to have chest pain and much coughing. On 11-24-xx, pt too ill to work and
	decided to file for SDI benefits. Pt states illness is not work connected and he does not receive sick pay.
	PE: Pt examined and complained of productive cough of 3 wks duration and chest pain. Chest x-rays
	confirmed dx-mucopurulent chronic bronchitis. Continue home rest and prescribed antibiotic medication. RTO
	12-7-xx. Pt will be capable of returning to work 12-8-xx.
	GP/mtf *Gerald Practon, MD*
12-07-xx	Established pt returns for F/U c bronchitis. Chest pain improved. Still running low grade temp c̄ productive cough.
	F/U CXR shows clearing. Recommended bed rest x 7d. Will extend disability to 12-15-xx at which time pt
	can resume reg work. No complications anticipated.
	GP/mtf *Gerald Practon, MD*

Fig. 10.3: Patient Record

Use this form if you became disabled **while employed** or if you became disabled **within four (4) weeks after termination of employment** OR if you became **disabled after having been unemployed for more than four (4) weeks**. Please answer all questions in Part A and questions 1 through 3 in Part B. Read all instructions on this form carefully. Health care providers must complete Part B on page 2.

PART A - CLAIMANT'S INFORMATION (Please Print or Type)

1. Last Name: _____ First Name: _____ MI: ____

2. Mailing Address (Street & Apt. #): _____

   City: _____ State: _____ Zip: _____ Country: _____

3. Daytime Phone #: _____ 4. Email Address: _____

5. Social Security #: _____ - ___ - _____ 6. Date of Birth: ___ - ___ - _____ 7. Gender: ☐ Male ☐ Female

8. My disability is (if injury, also state <u>how</u>, <u>when</u> and <u>where</u> it occurred): _____

   _____

9. I became disabled or became ineligible for Unemployment Insurance because of this disability on: ____ / ____ / _____

   I worked on that day: ☐ Yes ☐ No

   Have you recovered from this disability? ☐ Yes ☐ No   If Yes, what was the date you were able to work: ____ / ____ / _____

   Have you since worked for wages or profit? ☐ Yes ☐ No   If Yes, list dates: _____

10. Give name of last employer. If more than one employer during last eight (8) weeks, name all employers. Average Weekly Wage is based on all wages earned in last eight (8) weeks worked.

LAST EMPLOYER			PERIOD OF EMPLOYMENT		Average Weekly Wage (Include Bonuses, Tips, Commissions, Reasonable Value of Board, Rent, etc.)
Firm or Trade Name	Address	Phone Number	First Day	Last Day Worked	
			Mo. Day Yr.	Mo. Day Yr.	

OTHER EMPLOYER (during last eight (8) weeks)			PERIOD OF EMPLOYMENT		Average Weekly Wage (Include Bonuses, Tips, Commissions, Reasonable Value of Board, Rent, etc.)
Firm or Trade Name	Address	Phone Number	First Day	Last Day Worked	
			Mo. Day Yr.	Mo. Day Yr.	
			Mo. Day Yr.	Mo. Day Yr.	

11. My job is or was: _____ 12. Union Member: ☐ Yes ☐ No If "Yes": _____
    Occupation   Name of Union or Local Number

13. Were you claiming or receiving unemployment prior to this disability? ☐ Yes ☐ No

    If you did **not** claim or if you claimed but did **not** receive unemployment insurance benefits after LAST DAY WORKED, explain reasons fully: _____

    _____

14. For the period of disability covered by this claim:

    A. Are you <u>receiving</u> wages, salary or separation pay: ☐ Yes ☐ No

    B. Are you <u>receiving</u> or <u>claiming</u>:

       1. Workers' compensation for work-connected disability: ☐ Yes ☐ No

       2. Paid Family Leave: ☐ Yes ☐ No

       3. No-Fault motor vehicle accident (check box): ☐ Yes ☐ No or personal injury involving third party (check box): ☐ Yes ☐ No

       4. Long-term disability benefits under the Federal Social Security Act for this disability: ☐ Yes ☐ No

    IF "YES" IS CHECKED IN ANY OF THE ITEMS IN 14, COMPLETE THE FOLLOWING:

    I have: ☐ received ☐ claimed from: _____ for the period: ____ / ____ / _____ to: ____ / ____ / _____

15. In the year (52 weeks) **before** your disability began, have you received disability benefits for other periods of disability? ☐ Yes ☐ No

    If "Yes", fill in the following: Paid by: _____ from: ____ / ____ / _____ to: ____ / ____ / _____

16. In the year (52 weeks) **before** your disability began, have you received Paid Family Leave? ☐ Yes ☐ No

    If "Yes", fill in the following: Paid by: _____ from: ____ / ____ / _____ to: ____ / ____ / _____

I hereby claim Disability Benefits and certify that for the period covered by this claim I was disabled. If my disability began while I was unemployed, I certify that I had been unemployed for more than four (4) weeks. I have read the instructions on page 2 of this form and that the foregoing statements, including any accompanying statements are, to the best of my knowledge, true and complete.

_____   _____
Claimant's Signature   Date

An individual may sign on behalf of the claimant only if he or she is legally authorized to do so and the claimant is a minor, mentally incompetent or incapacitated. If signed by other than claimant, print information below and complete and submit Form OC-110A, Claimant's Authorization to Disclose Workers' Compensation Records.

_____   _____   _____
On behalf of Claimant   Address   Relationship to Claimant

DB-450 (9-17) Page 1 of 2

Fig. 10.4 (From New York State Workers' Compensation Board.)

Continued

Chapter **10** Disability Income Insurance and Disability Benefits Programs

PART B - HEALTH CARE PROVIDER'S STATEMENT (Please Print or Type)

THE HEALTH CARE PROVIDER'S STATEMENT MUST BE FILLED IN COMPLETELY. THE ATTENDING HEALTH CARE PROVIDER SHALL COMPLETE AND RETURN TO THE CLAIMANT WITHIN SEVEN (7) DAYS OF RECEIPT OF THIS FORM. For item 7-d, you must give estimated date. If disability is caused by or arising in connection with pregnancy, enter estimated delivery date in item 9. **INCOMPLETE ANSWERS MAY DELAY PAYMENT OF BENEFITS.**

1. Last Name: _____ First Name: _____ MI: ____

2. Gender: ☐ Male ☐ Female   3. Date of Birth: ____ / ____ / _____

4. Diagnosis/Analysis: _____ Diagnosis Code: _____

   a. Claimant's symptoms: _____

   b. Objective findings: _____

5. Claimant hospitalized?: ☐ Yes ☐ No   From: ____ / ____ / _____   To: ____ / ____ / _____

6. Operation indicated?: ☐ Yes ☐ No   a. Type _____   b. Date ____ / ____ / _____

7.	ENTER DATES FOR THE FOLLOWING	MONTH	DAY	YEAR
a	Date of your first treatment for this disability			
b.	Date of your most recent treatment for this disability			
c.	Date Claimant was unable to work because of this disability			
d.	Date Claimant will again be able to perform work (Even if considerable question exists, estimate date. Avoid use of terms such as unknown or undetermined.)			
e.	If pregnancy related, please check box and enter the date ☐ estimated delivery date OR ☐ actual delivery date			

8. In your opinion, is this disability the result of injury arising out of and in the course of employment or occupational disease?: ☐ Yes ☐ No   If "Yes", has Form C-4 been filed with the Board? ☐ Yes ☐ No

I certify that I am a:

_____
(Physician, Chiropractor, Dentist, Podiatrist, Psychologist, Nurse-Midwife)   Licensed or Certified in the State of   License Number

_____
Health Care Provider's Printed Name   Health Care Provider's Signature   Date

_____
Health Care Provider's Address   Phone #

CLAIMANT: READ THESE INSTRUCTIONS CAREFULLY

PLEASE NOTE: Do not date and file this form prior to your first date of disability. In order for your claim to be processed, Parts A and B must be completed.

1. If you are using this form because you became disabled **while employed** or you became disabled **within four (4) weeks after termination of employment**, your completed claim should be mailed **within thirty (30) days to your employer or your last employer's insurance carrier**. You may find your employer's disability insurance carrier on the Workers' Compensation Board's website using Employer Coverage Search.

2. If you are using this form because you became **disabled after having been unemployed for more than four (4) weeks**, your completed claim should be mailed to: **Workers' Compensation Board, Disability Benefits Bureau, 328 State Street, Schenectady, NY 12305**. If you answered "Yes" to question 14.B.3, please complete and attach Form DB-450.1.

If you have any questions about claiming disability benefits, you may contact the Board's Disability Benefits Bureau at (800) 353-3092. Additional information may be obtained at the Board's website: www.wcb.ny.gov, or you may write to the Disability Benefits Bureau at the address listed above.

DB-450 (9-17) Page 2 of 2

Fig. 10.4, cont'd

ASSIGNMENT 10.4 COMPLETE A STATE DISABILITY INSURANCE FORM

Performance Objective

Task: Complete a state disability insurance form and define patient record abbreviations.

Conditions: Use the patient's record (Fig. 10.5), a New York State Notice and Proof of Claim for Disability Benefits (Fig. 10.6), and a computer.

Standards: Time: _____minutes

               Accuracy: _____

               (Note: The time element and accuracy criteria may be given by your instructor.)

Directions:

1. Assume that the Claimant's Information has been completed satisfactorily by Mr. James T. Fujita (see Fig. 10.5). Complete the Health Care Provider's Statement (see Fig. 10.6) and date it December 15.

2. The patient was treated by Gaston Input, MD, 4567 Broad Ave, Woodland Hills, XY 12345 (Phone 555-486-9002) (license # C08001X).

After the instructor has returned your work to you, either make the necessary corrections and place your work in a three-ring notebook for future reference or, if you received a high score, place it in your portfolio for reference when applying for a job.

Abbreviations pertinent to this record:

pt _____   exam _____

hx _____   neg _____

WBC _____   imp _____

wk _____   SDI _____

Chapter **10** **Disability Income Insurance and Disability Benefits Programs**

PATIENT RECORD

Fujita	James	T.	03-27-54	M	555-677-2881
LAST NAME	FIRST NAME	MIDDLE NAME	BIRTH DATE	SEX	HOME PHONE

3538 South A Street	Woodland Hills	XY	12345
ADDRESS	CITY	STATE	ZIP CODE

555-499-6556	555-988-4100	555-677-2881	fujita@wb.net
CELL PHONE	PAGER NO.	FAX NO.	E-MAIL ADDRESS

567-XX-8898	M4387931
PATIENT'S SOC. SEC. NO.	DRIVER'S LICENSE

electrician Payoll No. 8834	Macy Electric Company
PATIENT'S OCCUPATION	NAME OF COMPANY

2671 North C Street, Woodland Hills, XY 12345	555-677-2346
ADDRESS OF EMPLOYER	PHONE

Mary J. Fujita	homemaker
SPOUSE OR PARENT	OCCUPATION

EMPLOYER	ADDRESS	PHONE

Atlantic Mutual Insurance Company, 111 South Main Street, Woodland Hills, XY 12345
NAME OF INSURANCE

F20015		James T. Fujita
POLICY/CERTIFICATE NO.	GROUP NO.	INSURED OR SUBSCRIBER

REFERRED BY: Cherry Hotta (aunt)

DATE	PROGRESS NOTES
12-07-XX	Today pt could not go to work and came for exam complaining of pain in abdomen, nausea, and no vomiting. Pt
	has hx of mesentery adenopathy. Exam neg except abdomen showed tenderness all over with voluntary guarding.
	WBC 10,000. Imp: Mesenteric adenitis. Advised strict bed rest at home and bland diet. To return in 1 wk. Will file
	for SDI benefits. Pt states illness is not work connected and he receives sick leave pay of $150/wk.
	GI/mtf *Gaston Input, MD*
12-15-xx	Exam showed normal nontender abdomen. No nausea. Pt tolerating food well. WBC 7,500. Pt will be capable of
	returning to work 12-22-xx.
	GI/mtf *Gaston Input, MD*

Fig. 10.5: Patient Record

New York State
NOTICE AND PROOF OF CLAIM FOR DISABILITY BENEFITS

Use this form if you became disabled **while employed** or if you became disabled **within four (4) weeks after termination of employment** OR if you became **disabled after having been unemployed for more than four (4) weeks**. Please answer all questions in Part A and questions 1 through 3 in Part B. Read all instructions on this form carefully. Health care providers must complete Part B on page 2.

PART A - CLAIMANT'S INFORMATION (Please Print or Type)

1. Last Name: _____ First Name: _____ MI: ___

2. Mailing Address (Street & Apt. #): _____

   City: _____ State: _____ Zip: _____ Country: _____

3. Daytime Phone #: _____ 4. Email Address: _____

5. Social Security #: _____ - ____ - _____ 6. Date of Birth: ___ - ___ - _____ 7. Gender: ☐ Male ☐ Female

8. My disability is (if injury, also state <u>how</u>, <u>when</u> and <u>where</u> it occurred): _____
   _____

9. I became disabled or became ineligible for Unemployment Insurance because of this disability on: ____ / ____ / _____

   I worked on that day: ☐ Yes ☐ No

   Have you recovered from this disability? ☐ Yes ☐ No   If Yes, what was the date you were able to work: ____ / ____ / _____

   Have you since worked for wages or profit? ☐ Yes ☐ No   If Yes, list dates: _____

10. Give name of last employer. If more than one employer during last eight (8) weeks, name all employers. Average Weekly Wage is based on all wages earned in last eight (8) weeks worked.

LAST EMPLOYER			PERIOD OF EMPLOYMENT		Average Weekly Wage (Include Bonuses, Tips, Commissions, Reasonable Value of Board, Rent, etc.)
Firm or Trade Name	Address	Phone Number	First Day	Last Day Worked	
			Mo. Day Yr.	Mo. Day Yr.	

OTHER EMPLOYER (during last eight (8) weeks)			PERIOD OF EMPLOYMENT		Average Weekly Wage (Include Bonuses, Tips, Commissions, Reasonable Value of Board, Rent, etc.)
Firm or Trade Name	Address	Phone Number	First Day	Last Day Worked	
			Mo. Day Yr.	Mo. Day Yr.	
			Mo. Day Yr.	Mo. Day Yr.	

11. My job is or was: _____ (Occupation) 12. Union Member: ☐ Yes ☐ No If "Yes": _____ (Name of Union or Local Number)

13. Were you claiming or receiving unemployment prior to this disability? ☐ Yes ☐ No

    If you did **not** claim or if you claimed but did **not** receive unemployment insurance benefits after LAST DAY WORKED, explain reasons fully. _____
    _____

14. For the period of disability covered by this claim:

    A. Are you <u>receiving</u> wages, salary or separation pay: ☐ Yes ☐ No

    B. Are you <u>receiving</u> or <u>claiming</u>:

       1. Workers' compensation for work-connected disability: ☐ Yes ☐ No

       2. Paid Family Leave: ☐ Yes ☐ No

       3. No-Fault motor vehicle accident (check box): ☐ Yes ☐ No or personal injury involving third party (check box): ☐ Yes ☐ No

       4. Long-term disability benefits under the Federal Social Security Act for this disability: ☐ Yes ☐ No

    IF "YES" IS CHECKED IN ANY OF THE ITEMS IN 14, COMPLETE THE FOLLOWING:

    I have: ☐ received ☐ claimed from: _____ for the period: ____ / ____ / _____ to: ____ / ____ / _____

15. In the year (52 weeks) **before** your disability began, have you received disability benefits for other periods of disability? ☐ Yes ☐ No

    If "Yes", fill in the following: Paid by: _____ from: ____ / ____ / _____ to: ____ / ____ / _____

16. In the year (52 weeks) **before** your disability began, have you received Paid Family Leave? ☐ Yes ☐ No

    If "Yes", fill in the following: Paid by: _____ from: ____ / ____ / _____ to: ____ / ____ / _____

I hereby claim Disability Benefits and certify that for the period covered by this claim I was disabled. If my disability began while I was unemployed, I certify that I had been unemployed for more than four (4) weeks. I have read the instructions on page 2 of this form and that the foregoing statements, including any accompanying statements are, to the best of my knowledge, true and complete.

_____   _____
Claimant's Signature   Date

An individual may sign on behalf of the claimant only if he or she is legally authorized to do so and the claimant is a minor, mentally incompetent or incapacitated. If signed by other than claimant, print information below and complete and submit Form OC-110A, Claimant's Authorization to Disclose Workers' Compensation Records.

_____   _____   _____
On behalf of Claimant   Address   Relationship to Claimant

DB-450 (9-17) Page 1 of 2

Fig. 10.6 (From New York State Workers' Compensation Board.)

Continued

PART B - HEALTH CARE PROVIDER'S STATEMENT (Please Print or Type)

THE HEALTH CARE PROVIDER'S STATEMENT MUST BE FILLED IN COMPLETELY. THE ATTENDING HEALTH CARE PROVIDER SHALL COMPLETE AND RETURN TO THE CLAIMANT WITHIN SEVEN (7) DAYS OF RECEIPT OF THIS FORM. For item 7-d, you must give estimated date. If disability is caused by or arising in connection with pregnancy, enter estimated delivery date in item 9. **INCOMPLETE ANSWERS MAY DELAY PAYMENT OF BENEFITS**.

1. Last Name: _____ First Name: _____ MI: ___

2. Gender: ☐ Male ☐ Female   3. Date of Birth: ___ / ___ / _____

4. Diagnosis/Analysis: _____ Diagnosis Code: _____

   a. Claimant's symptoms: _____

   _____

   b. Objective findings: _____

   _____

5. Claimant hospitalized?: ☐ Yes ☐ No   From: ___ / ___ / _____   To: ___ / ___ / _____

6. Operation indicated?: ☐ Yes ☐ No   a. Type _____   b. Date ___ / ___ / _____

7.	ENTER DATES FOR THE FOLLOWING	MONTH	DAY	YEAR
a	Date of your first treatment for this disability			
b.	Date of your most recent treatment for this disability			
c.	Date Claimant was unable to work because of this disability			
d.	Date Claimant will again be able to perform work (Even if considerable question exists, estimate date. Avoid use of terms such as unknown or undetermined.)			
e.	If pregnancy related, please check box and enter the date ☐ estimated delivery date OR ☐ actual delivery date			

8. In your opinion, is this disability the result of injury arising out of and in the course of employment or occupational disease?:
☐ Yes ☐ No   If "Yes", has Form C-4 been filed with the Board? ☐ Yes ☐ No

I certify that I am a:

_____   _____   _____
(Physician, Chiropractor, Dentist, Podiatrist, Psychologist, Nurse-Midwife)   Licensed or Certified in the State of   License Number

_____   _____   _____
Health Care Provider's Printed Name   Health Care Provider's Signature   Date

_____   _____
Health Care Provider's Address   Phone #

CLAIMANT: READ THESE INSTRUCTIONS CAREFULLY

PLEASE NOTE: Do not date and file this form prior to your first date of disability. In order for your claim to be processed, Parts A and B must be completed.

1. If you are using this form because you became disabled **while employed** or you became disabled **within four (4) weeks after termination of employment**, your completed claim should be mailed **within thirty (30) days to your employer or your last employer's insurance carrier**. You may find your employer's disability insurance carrier on the Workers' Compensation Board's website using Employer Coverage Search.

2. If you are using this form because you became **disabled after having been unemployed for more than four (4) weeks**, your completed claim should be mailed to: **Workers' Compensation Board, Disability Benefits Bureau, 328 State Street, Schenectady, NY 12305.** If you answered "Yes" to question 14.B.3, please complete and attach Form DB-450.1.

If you have any questions about claiming disability benefits, you may contact the Board's Disability Benefits Bureau at (800) 353-3092. Additional information may be obtained at the Board's website: www.wcb.ny.gov, or you may write to the Disability Benefits Bureau at the address listed above.

Notification Pursuant to the New York Personal Privacy Protection Law (Public Officers Law Article 6-A) and the Federal Privacy Act of 1974 (5 U.S.C. § 552a). The Workers' Compensation Board's (Board's) authority to request that claimants provide personal information, including their social security number, is derived from the Board's investigatory authority under Workers' Compensation Law (WCL) § 20, and its administrative authority under WCL § 142. This information is collected to assist the Board in investigating and administering claims in the most expedient manner possible and to help it maintain accurate claim records. Providing your social security number to the Board is voluntary. There is no penalty for failure to provide your social security number on this form; it will not result in a denial of your claim or a reduction in benefits. The Board will protect the confidentiality of all personal information in its possession, disclosing it only in furtherance of its official duties and in accordance with applicable state and federal law

HIPAA NOTICE - In order to adjudicate a workers' compensation claim or disability benefits claim, WCL 13-a(4)(a) and 12 NYCRR 325-1.3 require health care providers to regularly file medical reports of treatment with the Board and the insurance carrier or employer. Pursuant to 45 CFR 164.512 these legally required medical reports are exempt from HIPAA's restrictions on disclosure of health information.

Disclosure of Information: The Board will not disclose any information about your case to any unauthorized party without your consent. If you choose to have such information disclosed to an unauthorized party, you must file with the Board an original signed Form OC-110A, Claimant's Authorization to Disclose Workers' Compensation Records, or an original signed, notarized authorization letter. You may telephone your local WCB office to have Form OC-110A sent to you, or you may download it from our website, www.wcb.ny.gov. It can be found under Forms on the 'List of All Common Workers' Compensation Board Forms' web page. Mail the completed authorization form to the address listed above.

An employer or insurer, or any employee, agent, or person acting on behalf of an employer or insurer, who KNOWINGLY MAKES A FALSE STATEMENT OR REPRESENTATION as to a material fact in the course of reporting, investigation of, or adjusting a claim for any benefit or payment under this chapter for the purpose of avoiding provision of such payment or benefit SHALL BE GUILTY OF A CRIME AND SUBJECT TO SUBSTANTIAL FINES AND IMPRISONMENT.

DB-450 (9-17) Page 2 of 2

Fig. 10.6, cont'd

ASSIGNMENT 10.5 COMPLETE A STATE DISABILITY INSURANCE FORM

Performance Objective

Task: Complete a state disability insurance form and define patient record abbreviations.

Conditions: Use the patient's record (Fig. 10.7), a New York State Notice and Proof of Claim for Disability Benefits (Fig. 10.8), and a computer.

Standards: Time: _____minutes

               Accuracy: _____

               (Note: The time element and accuracy criteria may be given by your instructor.)

Directions:

1. Mr. Vincent P. Michael (see Fig. 10.7) is applying for state disability benefits. Complete the New York State Notice and Proof of Claim for Disability Benefits (Fig. 10.8) and date it September 22. Assume that the Claimant's Information has been completed satisfactorily by Mr. Michael. Remember that this is not a claim for payment to the physician, so no ledger card has been furnished for this patient.

2. The patient was treated by Brady Coccidioides, MD, 4567 Broad Ave, Woodland Hills, XY 12345 (Phone 555-486-9002) (license # C04821X).

After the instructor has returned your work to you, either make the necessary corrections and place your work in a three-ring notebook for future reference or, if you received a high score, place it in your portfolio for reference when applying for a job.

Abbreviations pertinent to this record:

Pt _____   exam _____

ESR _____   mm _____

hr _____   imp _____

CVA _____   adv _____

retn _____   wk _____

approx _____   L _____

PATIENT RECORD

Michael	Vincent	P.	05-17-55	M	555-567-9001
LAST NAME	FIRST NAME	MIDDLE NAME	BIRTH DATE	SEX	HOME PHONE

1529 1/2 Thompson Boulevard	Woodland Hills	XY	12345
ADDRESS	CITY	STATE	ZIP CODE

555-398-5677	555-311-0098	555-567-9001	michael@wb.net
CELL PHONE	PAGER NO.	FAX NO.	E-MAIL ADDRESS

562-XX-8888	E0034578
PATIENT'S SOC. SEC. NO.	DRIVER'S LICENSE

assembler "A"	Burroughs Corporation
PATIENT'S OCCUPATION	NAME OF COMPANY

5411 North Lindero Canyon Road, Woodland Hills, XY 12345	555-560-9008
ADDRESS OF EMPLOYER	PHONE

Helen J. Michael	homemaker
SPOUSE OR PARENT	OCCUPATION

EMPLOYER	ADDRESS	PHONE

Blue Shield	Vincent P. Michael
NAME OF INSURANCE	INSURED OR SUBSCRIBER

T8411981A	677899AT
POLICY/CERTIFICATE NO.	GROUP NO.

REFERRED BY: Robert T. Smith (friend)

DATE	PROGRESS NOTES
9-20-xx	Patient calls the office complaining of having had the flu, headache, dizziness, and of being tired. Pt unable to
	go to work today. Exam shows weakness of L hand. Pt exhibits light dysphasia and confusion. Pt is referred to
	XYZ Radiology for chest x-ray, frontal and lateral, and to the lab at College Hospital for ESR. Pt to return tomorrow
	at 11 AM for results.
	BC/mtf *Brady Coccidioides, MD*
9-21-xx	Chest x-rays show cardiomegaly and slight pulmonary congestion. ESR 46 mm/hr. Imp.
	Post flu syndrome, transient ischemic attack, possible CVA. Prescribed medication for the congestion and adv. pt.
	to take aspirin 1/day. Pt to stay off work and retn in 1 week. Approx. date of retn to work 10-16-xx.
	BC/mtf *Brady Coccidioides, MD*

Fig. 10.7: Patient Record

New York State
NOTICE AND PROOF OF CLAIM FOR DISABILITY BENEFITS

Use this form if you became disabled **while employed** or if you became disabled **within four (4) weeks after termination of employment** OR if you became **disabled after having been unemployed for more than four (4) weeks**. Please answer all questions in Part A and questions 1 through 3 in Part B. Read all instructions on this form carefully. Health care providers must complete Part B on page 2.

PART A - CLAIMANT'S INFORMATION (Please Print or Type)

1. Last Name: _____ First Name: _____ MI: ____

2. Mailing Address (Street & Apt. #): _____

   City: _____ State: ____ Zip: _____ Country: _____

3. Daytime Phone #: _____ 4. Email Address: _____

5. Social Security #: ____ - ___ - _____ 6. Date of Birth: ___ - ___ - ____ 7. Gender: ☐ Male ☐ Female

8. My disability is (if injury, also state <u>how</u>, <u>when</u> and <u>where</u> it occurred): _____

_____

9. I became disabled or became ineligible for Unemployment Insurance because of this disability on: ____ / ____ / _____

   I worked on that day: ☐ Yes ☐ No

   Have you recovered from this disability? ☐ Yes ☐ No   If Yes, what was the date you were able to work: ____ / ____ / _____

   Have you since worked for wages or profit? ☐ Yes ☐ No   If Yes, list dates: _____

10. Give name of last employer. If more than one employer during last eight (8) weeks, name all employers. Average Weekly Wage is based on all wages earned in last eight (8) weeks worked.

LAST EMPLOYER			PERIOD OF EMPLOYMENT		Average Weekly Wage (Include Bonuses, Tips, Commissions, Reasonable Value of Board, Rent, etc.)
Firm or Trade Name	Address	Phone Number	First Day	Last Day Worked	
			Mo. Day Yr.	Mo. Day Yr.	

OTHER EMPLOYER (during last eight (8) weeks)			PERIOD OF EMPLOYMENT		Average Weekly Wage (Include Bonuses, Tips, Commissions, Reasonable Value of Board, Rent, etc.)
Firm or Trade Name	Address	Phone Number	First Day	Last Day Worked	
			Mo. Day Yr.	Mo. Day Yr.	
			Mo. Day Yr.	Mo. Day Yr.	

11. My job is or was _____ 12. Union Member: ☐ Yes ☐ No If "Yes": _____
   Occupation   *Name of Union or Local Number*

13. Were you claiming or receiving unemployment prior to this disability? ☐ Yes ☐ No

   If you did **not** claim or if you claimed but did **not** receive unemployment insurance benefits after LAST DAY WORKED, explain reasons fully: _____

_____

14. For the period of disability covered by this claim:

   A. Are you <u>receiving</u> wages, salary or separation pay: ☐ Yes ☐ No

   B. Are you <u>receiving</u> or <u>claiming</u>:

      1. Workers' compensation for work-connected disability: ☐ Yes ☐ No

      2. Paid Family Leave: ☐ Yes ☐ No

      3. No-Fault motor vehicle accident (check box): ☐ Yes ☐ No or personal injury involving third party (check box): ☐ Yes ☐ No

      4. Long-term disability benefits under the Federal Social Security Act for this disability: ☐ Yes ☐ No

   IF "YES" IS CHECKED IN ANY OF THE ITEMS IN 14, COMPLETE THE FOLLOWING:

   I have: ☐ received ☐ claimed from: _____ for the period: ____ / ____ / _____ to: ____ / ____ / _____

15. In the year (52 weeks) **before** your disability began, have you received disability benefits for other periods of disability? ☐ Yes ☐ No

   If "Yes", fill in the following: Paid by: _____ from: ____ / ____ / _____ to: ____ / ____ / _____

16. In the year (52 weeks) **before** your disability began, have you received Paid Family Leave? ☐ Yes ☐ No

   If "Yes", fill in the following: Paid by: _____ from: ____ / ____ / _____ to: ____ / ____ / _____

I hereby claim Disability Benefits and certify that for the period covered by this claim I was disabled. If my disability began while I was unemployed, I certify that I had been unemployed for more than four (4) weeks. I have read the instructions on page 2 of this form and that the foregoing statements, including any accompanying statements are, to the best of my knowledge, true and complete.

_____   _____
Claimant's Signature   Date

An individual may sign on behalf of the claimant only if he or she is legally authorized to do so and the claimant is a minor, mentally incompetent or incapacitated. If signed by other than claimant, print information below and complete and submit Form OC-110A, Claimant's Authorization to Disclose Workers' Compensation Records.

_____   _____   _____
On behalf of Claimant   Address   Relationship to Claimant

DB-450 (9-17) Page 1 of 2

Fig. 10.8. (From New York State Workers' Compensation Board)

Continued

Chapter **10** Disability Income Insurance and Disability Benefits Programs

PART B - HEALTH CARE PROVIDER'S STATEMENT (Please Print or Type)

THE HEALTH CARE PROVIDER'S STATEMENT MUST BE FILLED IN COMPLETELY. THE ATTENDING HEALTH CARE PROVIDER SHALL COMPLETE AND RETURN TO THE CLAIMANT WITHIN SEVEN (7) DAYS OF RECEIPT OF THIS FORM. For item 7-d, you must give estimated date. If disability is caused by or arising in connection with pregnancy, enter estimated delivery date in item 9. **INCOMPLETE ANSWERS MAY DELAY PAYMENT OF BENEFITS.**

1. Last Name: _____ First Name: _____ MI: ___

2. Gender: ☐ Male ☐ Female   3. Date of Birth: ___ / ___ / _____

4. Diagnosis/Analysis: _____ Diagnosis Code: _____

   a. Claimant's symptoms: _____

   b. Objective findings: _____

5. Claimant hospitalized?: ☐ Yes ☐ No   From: ___ / ___ / _____   To: ___ / ___ / _____

6. Operation indicated?: ☐ Yes ☐ No   a. Type _____   b. Date ___ / ___ / _____

7.	ENTER DATES FOR THE FOLLOWING	MONTH	DAY	YEAR
a	Date of your first treatment for this disability			
b.	Date of your most recent treatment for this disability			
c.	Date Claimant was unable to work because of this disability			
d.	Date Claimant will again be able to perform work (Even if considerable question exists, estimate date. Avoid use of terms such as unknown or undetermined.)			
e.	If pregnancy related, please check box and enter the date ☐ estimated delivery date OR ☐ actual delivery date			

8. In your opinion, is this disability the result of injury arising out of and in the course of employment or occupational disease?: ☐ Yes ☐ No   If "Yes", has Form C-4 been filed with the Board? ☐ Yes ☐ No

I certify that I am a:

_____   _____   _____
(Physician, Chiropractor, Dentist, Podiatrist, Psychologist, Nurse-Midwife)   Licensed or Certified in the State of   License Number

_____   _____   _____
Health Care Provider's Printed Name   Health Care Provider's Signature   Date

_____   _____
Health Care Provider's Address   Phone #

CLAIMANT: READ THESE INSTRUCTIONS CAREFULLY

PLEASE NOTE: Do not date and file this form prior to your first date of disability. In order for your claim to be processed, Parts A and B must be completed.

1. If you are using this form because you became disabled **while employed** or you became disabled **within four (4) weeks after termination of employment**, your completed claim should be mailed **within thirty (30) days to your employer or your last employer's insurance carrier.** You may find your employer's disability insurance carrier on the Workers' Compensation Board's website using Employer Coverage Search.

2. If you are using this form because you became **disabled after having been unemployed for more than four (4) weeks**, your completed claim should be mailed to: **Workers' Compensation Board, Disability Benefits Bureau, 328 State Street, Schenectady, NY 12305.** If you answered "Yes" to question 14.B.3, please complete and attach Form DB-450.1.

If you have any questions about claiming disability benefits, you may contact the Board's Disability Benefits Bureau at (800) 353-3092. Additional information may be obtained at the Board's website: www.wcb.ny.gov, or you may write to the Disability Benefits Bureau at the address listed above.

DB-450 (9-17) Page 2 of 2

Fig. 10.8, cont'd

11 Medical Documentation and the Electronic Health Record

Cheryl Fassett

KEY TERMS

Your instructor may wish to select some words pertinent to this chapter for a test. For definitions of the terms, further study, and/or reference, the words, phrases, and abbreviations may be found in the glossary at the end of the Textbook. Key terms for this chapter follow.

acute
attending physician
chief complaint
chronic
clinical documentation improvement
cloned note
computed tomography
concurrent care
concurrent review
consultation
consulting physician
continuity of care
counseling
critical care
deep
degaussing
documentation
electronic health record
emergency care
eponym
established patient
external audit
family history
gross examination
health record
high complexity
history of present illness
internal review
laboratory services
lateral
legible
magnetic resonance imaging
medial
medical decision making
medical necessity
microscopy
modality

morbidity
mortality
new patient
non-physician practitioner
occupational therapy
ordering provider
past history
pathology
physical examination
physical therapy
preoperative
prepayment (prospective) audit
postoperative
primary care provider
prone
prospective review
proximal
query
referral
referring provider
resident physician
retrospective review or audit
review of systems
social history
speech-language pathology
subacute
subpoena
subpoena duces tecum
superficial
supine
teaching physician
transfer of care
treating, or performing, provider
ultrasound
x-ray
zeroization

KEY ABBREVIATIONS

See how many abbreviations and acronyms you can translate and then use this as a handy reference list. Definitions for the key abbreviations are located near the back of the Textbook in the glossary.

ARRA _____

CC _____

CDI _____

CCU _____

119

CT _____   PCP _____

dx or Dx _____   PE or PX _____

ED or ER _____   PFSH _____

EHR _____   PH _____

E/M _____   POMR system _____

EMR _____   Preop _____

FH _____   Postop _____

HIM _____   RCU _____

HIV _____   RLQ _____

HPI _____   ROS _____

ICU _____   RUQ _____

LLQ _____   SH _____

LUQ _____   SOAP style _____

MDM _____   SOR system _____

MRI _____   U/S _____

PACU _____   WNL _____

PERFORMANCE OBJECTIVES

The student will be able to:

- Define and spell the key terms and key abbreviations for this chapter, given the information from the *Textbook* glossary, within a reasonable time period and with enough accuracy to obtain a satisfactory evaluation.

- Answer the fill in the blank, mix and match, multiple choice, and true/false review questions after reading the chapter, with enough accuracy to obtain a satisfactory evaluation.

- Abstract subjective and objective data from patient records, within a reasonable time period and with enough accuracy to obtain a satisfactory evaluation.

- Review a patient record and obtain answers to questions about the documentation presented, within a reasonable time period and with enough accuracy to obtain a satisfactory evaluation.

STUDY OUTLINE

Part I Fill in the Blank

Review the objectives, key terms, glossary definitions to key terms, chapter information, and figures before completing the following review questions.

1. Written or graphic information about patient care is termed a/an _____.

2. List the two types of health record systems that can be used in a medical practice.

   a. _____

   b. _____

3. The difference between an EMR and an EHR is that the _____ is an individual physician's record of the patient's care, whereas the _____ is all of the patient's health records, from many different information systems and providers.

4. The greatest advantage of an EHR system is the improvement of quality of care and patient safety through the _____ of medical records between providers and other health care organizations.

5. What is the Centers for Medicare and Medicaid Services (CMS) definition of *legible documentation?*

   _____

   _____

6. What are the three requirements for all types of documentation?

   _____

7. Medicare administrative contractors have _____ to access a medical practice without an appointment or search warrant to conduct a review of documentation, audits, and evaluations.

8. A _____ is a writ requiring the appearance of a witness at a trial or other proceeding.

9. Define the following terms in relationship to billing.

   a. New patient _____

   _____

   b. Established patient _____

   _____

10. Explain the difference between a consultation and the referral of a patient.

    a. Consultation:

    _____

    _____

    b. Referral:

    _____

    _____

11. If more than one service provider are both treating the same condition in a patient, the case involves _____.

12. An emergency medical condition, as defined by Medicare, is a medical condition manifesting itself by _____ of _____ such that the absence of immediate medical attention could reasonably be expected to result in placing the patient's health in serious jeopardy, serious impairment to body functions, or serious dysfunction of any body organ or part.

13. For EHRs, how should an insurance billing specialist correct an error on a patient's record?

    _____

14. For paper-based records, how should an error be corrected on a patient's record?
_____

15. What are the components of complete documentation outlined by CMS for E/M services?

   a. _____

   b. _____

   c. _____

   d. _____

   e. _____

   f. _____

16. List the eight descriptive elements that can be documented in the HPI.

   a. _____

   b. _____

   c. _____

   d. _____

   e. _____

   f. _____

   g. _____

   h. _____

17. List four of the body systems that are recognized for the reporting of the review of systems (ROS).

   a. _____

   b. _____

   c. _____

   d. _____

18. An effective method of records disposal that writes repeated sequences of ones and zeros over protected information is called _____.

19. Medical decision making (MDM) is the process performed after taking the patient's history and performing the examination, which results in a/an _____.

20. A type of review conducted by hospital facilities for inpatient stays is a _____ review.

21. Write the definition of the following terms that are found in anesthesia records:

   local anesthesia _____

   moderate sedation _____

   regional anesthesia _____

   general anesthesia _____

   arterial line _____

   central line _____

   swan-ganz _____

   nerve block _____

Chapter **11** **Medical Documentation and the Electronic Health Record**

Part II Mix and Match

22. Match the following terms in the right column with their descriptions, and fill in the blank with the appropriate letter.

_____ Renders a service to a patient

_____ Directs selection, preparation, and administration of tests, medication, or treatment

_____ Legally responsible for the care and treatment given to a patient in the facility setting

_____ Gives an opinion regarding a specific problem that is requested by another doctor

_____ Sends the patient for tests or treatment or to another doctor for consultation

_____ Oversees care of patients in managed care plans and refers patients to see specialists when needed

_____ Responsible for training and supervising medical students

_____ Clinical nurse specialist or licensed social worker who treats a patient for a specific medical problem and uses the results of a diagnostic test in managing a patient's medical problem

_____ Performs one or more years of training in a specialty area while working at a hospital (medical center)

a. Attending physician

b. Consulting physician

c. Non-physician practitioner

d. Ordering physician

e. Primary care provider

f. Referring provider

g. Resident physician

h. Teaching physician

i. Treating or performing provider

23. Place the appropriate letter on a blank line before the phrase.

_____ internal or closer to the center of the body

_____ nearer the point of attachment

_____ toward the sides

_____ external or closer to the surface

_____ farther from the point of attachment

_____ toward the center

a. lateral

b. medial

c. distal

d. proximal

e. superficial

f. deep

24. Place the appropriate letter on a blank line before the phrase.

_____ produces a cross-section image of ligaments, the brain, spinal cord and other internal organs

_____ a series of x-rays to visualize a cross-section of the body

_____ uses sound waves to visualize internal structures

_____ visualizes solid, dense internal structures like bone

_____ assists patients with communication deficits

_____ focuses on improving strength, mobility, range of motion and flexibility

_____ evaluates performance deficits in day-to-day activities

a. ultrasound

b. x-ray

c. CT

d. MRI

e. physical therapy

f. occupational therapy

g. speech-language pathology

Part III Multiple Choice

Choose the best answer.

25. Chart chasing is eliminated when using which type of record system?
    a. Paper-based
    b. EHR
    c. Problem-oriented
    d. Integrated record

26. Regarding the SOAP style of documentation that a physician uses to chart a patient's progress in the health record, SOAP stands for:
    a. signature, observation, assessment, and progress.
    b. subjective, objective, assessment, and plan.
    c. symptoms, objective findings, and professional services.
    d. subjective, opinions, assistance, and present illness.

27. A patient comes into the office for treatment of a cold. He does not return, because he is dissatisfied with Dr. Practon's treatment. How long should the office keep his records when he obviously will not return?
    a. 10 years from the date of the patient's first visit
    b. 6 years from the last date of service
    c. 90 days
    d. It is not necessary to retain the records.

28. Which of these providers would be considered to be a non-physician practitioner?
    a. speech therapist
    b. social worker
    c. audiologist
    d. all of the above

29. A tool used by a clinical documentation specialist is a/an:
    a. subpoena.
    b. query.
    c. EHR.
    d. history and physical.

30. Critical care is rendered in:
    a. the coronary care unit.
    b. the intensive care unit.
    c. the emergency room.
    d. all of the above.

31. Verification of successful backups by comparing original records with copied records should be performed:
    a. once a day.
    b. once a week.
    c. once a month.
    d. once a year.

32. An acceptable method for ensuring that electronic protected health information (ePHI) cannot be recovered from a hard drive that is being disposed of is by:
    a. deletion of files.
    b. formatting drives.
    c. degaussing the drives.
    d. none of the above.

33. What part of the history would contain information on the patient's tobacco use?
    a. past history
    b. family history
    c. social history

34. If a provider states in his dictation that the patient appears to be a healthy 52-year-old, what part of the examination would this be?
    a. constitutional
    b. chief complaint
    c. psychiatric

35. What term is used to refer to a condition that persists over a long period of time?
    a. subacute
    b. acute
    c. chronic

36. If a patient saw a provider within the same practice and specialty five years ago, what type of patient would they be?
    a. established patient
    b. new patient
    c. terminated patient

37. What term refers to the upper middle region of the abdomen?
    a. inguinal
    b. umbilical
    c. epigastric

Chapter **11 Medical Documentation and the Electronic Health Record**

Part IV True/False

Write "T" or "F" in the blank line to indicate whether you think the statement is true or false.

_____ 38. A patient's hospital discharge summary contains the discharge diagnosis but not the admitting diagnosis.

_____ 39. An eponym should not be used when a comparable anatomic term can be used in its place.

_____ 40. Assigned claims for Medicaid and Medicare must be kept for 10 years.

_____ 41. During a prospective review or prebilling audit, all procedures or services and diagnoses listed on the encounter form must match the data on the insurance claim form.

_____ 42. Willful disregard of a subpoena is punishable as contempt of court.

_____ 43. Based on Health Insurance Portability and Accountability Act (HIPAA), covered entities must retain medical records for a period of at least 4 years.

_____ 44. Under the False Claims Act, a claim must be filed within 3 years of the date of service.

_____ 45. If a patient fails to make payment on an overdue account, the physician has the right to formally withdraw from providing care to the patient.

_____ 46. It is advisable to maintain pediatric health records 3-4 years beyond the patient's age of maturity.

_____ 47. Deleting files or formatting the hard drive is sufficient to keep electronic protected health information from being accessed.

ASSIGNMENT 11.2 CRITICAL THINKING: SOLVE AN OFFICE PROBLEM

Answer questions after reviewing the case study using your critical thinking skills. Record your answer on the blank lines.

1. A patient comes into the office for treatment. He does not return because he is dissatisfied with Dr. Practon's treatment. Is it necessary to keep his records when he obviously will not return? _____

   Why? _____

   _____

2. A coding specialist is abstracting information from a provider's office note. Information in the exam conflicts with information in the both the history and the final impressions documented. What should the coding specialist do? _____

   _____

   _____

ASSIGNMENT 11.3 ABSTRACT SUBJECTIVE OBSERVATIONS AND OBJECTIVE FINDINGS FROM PATIENT RECORDS

List subjective observations and objective findings after reading each of the case studies.

Case Study 1 Mrs. Smith is 25 years old and was brought into the emergency department of College Hospital with complaints of difficulty breathing and chest pain. Her vital signs show an elevated temperature of 101 °F and pulse rate of 90. Respirations are labored at 30 per minute. Blood pressure is 140/80. Her skin is warm and diaphoretic (perspiring). She states, "This condition has been going on for the past three days."

Subjective observations: _____

Objective findings: _____

Case Study 2 Mr. Jones is 56 years old and was admitted to the hospital with chest pain. Upon examination, patient had elevated pulse and blood pressure. His skin is cold and clammy.

Subjective observations: _____

Objective findings: _____

Case Study 3 Sally Salazar, a 6-year-old Hispanic girl, is brought into the pediatrician's office with a suspected fracture of the right arm. Sally states she was "running at school, tripped on my shoelace, and fell." She tells the provider her "arm hurts," points out how "funny my arm looks," and starts to cry. Sally is cradling her arm against her body and is unwilling to let go because "it's going to fall off." The provider notes her arm looks disfigured and is covered with dirt.

Subjective observations: _____

Objective findings: _____

Case Study 4 A frail 91 year old female is brought to the ED by her daughter. Patient agitated. Claiming someone at the nursing home is trying to kill her. Patient claims she is sick every night after dinner. Daughter clarifies that the patient had some dry heaves but did not actually vomit. Upon exam, provider notes patient is afebrile and abdomen is not tender to palpation. There is no abdominal distention and bowel sound can be heard in all quadrants.

Subjective observations: _____

Objective findings: _____

ASSIGNMENT 11.4 REVIEW OF A PATIENT RECORD

In many instances, when developing the skill of reviewing a patient record, you may need critical thinking in addition to efficient use of reference books. Answer only those questions you think can be justified by the documentation presented in the patient's record. Because the content of each record is variable, you may or may not have answers to all eight questions.

Answer the questions by recording on the blank lines the documentation found identifying the components from the patient's record.

If your answers vary, perhaps you have a reason for them that may or may not be valid. List your reasons in the response section. Differences may be reviewed with your instructor privately or via class discussion.

Patient Record

10-21-20xx
HPI
This new pt is an 80-year-old white male who has had problems with voiding since 9-5-20xx.
During the night, the pt had only 50 mL output and was catheterized this morning because of his poor urinary output (200 mL). He was thought to have a distended bladder; he complains of pressure in the suprapubic region. He has not had any gross hematuria. He has difficulty voiding, especially lying down. His voiding pattern is improved while standing and sitting.

Gene Ulibarri, MD

1. Location: In what body system is the sign or symptom occurring?

   Response: _____

2. Quality: Is the symptom or pain burning, gnawing, stabbing, pressure-like, squeezing, fullness?

   Response: _____

3. Severity: In this case, how would you rank the symptom (how was distress relieved) or pain (slight, mild, severe, persistent)?

   Response: _____

4. Duration: How long has the symptom been present, or how long does it last?

   Response: _____

5. Timing: When does(do) a sign(s) or symptom(s) occur (AM, PM, after or before meals)?

   Response: _____

6. Context: Is the pain/symptom associated with big meals, dairy products, etc.?

   Response: _____

7. Modifying factors: What actions make symptoms worse or better?

   Response: _____

8. Associated signs and symptoms: What other system or body area produces complaints when the presenting problem occurs? (Example: Chest pain leads to shortness of breath.)

   Response: _____

Chapter **11** **Medical Documentation and the Electronic Health Record**

ASSIGNMENT 11.5 REVIEW AN OPERATIVE REPORT

Using information in the textbook and the figures referenced, answer the following questions.

CASE 1: Fig. 11.1

1. What is noted as the indication for surgery? _____

   _____

2. What approach was used? _____

3. What type of anesthesia was used? _____

4. Using the internet, what is a EndoGIA? _____

5. Using the internet, what is an EndoCatch? _____

6. Were there complications during the surgery? _____

CASE 2: Fig. 11.2

1. What were the indications for this procedure? _____

   _____

2. Were there any issues during the procedure? _____

   _____

3. What are the risks of the procedure? _____

   _____

4. Using the internet, what is an INR and why would the provider need to be aware of it? _____

   _____

   _____

5. What are the provider's postoperative care directions? _____

   _____

6. What is missing from this documentation? _____

   _____

PATIENT: Molly Jones
DOB: 06/08/20XX
MRN: 829108B
DATE OF SERVICE: 02/28/20XX

PREOPERATIVE DIAGNOSIS: Acute appendicitis.
POSTOPERATIVE DIAGNOSIS: Acute appendicitis.

PROCEDURE: Laparoscopic appendectomy.

ANESTHESIA: General endotracheal.

INDICATIONS: Patient is a pleasant 17-year-old female who presented to the hospital with acute onset of right lower quadrant pain. History as well as signs and symptoms are consistent with acute appendicitis as was her CAT scan. I evaluated the patient in the emergency room and recommended that she undergoes the above-named procedure. The procedure, purpose, risks, expected benefits, potential complications, alternative forms of therapy were discussed with her and her parents and they were agreeable with surgery.

FINDINGS: Patient was found to have acute appendicitis. The appendix itself was noted to have a significant inflammation. There was no evidence of perforation of the appendix.

TECHNIQUE: The patient was placed in a supine position. After appropriate anesthesia was obtained and sterile prep and drape completed, a #10 blade scalpel was used to make a curvilinear infraumbilical incision. Through this incision, a Veress needle was utilized to create a CO pneumoperitoneum of 15 mmHg. The Veress needle was then removed. A 10 mm trocar was then introduced through this incision into the abdomen. A video laparoscope was then inserted and the above noted gross findings were appreciated upon evaluation.

A 5 mm port was then placed in the right upper quadrant. This was done under direct visualization and a blunt grasper was utilized to mobilize the appendix. Next, a 12 mm port was placed in the left lower quadrant lateral to the rectus musculature under direct visualization. Through this port, the dissector was utilized to create a small window in the mesoappendix. Next, an EndoGIA with GI staples was utilized to fire across the base of the appendix, which was done noting it to be at the base of the appendix. Next, staples were changed to vascular staples and the mesoappendix was then cut and vessels were then ligated with vascular staples. Two 6 X-loupe wires with EndoGIA were utilized in this prior portion of the procedure. Next, an EndoCatch was placed through the 12 mm port and the appendix was placed within it. The appendix was then removed from the 12 mm port site and taken off the surgical site. The 12 mm port was then placed back into the abdomen and CO pneumoperitoneum was recreated. The base of the appendix was reevaluated and noted to be hemostatic. Aspiration of warm saline irrigant then done and noted to be clear. There was a small adhesion apperciated in the region of the surgical site. This was taken down with blunt dissection without difficulty. There was no evidence of other areas of disease. Upon re-exploration with a video laparoscope in the abdomen and after this noting the appendix base to be hemostatic and intact. The instruments were removed from the patient and the port sites were then taken off under direct visualization. The CO pneumoperitoneum was released into the air and the fascia was approximated in the 10 mm and 12 mm port sites with #0 Vicryl ligature x2. Marcaine 0.25% was then utilized in all three incision sites and #4-0 Vicryl suture was used to approximate the skin and all three incision sites. Steri-Strips and sterile dressings were applied. The patient tolerated the procedure well and was taken to PACU in stable condition. She will be admitted overnight and monitored on IV antibiotics, pain medications, and return to diet.

Electronically signed by: Rebekah Mallard, MD 02/28/20XX 14:25

Fig. 11.1

PATIENT: Marion Banks
DOB: 10/25/19XX
MRN: 55-826
DATE OF SERVICE: 05/22/20XX

PROCEDURE: Upper endoscopy with the removal of food impaction.
ANESTHESIA: Monitored Anesthesia Care, Dr. Xander

HISTORY OF PRESENT ILLNESS: A 92-year-old lady with a history of dysphagia on and off for two years. She came this morning with complaints of inability to swallow anything including her saliva. This started almost a day earlier. She was eating lunch and had beef stew and suddenly noticed inability to finish her meal and since then has not been able to eat anything. She is on Coumadin and her INR is 2.5.

OPERATIVE NOTE: Informed consent was obtained from the patient. The risks of aspiration, bleeding, perforation, infection, and serious risk including the need for surgery and ICU stay particularly in view of food impaction for almost a day was discussed. Daughter was also informed about the procedure and risks. Conscious sedation initially was administered with Versed 2 mg and 175 mcg of fentanyl. The scope was advanced into the esophagus and showed liquid and solid particles from the mid esophagus all the way to the distal esophagus. There was a meat bolus in the distal esophagus. This was visualized after clearing the liquid material and small particles of what appeared to be carrots. The patient, however, as not tolerating the conscious sedation. Hence, Dr. Xander was consulted and we continued the procedure with propofol sedation.

The scope was reintroduced into the esophagus after propofol sedation. Initially, a Roth net was used and some small amounts of soft food in the distal esophagus was removed with the Roth net. Then, a snare was used to cut the meat bolus into pieces, as it was very soft. Small pieces were grabbed with the snare and pulled out. Thereafter, the residual soft meat bolus was passed into the stomach along with the scope, which was passed between the bolus and the esophageal wall carefully. The patient had a severe bruising and submucosal hemorrhage in the esophagus possibly due to longstanding bolus impaction and Coumadin therapy. No active bleeding was seen. There was a distal esophageal stricture, which caused slight resistance to the passage of the scope into the stomach. As this area was extremely inflamed, a di-latation was not attempted.

IMPRESSION: Distal esophageal stricture with food impaction, treated as described above.

RECOMMENDATIONS: IV Protonix 40 mg q.12h. Clear liquid diet for 24 hours. If the patient is stable, thereafter she may take a soft pureed diet only until the next endoscopy, which will be scheduled in three to four weeks. She should take Prevacid SoluTab 30 mg b.i.d on discharge.

Fig. 11.2

Using Fig. 11.3 and information in the textbook, answer the following questions.

1. Why did the patient need a CT? _____

_____

2. What type of contrast was used? _____

3. Should the provider be concerned about the aneurysm? _____

_____

4. What is missing from this documentation? _____

_____

PATIENT: Roger Miller
DOB: 07/04/19XX
MRN: 253-675
DATE OF SERVICE: 3/31/20XX

EXAM: CT Abdomen & Pelvis W&WO Contrast

REASON FOR EXAM: Status post aortobiiliac graft repair.

TECHNIQUE: 5 mm spiral thick spiral CT scanning was performed through the entire abdomen and pelvis utilizing the intravenous dynamic bolus contrast enhancement. No oral or rectal contrast were utilized. Comparison is made with the prior CT abdomen and pelvis dated 10/20/20XX. There have been no significant changes in the size of the abdominal aortic aneurysm centered roughly at the renal artery origin level which has dimensions of 3.7 cm transversely x 3.4 AP. Just below this level is the top of the endoluminal graft repair with numerous surrounding surgical clips. The size of the native aneurysm component at this level is stable at 5.5 cm in diameter with mural thrombus surrounding the enhancing endoluminal. There is no abnormal entrance of the contrast agent into the mural thrombus to indicate an endoluminal leak. Further distally, there is an extension of the graft into both proximal common iliac arteries without evidence for the endoluminal leak at this level either. No exoluminal leakage is identified at any level. There is no retroperitoneal hematoma present. The findings are unchanged from the prior exam.

The liver, spleen, pancreas, adrenals, and right kidney are unremarkable with moderate diffuse atrophy of the pancreas is present. There is advanced atrophy of the left kidney. No hydronephrosis is present. No acute findings are identified elsewhere in the abdomen.

The lung bases are clear.

Concerning the remainder of the pelvis, no acute pathology is identified. There is a prominent streak artifact from the left total hip replacement. There is diffuse moderate sigmoid diverticulosis without evidence for diverticulitis. The bladder grossly appears normal. A hysterectomy has been performed.

IMPRESSION:
1. No complications were identified regarding endoluminal aortoiliac graft repair as described. The findings are stable compared to the study of 10/20/20XX.
2. Stable mild aneurysm of aortic aneurysm, centered roughly at renal artery level.
3. No other acute findings were noted.
4. Advanced left renal atrophy.

Electronically signed by Maxine Sandell, MD, 3/31/20XX, 22:45

Fig. 11.3

ASSIGNMENT 11.7 REVIEW PATHOLOGY/LABORATORY REPORT

Using Fig. 11.4 and information in the textbook, answer the following questions.

1. What information is listed that identifies the patient? _____

_____

2. What additional information would complete this report? _____

_____

3. From the impressions, have the carcinoma cells spread? _____

_____

PATIENT: Maxwell Harper
DOB: 8/2/19XX
MRN: 1116895
DATE OF SERVICE: 8/5/20XX

ORDERING PROVIDER: Elias Stern, MD

CLINICAL HISTORY: Patient is a 37-year-old male with a history of colectomy for adenoma. During his preop evalution, it was noted that he had a lesion on his chest x-ray. CT scan of the chest confirmed a left lower mass.

SPECIMEN: Lung, left lower lobe resection.

IMMUNOHISTOCHEMICAL STUDIES: Tumor cells shows no reactivity with cytokeratin AE1/AE3. No significant reactivity with CAM5.2 and no reactivity with cytokeratin-20 are seen. Tumor cells show partial reactivity with cytokertatin-7. PAS with diastase demonstrates no convincing intracytoplasmic mucin. No neuroendocrine differentiation is demonstrated with synaptophysin and chromogranin stains. Tumor cells show cytoplasmic and nuclear reactivity with S100 antibody. No significant reactivity is demonstrated with melanoma marker HMB-45 or Melan-A. Tumor cell nuclei (spindle cell and pleomorphic/giant cell carcinoma components) show nuclear reactivity with thyroid transcription factor marker (TTF-1). The immunohistochemical studies are consistent with primary lung sarcomatoid carcinoma with pleomorphic/giant cell carcinoma and spindle cell carcinoma components.

FINAL DIAGNOSIS:
Histologic Tumor Type: Sarcomatoid carcinoma with areas of pleomorphic/giant cell carcinoma and spindle cell carcinoma.
Tumor Size: 2.7×2.0×1.4 cm.
Visceral Pleura Involvement: The tumor closely approaches the pleural surface but does not invades the pleura.
Vascular Invasion: Present.
Margins: Bronchial resection margins and vascular margins are free of tumor.
Lymphs Nodes: Metastatic sarcomatoid carcinoma into one of four hilar lymph nodes.
Pathologic Stage: pT1N1MX.

Electronically signed: Hope Lightman, MD; Main Street Labs; 08/03/20XX 14:22

Fig. 11.4

Using Fig. 11.5 and information in the textbook, answer the following questions.

1. What types of evaluation does the therapist perform? _____
_____

2. What is the time frame for the short and long term goals? _____
_____

3. What types of modalities are planned? _____
_____

4. As therapy progresses, what other documentation should be included in the record? _____
_____

Chapter **11 Medical Documentation and the Electronic Health Record**

PATIENT: Mary Mack
DOB: 12/23/19XX

MRN: 5264-888
DATE OF SERVICE: 1/2/20XX

REFERRING PROVIDER: Dr. Frank Meade
DIAGNOSIS: Low back pain and degenerative lumbar disk.

HISTORY: The patient is a 59-year-old female, who was referred to Physical Therapy, secondary to low back pain and degenerative disk disease. The patient states she has had a cauterization of some sort to the nerves in her low back to help alleviate with painful symptoms. The patient states that this occurred in October 20XX The patient has a history of low back pain, secondary to a fall that originally occurred in 20XX. The patient states that she slipped on a newly waxed floor and fell on her tailbone and low back region. The patient then had her second fall in March 20XX. The patient states that she was walking and lost her footing and states that she fell more due to weakness in her lower extremities rather than loss of balance.

PAST MEDICAL HISTORY: No significant past medical history.

PAST SURGICAL HISTORY: The patient has a past surgical history of appendectomy and hysterectomy.

MEDICATIONS:
1. TriCor.
2. The patient is also taking ibuprofen 800 mg occasionally as needed for pain management. The patient states she rarely takes this and does not like to take pain medication if at all possible.

SOCIAL HISTORY: The patient states she lives in a single-level home with her husband, who is in good health and is able to assist with any tasks or activities the patient is having difficulty with. The patient rates her general health as excellent and denies any smoking and reports very occasional alcohol consumption. The patient does state that she has completed exercises on a daily basis of one to one and a half hours a day. However, has not been able to complete these exercise routine since approximately June 20XX, secondary to back pain. The patient is working full-time as a project manager and is required to do extensive walking at various periods during a workday.

MEDICAL IMAGING: The patient states that she has had an MRI recently performed; however, the results are not available at the time of the evaluation. The patient states she is able to bring the report in upon the next visit.

SUBJECTIVE: The patient rates her pain at 7/10 on a Pain Analog Scale, 0-10, 10 being worse. The patient describes her pain as a deep aching, primarily on the right lower back and gluteal region. Aggravating factors include stairs and prolonged driving, as well as general limitations with home tasks and projects. The patient states she is a very active individual and is noticing extreme limitations with the ability to complete home tasks and projects she used to be able to complete.

NEUROLOGICAL SYMPTOMS: The patient reports having occasional shooting pains in the lower extremities. However, these are occurring less frequently and is now occurring more frequently in the right versus the left lower extremity when they do occur.

FUNCTIONAL ACTIVITES AND HOBBIES: Include exercising and gerneral activites.

PATIENTS' GOAL: The patient would like to improve her overall body movements and return to daily exercise routine as able and well-maintaining safety.

Fig. 11.5

OBJECTIVE: Upon observation, the patient ambulates independently without the use of an assistive device. However, does present with a mild limp and favoring the left lower extremity after extensive standing and walking activity. The patient does have mild difficulty transferring from the seated position to standing. However, once is upright, the patient denies any increased pain or symptoms.

ACTIVE RANGE OF MOTION OF LUMBAR SPINE: Forward flexion is 26 cm, fingertip to the floor, lateral side bend, fingertip to the floor is 52.5 cm bilaterally.

STRENGTH: Strength is grossly 4/5. The patient denies any significant tenderness to palpation. However, does have a mild increase in tenderness on the right versus left. A six-minute walk test revealed painful symptoms and achiness occurring after approximately 400 feet of walking. The patient was able to continue; however, stopped after 700 feet. There were two minutes remaining in the six-minute walk test. The patient does have tight hamstrings as well as a negative slump test.

ASSESSMENT: The patient would benefit from skilled physical therapy intervention in order to address the following problem list.

PROBLEMS LIST:
1. Increased pain.
2. Decreased ability to complete tasks and hobbies.
3. Decreased lumbar range of motion.

SHORT-TERM GOALS TO BE COMPLETED IN THREE WEEKS:
1. The patient will demonstrate independence with a home exercise program.
2. The patient will report max pain of 5/10 in a 24-hour period without medication use.
3. The patient will tolerate 1000 feet of walking and complete a six-minute walk test, without a significant increase in pain.

LONG-TERM GOALS TO BE COMPLETED IN SIX WEEKS:
The patient will return to a full daily exercise routine without an increase in pain and maintain safety.

PROGNOSIS: Prognosis is good for the above-stated goals, with compliance with a home exercise program and therapy treatments.

PLAN OF CARE: The patient is to be seen three times a week for six weeks for the following:
1. Therapeutic exercise with the home exercise program.
2. Modalities to includes ice, heat, ultrasound, electrical stimulation in order to reduce pain and inflammation.
3. Manual therapy to include soft tissue mobilization and joint mobilization as needed in order to promote increased mobility and decreased muscle tightness.

I have discussed the plan of care with the patient as well as the findings of the evaluations. The patient reports understanding and agrees to be compliant with physical therapy intervention.

Electronically signed: Michelle Rodriguez, PT
01/02/20XX, 08:30

Fig. 11.5, cont'd

Chapter **11 Medical Documentation and the Electronic Health Record**

12 Diagnostic Coding

Cheryl Fassett

KEY TERMS

Your instructor may wish to select some words pertinent to this chapter for a test. For definitions of the terms, further study, and/or reference, the words, phrases, and abbreviations may be found in the glossary at the end of the Textbook. Key terms for this chapter follow.

adverse effect
benign tumor
carcinoma in situ
chief complaint
combination code
complication
computer-assisted coding
conventions
eponym
essential modifiers
etiology
exacerbation
Excludes 1
Excludes 2
external causes of morbidity
International Classification of Diseases, Tenth Revision, Clinical Modification
International Classification of Diseases, Tenth Revision, Procedure Coding System
intoxication
late effect
laterality
malignant tumor
manifestation

medical necessity
metastasis
morbidity
mortality
neoplasm
nonessential modifiers
not elsewhere classifiable
not otherwise specified
Official Guidelines for Coding and Reporting
ordinality of encounter
placeholder
poisoning
primary diagnosis
principal diagnosis
prophylaxis
residual subcategories
rule out
secondary diagnosis
sequela
sequencing
status asthmaticus
syndrome
Uncertain Behavior
Z codes

KEY ABBREVIATIONS

AHA _____

AHIMA _____

CAC _____

CC _____

CPT _____

DM _____

HIV _____

ICD-10-CM _____

ICD-10-PCS _____

ICD-11 _____

MRI _____

NCHS _____

NEC _____

NOS _____

SNOMED CT _____

WHO _____

PERFORMANCE OBJECTIVES

The student will be able to:

- Define and spell the key terms and key abbreviations for this chapter, given the information from the textbook glossary, within a reasonable time period and with enough accuracy to obtain a satisfactory evaluation.

- Answer the fill-in-the-blank, multiple choice, and true/false review questions after reading the chapter, with enough accuracy to obtain a satisfactory evaluation.

- Indicate main terms, subterms, subterms to subterms, and carryover lines, given a section of a page from the ICD-10-CM codebook, with enough accuracy to obtain a satisfactory evaluation.

- Answer questions, given a section of a page from the ICD-10-CM codebook, with enough accuracy to obtain a satisfactory evaluation.

- Select the correct diagnostic code numbers and given diagnoses, and locate the conditions using Volumes 1 and 2 of the ICD-10-CM codebook, with enough accuracy to obtain a satisfactory evaluation.

- Select the correct diagnostic code numbers, given a series of scenarios and diagnoses, using Volumes 1 and 2 of the ICD-10-CM codebook, with enough accuracy to obtain a satisfactory evaluation.

STUDY OUTLINE

Diagnosis Coding Overview
International Classification of Diseases
  History
  ICD-10 Diagnosis and Procedure Codes
  Selection of a Coding Manual
Assigning a Diagnosis Code
  Sequencing of Diagnostic Codes
  Admitting Diagnoses
  Medical Necessity
Organization and Format of ICD-10-CM
  Alphabetic Index to Diseases and Injuries
  Tabular List of Diseases and Injuries
Official Coding Guidelines for ICD-10-CM
  Diagnostic Codebook Conventions
  Placeholder Character
  Other and Unspecified Codes
  Punctuation and Symbols
  Includes Notes
  Excludes Notes
  "And" and "With"
  "See" and "See Also"
  Default Code
  Gender and Age Codes
General Coding Guidelines
  Locating a Code in the ICD-10-CM
  Level of Detail in Coding
  Signs and Symptoms
  Multiple Coding for a Single Condition
  Acute, Subacute and Chronic Conditions
  Combination Code
  Sequela
  Impending or Threatened Condition
  Reporting the Same Diagnosis Code More Than Once
  Laterality

  Documentation for Body Mass Index and Pressure
    Ulcer Stages
  Syndromes
  Documentation of Complications of Care
Chapter-Specific Coding Guidelines
  Human Immunodeficiency Virus
  Neoplasms
  Coding of Diabetes Mellitus
  Circulatory System Conditions
  Respiratory Conditions
  Pregnancy, Delivery, or Abortion
  Injury, Poisoning, and Other Consequences of External
    Causes
  External Causes of Morbidity
  Factors Influencing Health Status and Contact with
    Health Services
Diagnostic Coding and Reporting Guidelines for
  Outpatient Services
  Outpatient Surgery
  Uncertain Diagnosis
  Chronic Disease
  Code All Documented Conditions That Coexist
  Patients Receiving Diagnostic Services Only
  Preoperative Evaluations
  General Medical Examinations with Abnormal Findings
Coding and Reporting Guidelines for Inpatient
  Hospital Care
  Signs and Symptoms
  Uncertain Diagnosis
  Admission after Outpatient Surgery
  Admission for Rehabilitation
Computer-Assisted Coding
The Future of Diagnosis Coding

Part I Fill in the Blank on ICD-10-CM

Review the objectives, key terms, and chapter information before completing the following review questions.

1. When submitting insurance claims for patients seen by a health care organization office or in an outpatient hospital setting, the _____ diagnosis is listed first, but in the inpatient hospital setting, the _____ diagnosis is used.

2. Claims to insurance carriers often are denied because of lack of _____, which indicates that the procedure provided was not payable for the diagnosis submitted.

3. Diagnosis coding for services provided by a health care organization are reported using ICD-10-CM effective with dates of service _____.

4. The abbreviation ICD-10-CM means _____.

5. The official version of the International Classification of Disease (ICD) was developed by the _____ _____.

6. One of the benefits of adopting the ICD-10-CM coding system is much greater _____, including laterality.

7. Diagnosis codes must be _____ correctly on an insurance claim so that the reason for medical services and the severity of the disease can be understood.

8. ICD-10-CM is the standard code set required under _____ legislation and must be used by covered entities when assigning diagnostic codes.

9. Volume 2, Diseases, is a/an _____ index or listing of terms.

10. Volume 1, Diseases, is a/an _____ listing of code numbers.

11. When using the ICD-10-CM coding system, the _____ is used as a placeholder to save space for future code expansion.

12. Conventions are _____ used in the diagnostic code books to assist in the selection of correct codes for the diagnosis encountered.

13. The abbreviation NEC appearing in the ICD-10-CM codebook means _____.

14. _____ are used to enclose synonyms in the Tabular List.

15. If a condition is documented in the medical record, but it is not specified as to whether the condition is acute or chronic, then the _____ code should be assigned.

16. When selecting a code that corresponds with the condition stated in the medical record, the coder should first locate the term in the _____ and then confirm the code in the _____.

17. The instructional note _____ listed in the Tabular List assists the coder as to when it is appropriate to report a secondary code.

18. A condition that is produced after the acute phase of an illness is listed as the main term _____ in the Alphabetic Index.

19. When reporting a condition that affects the left side of the patient, the character _____ is reported to indicate laterality.

20. The Neoplasm Table has column headings for _____, _____, _____, and _____.

21. In juvenile diabetes, the patient's _____ does not function and produce enough insulin.

22. When coding for diabetes in pregnancy, a code from category _____ is assigned as the primary diagnosis.

23. _____ hypertension is indicative of a life-threatening condition.

24. Full-term uncomplicated _____ deliveries are always reported with the code O80.

25. When reporting accidents and injuries, a seventh character of "A" identifies that the encounter is _____.

26. Additional external cause codes are _____ when reporting poisonings using combination codes from T36 through T65.

27. If documentation states that the incident related to a poisoning was a suspected suicide attempt, the code would be reported from the column titled _____.

28. If a patient falls and fractures his or her wrist, the fracture code is the primary code, followed by a/an _____ code to explain how the accident occurred.

29. When a person encounters health services to receive a vaccination, the diagnosis is reported with a/an _____.

Part II Multiple Choice on ICD-10-CM

Choose the best answer.

30. The consequences of inaccurate assignment of diagnostic codes include:
    a. delay in payment of claim.
    b. denial of claim.
    c. change in level of reimbursement.
    d. all of the above.

31. Diagnosis codes should be reported to the highest level of:
    a. specificity.
    b. medical necessity.
    c. etiology.
    d. laterality.

32. When a provider makes a hospital visit, the encounter should be reported with a diagnosis code that represents:
    a. the reason the patient was admitted to the hospital.
    b. the condition the provider evaluated and treated during the encounter.
    c. the condition that was requested by the admitting physician.
    d. the final discharge diagnosis.

33. To determine the diagnosis codes that would support medical necessity of a specific procedure, such as magnetic resonance imaging (MRI), under Medicare guidelines, the coder should consult:
    a. *Current Procedural Terminology* (CPT) guidelines.
    b. local coverage determinations (LCDs) and national coverage determinations (NCDs).
    c. all of the above.
    d. none of the above.

34. Passage of which legislation, in 1988, placed requirements on physicians to report appropriate diagnosis codes on all claims to Medicare?
    a. Affordable Care Act
    b. Health Insurance Portability and Accountability Act (HIPAA)
    c. American Recovery and Reinvestment Act
    d. Medicare Catastrophic Coverage Act

35. ICD-10-PCS (Procedure Coding System) was developed by 3M Health Information Systems under contract with the:
    a. National Center for Health Statistics.
    b. World Health Organization.
    c. Centers for Disease Control.
    d. Centers for Medicare and Medicaid Services.

36. Annual updates to ICD-10-CM are published:
    a. by the AMA and AHA.
    b. by the AHA and AHIMA.
    c. by the AHA, AHIMA, and US Printing Office.
    d. by the AMA, AHA, AHIMA, and US Printing Office.

37. The Alphabetic Index to Diseases and Injuries is placed:
    a. after Volume 1, the Tabular Index.
    b. first in the coding manual.
    c. after the Table of Drugs and Chemicals.
    d. after the Index to External Causes.

38. How many chapters does the Tabular List contain?
    a. 17
    b. 17 with two supplementary classifications
    c. 19
    d. 21

39. When two diagnoses are classified with a single code, it is referred to as:
    a. a combination code.
    b. a manifestation.
    c. an external cause code.
    d. a Z code.

40. An essential modifier is also referred to as a:
    a. main term.
    b. nonessential modifier.
    c. subterm.
    d. convention.

41. The equivalent of unspecified is:
    a. NEC.
    b. NOS.

c. nonessential.
d. secondary.

42. When reporting outpatients' services, signs and symptoms are acceptable for reporting purposes:
a. in all situations.
b. in addition to the definitive diagnosis.
c. when a definitive diagnosis has not been determined.
d. under no circumstances.

43. When conditions documented as "threatened" are referenced in the Alphabetic Index and there is no entry for the threatened condition, report:
a. with signs and symptoms.
b. as if the patient has the condition.
c. the existing underlying condition.
d. all of the above.

44. When reporting laterality, the final character "3" is reported to indicate:
a. right side.
b. left side.
c. bilateral.
d. unspecified.

45. When reporting an encounter for testing of human immunodeficiency virus (HIV), the code should be assigned as:
a. B20.
b. R75.
c. Z11.4.
d. Z21.

46. When fractures are documented, but there is no indication of whether the fracture is open or closed,
a. report as closed.
b. report as open.
c. it does not matter if it is reported as open or closed.
d. report as unspecified.

47. When identifying the total body surface area of a burn, the front torso is considered as:
a. 1%.
b. 9%.
c. 18%.
d. 36%.

48. Why are external cause codes used?
a. To generate additional revenue
b. To establish injury prevention programs
c. All of the above
d. None of the above

Part III True/False

Write "T" or "F" in the blank to indicate whether you think the statement is true or false.

_____ 49. Diagnoses that relate to the patient's previous medical problem must always be reported.

_____ 50. The concept of "principal diagnosis" is applicable to outpatient and inpatient cases.

_____ 51. The diagnosis coding system is designed to provide statistical mortality rate data that include information about the causes of diseases.

_____ 52. Appropriate diagnosis coding can mean the financial success or failure of a health care organization.

_____ 53. ICD-10 was published by the World Health Organization (WHO) and clinically modified by the Centers for Medicare and Medicaid Services (CMS).

_____ 54. The Alphabetic Index contains the Table of Drugs and Chemicals.

_____ 55. ICD-10-CM codes can contain up to seven characters.

_____ 56. Signs and symptoms that are not typically associated with a disease process should be reported when documented when coding for outpatient services.

_____ 57. When a person who is not currently sick encounters health services for some specific purpose, such as to receive a vaccination, a Z code is used.

_____ 58. *Code conventions* are rules or principles for determining a diagnostic code when using a diagnostic code book.

_____ 59. Annual ICD-10-CM code revisions must be in place and in use by January 1 each year.

_____ 60. An external cause code may never be sequenced as the primary diagnosis in the first position.

Performance Objective

Task: Answer questions pertaining to categories G00-G09 of ICD-10-CM, Volume 2.

Conditions: Use the abstracted section from ICD-10-CM, Volume 2, and a pen or a pencil.

Standards: Time: _____ minutes

            Accuracy: _____

            (Note: The time element and accuracy criteria may be given by your instructor.)

Directions: Refer to a section from a page of ICD-10-CM, Volume 2 (Fig. 12.1), and answer questions pertaining to categories G00 through G09.

1. Locate the section title. _____

2. Place an X in front of each of the following diagnostic statements included in category code G00 and its subcategories.

    _____ bacterial leptomeningitis

    _____ bacterial meningitis

    _____ bacterial meningomyelitis

    _____ leptospirosis

    _____ tuberculous meningitis

    _____ meningoencephalitis

    _____ bacterial arachnoiditis

3. Refer to the *Exclusion* 1 note located under category code G01, titled "Meningitis in bacterial diseases classified elsewhere." Place an X in front of the following code number(s) that are excluded.

    _____ gonococcal meningitis A54.81

    _____ meningitis as a result of measles (B05.1)

    _____ meningitis in neurosyphilis (A52.13)

    _____ *Hemophilus* meningitis (G00.0)

    _____ meningitis as a result of candidal meningitis (B37.5)

    _____ Lyme disease (A69.21)

4. Place an X in front of each of the following diagnostic statements included in category code G04 and its subcategories.

    _____ meningomyelitis

    _____ meningoencephalitis

    _____ pyogenic meningitis

    _____ epidemic meningitis

    _____ tuberculous meningitis

    _____ acute ascending myelitis

5. Write the code numbers for category G04.0 that require a fifth digit.

_____

```
INFLAMMATORY DISEASES OF THE CENTRAL NERVOUS SYSTEM (G00-G09)

● G00 Bacterial meningitis, not elsewhere classified
        An infection of the cerebrospinal fluid surrounding the spinal
          cord and brain.
   [Includes]   bacterial arachnoiditis
                bacterial leptomeningitis
                bacterial meningitis
                bacterial pachymeningitis
   [Excludes1]  bacterial:
                  meningoencephalitis (G04.2)
                  meningomyelitis (G04.2)
   G00.0 Hemophilus meningitis
          Meningitis due to Hemophilus influenzae
   G00.1 Pneumococcal meningitis
          Meningitis due to Streptococcal pneumoniae
   G00.2 Streptococcal meningitis
          Use additional code to further identify organism
            (B95.0-B95.5)
   G00.3 Staphylococcal meningitis
          Use additional code to further identify organism
            (B95.61-B95.8)
   G00.8 Other bacterial meningitis
          Meningitis due to Escherichia coli
          Meningitis due to Friedländer bacillus
          Meningitis due to Klebsiella
          Use additional code to further identify organism
            (B96.-)
   ▪ G00.9 Bacterial meningitis, unspecified
          Meningitis due to gram-negative bacteria,
            unspecified
          Purulent meningitis NOS
          Pyogenic meningitis NOS
          Suppurative meningitis NOS

●▶ G01 Meningitis in bacterial diseases classified elsewhere

        Code first underlying disease
   [Excludes1]  meningitis (in):
                  gonococcal (A54.81)
                  leptospirosis (A27.81)
                  listeriosis (A32.11)
                  Lyme disease (A69.21)
                  meningococcal (A39.0)
                  neurosyphilis (A52.13)
                  tuberculosis (A17.0)
                  meningoencephalitis and meningomyelitis
                    in bacterial diseases classified
                    elsewhere (G05)
```

Fig. 12.1

Chapter **12 Diagnostic Coding**

● ▶ **G02   Meningitis in other infectious and parasitic diseases classified elsewhere**
    Code first underlying disease, such as:
        African trypanosomiasis (B56.-)
        poliovirus infection (A80.-)
    Excludes1   candidal meningitis (B37.5)
            coccidioidomycosis meningitis (B38.4)
            cryptococcal meningitis (B45.1)
            herpesviral [herpes simplex] meningitis
                (B00.3)
            infectious mononucleosis complicated
                by meningitis (B27.- with fourth
                character 2)
            measles complicated by meningitis (B05.1)
            meningoencephalitis and meningomyelitis
                in other infectious and parasitic diseases
                classified elsewhere (G05)
            mumps meningitis (B26.1)
            rubella meningitis (B06.02)
            varicella [chickenpox] meningitis (B01.0)
            zoster meningitis (B02.1)

● **G03   Meningitis due to other and unspecified causes**
    Includes   arachnoiditis NOS
            leptomeningitis NOS
            meningitis NOS
            pachymeningitis NOS
    Excludes1   meningoencephalitis (G04.-)
            meningomyelitis (G04.-)
    G03.0   Nonpyogenic meningitis
        Aseptic meningitis
        Nonbacterial meningitis
    G03.1   Chronic meningitis
    G03.2   Benign recurrent meningitis [Mollaret]
    G03.8   Meningitis due to other specified causes
    ■ **G03.9   Meningitis, unspecified**
        Arachnoiditis (spinal) NOS

● **G04   Encephalitis, myelitis and encephalomyelitis**
    Includes   acute ascending myelitis
            meningoencephalitis
            meningomyelitis
    Excludes1   encephalopathy NOS (G93.40)
    Excludes2   acute transverse myelitis (G37.3-)
            alcoholic encephalopathy (G31.2)
            benign myalgic encephalomyelitis (G93.3)
            multiple sclerosis (G35)
            subacute necrotizing myelitis (G37.4)
            toxic encephalitis (G92)
            toxic encephalopathy (G92)
    ● **G04.0   Acute disseminated encephalitis and encephalomyelitis (ADEM)**
        Excludes1   acute necrotizing hemorrhagic
                encephalopathy (G04.3-)
            other noninfectious acute disseminated
                encephalomyelitis (noninfections ADEM)
                (G04.81)
        G04.00   Acute disseminated encephalitis and encephalomyelitis, unspecified

G04.01   Postinfectious acute disseminated encephalitis and encephalomyelitis (postinfectious ADEM)
    Excludes1   post chickenpox encephalitis
                (B01.1)
            post measles encephalitis
                (B05.0)
            post measles myelitis (B05.1)
G04.02   Postimmunization acute disseminated encephalitis, myelitis and encephalomyelitis
    Encephalitis, post immunization
    Encephalomyelitis, post immunization
    Use additional code to identify the
        vaccine (T50.A-, T50.B-, T50.Z-)
G04.1   Tropical spastic paraplegia
G04.2   Bacterial meningoencephalitis and meningomyelitis, not elsewhere classified
● **G04.3   Acute necrotizing hemorrhagic encephalopathy**
    Sudden and severe CNS disease with pathology of hemorrhages and necrosis of white matter
    Excludes1   acute disseminated encephalitis and
                encephalomyelitis (G04.0-)
    G04.30   Acute necrotizing hemorrhagic encephalopathy, unspecified
    G04.31   Postinfectious acute necrotizing hemorrhagic encephalopathy
    G04.32   Postimmunization acute necrotizing hemorrhagic encephalopathy
        Use additional code to identify vaccine
            (T50.A-, T50.B-, T50.Z-)
    G04.39   Other acute necrotizing hemorrhagic encephalopathy
        Code also underlying etiology, if
            applicable
● **G04.8   Other encephalitis, myelitis and encephalomyelitis**
    Code also any associated seizure (G40.-, R56.9)
    G04.81 Other encephalitis and encephalomyelitis
        Noninfectious acute disseminated
            encephalomyelitis (noninfectious
            ADEM)
    G04.89 Other myelitis
● **G04.9   Encephalitis, myelitis and encephalomyelitis, unspecified**
    ■ **G04.90   Encephalitis and encephalomyelitis, unspecified**
        Ventriculitis (cerebral) NOS
    ■ **G04.91   Myelitis, unspecified**

Fig. 12.1, cont'd

In this chapter, the points awarded for assignments that require diagnostic codes are 1 point for each correct digit.

ASSIGNMENT 12.3 OBTAIN GENERAL DIAGNOSTIC CODES FOR CONDITIONS

Performance Objective

Task: Locate the correct diagnostic code for each diagnosis listed.

Conditions: Use a pen or a pencil and ICD-10-CM diagnostic codebook.

Standards: Time: _____ minutes

                   Accuracy: _____

                   (Note: The time element and accuracy criteria may be given by your instructor.)

Directions: Using the ICD-10-CM codebook, read each diagnosis and locate the condition in Volume 2, the Alphabetic Index. Then go to Volume 1, to the Tabular List of Diseases. Match the definition as closely as possible to the written description and assign the correct code, entering it on the blank line.

Problems	ICD-10-CM Codes
1. Breast mass	_____
2. *Klebsiella* pneumonia	_____
3. Acute lateral wall myocardial infarction; initial episode	_____
4. Acute cerebrovascular accident	_____
5. Atherosclerotic cardiovascular disease	_____
6. Dyspnea, rule out (R/O) cystic fibrosis	_____
7. Ileitis	_____
8. Osteoarthritis of elbow	_____
9. Tinnitus	_____
10. Acute exacerbation of chronic asthmatic bronchitis	_____

Performance Objective

Task: Locate the correct diagnostic code for each case scenario.

Conditions: Use a pen or a pencil and ICD-10-CM diagnostic code book.

Standards: Time: _____ minutes

                   Accuracy: _____

                   (Note: The time element and accuracy criteria may be given by your instructor.)

Directions: This exercise will give you experience in basic diagnostic coding for physicians' insurance claims. First list the ICD-10-CM code for the diagnosis, condition, problem, or other reason for the admission and/or encounter (visit) shown in the medical record to be chiefly responsible for the services provided. Then list additional diagnostic codes that describe any coexisting conditions that affect patient care. Always assign codes to their highest level of specificity—the more digits, the more specific. Do not code probable, R/O, suspected, or questionable conditions. Assign the correct code(s), entering it (them) on the blank line.

Problems   **ICD-10-CM Codes**

Problem 1. A patient, Mrs. Jennifer Hanson, calls Dr. Input's office stating she has blood in her   _____
stool. Dr. Input suspects a gastrointestinal bleed and tells Mrs. Hanson to come in immediately.
It is discovered that the reason for the blood in the stool is a bleeding duodenal ulcer. Code the
diagnosis to be listed on the insurance claim for the office visit.

Problem 2. a. Jason Belmen comes in with a fractured humerus. He also has a chronic obstructive   _____
     pulmonary disease (COPD), which is not treated. Code the diagnosis.

     b. Assume Mr. Belmen needs general anesthesia for open reduction of the fractured   _____
     humerus. The COPD could now be considered a risk factor. List the diagnostic code
     in the second part of this scenario.

Problem 3. Margarita Sanchez came into the office for removal of sutures. Code the diagnosis.   _____

Problem 4. A patient, George Martin, has benign prostatic hypertrophy (BPH). He is seen for   _____
catheterization because of urinary retention. Code the primary and secondary diagnoses for
the office visit. (Note: BPH is an enlargement of the prostate gland, caused by overgrowth of
androgen-sensitive glandular elements, which occurs naturally with aging.)

Problem 5. Mia Bartholomew is seen in the office complaining of a sore throat. A throat culture   _____
is done, and the specimen is sent to an outside laboratory for a culture and sensitivity study to
determine the presence of *Streptococcus*. List the diagnostic code the physician would use if
the insurance claim is submitted before the results are known. List the diagnostic code used
if the physician submits the insurance claim after the laboratory report is received indicating
Streptococcus is present.

ASSIGNMENT 12.5 CODE DIAGNOSES USING Z CODES

Performance Objective

Task: Locate the correct diagnostic code for each case scenario.

Conditions: Use a pen or a pencil and ICD-10-CM diagnostic codebook.

Standards: Time: _____ minutes

                        Accuracy: _____

                        (Note: The time element and accuracy criteria may be given by your instructor.)

Directions: In this exercise, you will be reviewing Z codes in the ICD-10-CM codebook. Assign the correct code, entering it on the blank line. These are some keywords under which Z codes may be located in Volume 2:

admission	checking/checkup	donor	insertion of	status post
aftercare	conflict	evaluation	maintenance	vaccination
attention to	contact	examination	observation	
border	contraception	fitting of	person with	
care of	counseling	follow-up	problem with	
carrier	dialysis	history of	screening	

Problems   ICD-10-CM Codes

1. Kathy Osborn, a patient, is seen in the office for an annual checkup with no abnormal
   findings.   _____

2. Daniel Matsui is seen in the office for adjustment of a lumbosacral corset.   _____

3. Philip O'Brien comes into the office to receive a prophylactic flu shot.   _____

4. Bernadette Murphy is seen in the office for a pregnancy test; the result is positive.   _____

5. Michiko Fujita is seen in the office for a fractured rib. No x-rays are taken because
   Mrs. Fujita thinks she is pregnant.   _____

6. Dr. Perry Cardi sees Kenneth Pickford in the office for a cardiac pacemaker adjustment.
   The pacemaker was implanted because of sick sinus syndrome.   _____

7. Frank Meadows returns for follow-up, postoperative transurethral prostatic resection
   (TURP) for prostate cancer after treatment has been completed.   _____

Performance Objective

Task:	Locate the correct diagnostic code for each diagnosis listed.
Conditions:	Use a pen or a pencil and ICD-10-CM diagnostic code book.
Standards:	Time: _____ minutes
	Accuracy: _____
	(Note: The time element and accuracy criteria may be given by your instructor.)

Directions: In this exercise, you will be reviewing diagnostic codes in the ICD-10-CM codebook involving neoplasms. Assign the correct code, entering it on the blank line.

Problems	ICD-10-CM Codes
1. Leiomyoma, uterus.	_____
2. Ewing's sarcoma, forearm.	_____
3. Adenocarcinoma, right breast, central portion, female.	_____
4. Dyspnea resulting from carcinoma of the breast, female with metastasis to the upper lobe, right lung.	_____
5. Patient is seen for a yearly examination 1 year after a mastectomy for breast cancer; she is disease-free at this time.	_____

ASSIGNMENT 12.7 CODE DIAGNOSES FOR PATIENTS WITH DIABETES

Performance Objective

Task:	Locate the correct diagnostic code for each diagnosis listed.
Conditions:	Use a pen or a pencil and ICD-10-CM diagnostic code book.
Standards:	Time: _____ minutes
	Accuracy: _____
	(Note: The time element and accuracy criteria may be given by your instructor.)

Directions: In this exercise, you will review diagnostic codes in the ICD-10-CM code book involving cases of patients with diabetes. The diabetes codes are combination codes that include the type of diabetes, the body system affected, and the complications affecting that body system. Use as many codes as are necessary to describe all of the complications of the disease. Assign as many codes from categories E08 through E13 as needed to identify all of the associated conditions that the patient has.

Example: If a patient with type 2 uncontrolled diabetes is treated for a skin ulcer on the lower extremity, look up "diabetes" in Volume 2 and find the subterm "with skin ulcer." The diabetes code listed is E11.622. Go to Volume 1 and verify. Volume 1 instructs you to "*use additional code to identify site of ulcer*" (L97.-, L98.-). The additional code L97.809 is selected, as it describes "Nonpressure chronic ulcer of other part of unspecified lower leg with unspecified severity."

Always verify all codes in Volume 1 before assigning them. Assign the correct code(s) for each case involving diabetes, entering it (them) on the blank line.

Problems	ICD-10-CM Codes
1. Diabetes mellitus.	_____
2. Type 2, non-insulin-dependent diabetes mellitus with neuropathy.	_____
3. Diabetic gangrene (type 1 diabetes).	_____
4. Type 2 diabetes with cataract.	_____
5. Type 1 diabetes with diabetic polyneuropathy and retinopathy.	_____

ASSIGNMENT 12.8 CODE DIAGNOSES FOR PATIENTS WITH HYPERTENSION

Performance Objective

Task: Locate the correct diagnostic code for each diagnosis listed.

Conditions: Use a pen or a pencil and ICD-10-CM diagnostic codebook.

Standards: Time: _____ minutes

                          Accuracy: _____

                          (Note: The time element and accuracy criteria may be given by your instructor.)

Directions: In this exercise, you will review diagnostic codes in the ICD-10-CM codebook involving patients who have hypertension. To begin coding, look in Volume 2 under "hypertension." Assign the correct code(s) for each case, entering it (them) on the blank line.

Problems	ICD-10-CM Codes
1. High blood pressure reading.	_____
2. Malignant hypertension.	_____
3. Hypertension complicating pregnancy.	_____
4. Hypertension with kidney disease.	_____
5. Hypertension as a result of arteriosclerotic cardiovascular disease (ASCVD) and systolic congestive heart failure (CHF).	_____
6. Myocarditis and CHF as a result of malignant hypertension.	_____

ASSIGNMENT 12.9 CODE DIAGNOSES FOR INJURIES, FRACTURES, BURNS, LATE EFFECTS, AND COMPLICATIONS

Performance Objective

Task: Locate the correct diagnostic code for each diagnosis listed.

Conditions: Use a pen or a pencil and ICD-10-CM diagnostic codebook.

Standards: Time: _____ minutes

Accuracy: _____

(Note: The time element and accuracy criteria may be given by your instructor.)

Directions: In this exercise, you will review diagnostic codes from the ICD-10-CM codebook involving patients who have suffered injuries, burns, fractures, and late effects. Here are some guidelines for coding injuries, fractures, burns, late effects, and complications.

Injuries

When coding injuries, assign separate codes for each injury unless a combination code is provided, in which case the combination code is assigned. The code for the most serious injury, as determined by the provider and the focus of treatment is sequenced first.

Fractures

Fractures are presumed to be closed unless otherwise specified. Fracture not indicated, whether displaced or not displaced, should be coded as displaced.

Burns

Multiple burns at the same site, but of different degrees, are coded to the most severe degree.

Code the extent of body surface involved (percentage of body surface), when specified, as an additional code.

Late Effects

A residual, late effect is defined as the current condition resulting from a previous acute illness or injury that is no longer the current problem. Late effects are coded using the residual or late effect as the primary diagnosis. The cause of the residual or late effect is coded second.

Complications

For conditions resulting from the malfunction of internal devices, use the subterm "mechanical" found under the main term "complication."

Postoperative complications are sometimes found under the subterm "postoperative," which appears under the main term identifying the condition. If not found there, look for a subterm identifying the type of procedure, type of complication, or surgical procedure under the main term "complication."

Problems   ICD-10-CM Codes

1. Supracondylar fracture of the right femur with intracondylar extension of the lower end; initial encounter _____

2. Fracture of the left humerus and left foot; subsequent encounter. _____

3. Comminuted fracture of left radius and ulna, not displaced; initial encounter. _____

4. Pathologic fracture of the right hip caused by drug-induced osteoporosis; initial encounter for fracture. _____

5. Lacerations of the upper arm with embedded glass; initial encounter. _____

6. Burns on the face and neck; sequela. _____

7. Second- and third-degree burns on chest wall; 20% of the body involved, 10% third-degree; initial encounter. _____

8. Bursitis of the knee resulting from crushing injury to the knee 1 year ago. _____

Performance Objective

Task: Locate the correct diagnostic code for each case scenario.

Conditions: Use pen or pencil and ICD-10-CM diagnostic codebook.

Standards: Time: _____ minutes

                 Accuracy: _____

                 (Note: The time element and accuracy criteria may be given by your instructor.)

Directions: In this exercise, you will review diagnostic codes from the ICD-10-CM codebook involving patients who have conditions involving pregnancy and delivery, and newborn infants.

For the supervision of a normal pregnancy, turn to Volume 2 and look up "pregnancy." This is a long category. Look up the subterm "supervision" and find the sub-subterm "normal" (NEC Z34.8-) and "first" (Z34.0-). Check Volume 1 to verify these codes. Also see code Z33.1, "pregnancy state, incidental." This code is used in the second position to tell the insurance carrier that the patient is pregnant in addition to any other diagnosis.

If a patient has complications, turn to Volume 2 and look under the main term "pregnancy." Find the subterm "complicated by" and find the sub-subterm stating the complication. These are codes from ICD-10-CM Chapter 15: "Pregnancy, Childbirth, and Puerperium" (O00-O9a).

Delivery in a completely normal case is coded O80 and is listed under the main term "delivery, uncomplicated." *Normal* is described as "delivery requiring minimal or no assistance, with or without episiotomy, without fetal manipulation (e.g., rotation version) or instrumentation (forceps) of a spontaneous, cephalic, vaginal, full-term, single, live-born infant." This code is for use as a single diagnosis code and is not to be used with any other code from Chapter 15.

When coding deliveries, always include a code for the status of the infant. Look up "outcome of delivery" in Volume 2, and you will find various Z37 codes listing possible outcomes. These codes would be listed as secondary codes on the insurance claim form for the delivery.

On the insurance claim form for the newborn, turn to "newborn" in Volume 2. You will find codes from Z38.0 to Z38.8 describing the birth of the newborn. Use these codes in the first position when billing for services for the newborn infant.

Assign the correct code(s) for each case, entering it (them) on the blank line.

Problems	**ICD-10-CM Codes**
1. A pregnant patient who is due to deliver in 6 weeks presents in the office with preeclampsia.	_____
2. A patient presents with a chief complaint of severe episodes of pain and vaginal hemorrhage. The physician determines that the patient has an incomplete spontaneous abortion complicated by excessive hemorrhage; she was 6 weeks pregnant.	_____
3. A patient comes in who is diagnosed with a kidney stone; the patient is pregnant.	_____
4. A patient has delivered twins, both live born with cephalopelvic disproportion, which caused an obstruction. Code the mother's chart.	_____

ASSIGNMENT 12.11 CODE DIAGNOSES USING TABLE OF DRUGS AND CHEMICALS

Performance Objective

Task: Locate the correct diagnostic code for each diagnosis listed.

Conditions: Use a pen or a pencil and the ICD-10-CM diagnostic codebook.

Standards: Time: _____ minutes

                     Accuracy: _____

                     (Note: The time element and accuracy criteria may be given by your instructor.)

Directions: In this exercise, you will be reviewing diagnostic codes from the ICD-10-CM codebook involving patients who may have had an adverse effect from ingesting a toxic substance. Read the definitions for poisoning and drug intoxication in the *Textbook*.

Injury codes T36 through T65 are combination codes that include the substances related to adverse effects, poisonings, toxic effects, and underdosing, as well as the external cause. No additional external cause code is required to report poisonings, toxic effects, adverse effects, or underdosing codes.

A code from categories T36 through T65 is sequenced first, followed by the code or codes that specify the nature of the adverse effect, poisoning, or toxic effect.

Assign the correct code(s) for each case and enter it (them) on the blank line.

Problems	ICD-10-CM Codes
1. Light-headedness caused by digitalis intoxication; initial encounter. The patient took the digitalis as prescribed.	_____
2. Treatment of a rash after an initial dose of penicillin is given.	_____
3. Initial encounter for accidental overdose of Demerol.	_____
4. A 20-month-old baby accidentally ingests approximately 15 aspirin and is severely nauseated.	_____
5. A patient presents in the physician's office with a vague complaint of not feeling well. The physician notices that the patient has ataxia (a staggering gait). After reviewing the patient's history, the physician determines the ataxia is caused by the meprobamate the patient is taking as directed.	_____
6. Initial visit for internal bleeding: abnormal reaction to a combination of chloramphenicol and warfarin (Coumadin).	_____

13 Procedural Coding

Cheryl Fassett

KEY TERMS

Your instructor may wish to select some words pertinent to this chapter for a test. For definitions of the terms, further study, and/or reference, the words, phrases, and abbreviations may be found in the glossary at the end of the textbook. *Key terms for this chapter follow.*

bilateral
bundled codes
comorbidity
comprehensive code
conversion factor
Current Procedural Terminology
customary fee
downcoding
durable medical equipment
emergency department
fee schedule
geographic practice cost indices
global surgery policy
Healthcare Common Procedure Coding System
modifiers

mutually exclusive code edits
National Correct Coding Initiative
never event
physical status modifiers
procedure code numbers
professional component
qualifying circumstances
reasonable fee
relative value studies
relative value unit
resource-based relative value scale
technical component
unbundling
upcoding
usual, customary, and reasonable

KEY ABBREVIATIONS

See how many abbreviations and acronyms you can translate and then use this as a handy reference list. Definitions for the key abbreviations are located near the back of the textbook in the glossary.

CF _____

CPT _____

DME _____

ECG _____

ED _____

E/M _____

EOB _____

FTC _____

GAF _____

GPCIs _____

HCPCS _____

NCCI _____

PC _____

PS _____

QC _____

RBRVS _____

RVS _____

RVU _____

TC _____

UCR _____

PERFORMANCE OBJECTIVES

The student will be able to:

- Define and spell the key terms and key abbreviations for this chapter, given the information from the textbook glossary, within a reasonable time period and with enough accuracy to obtain a satisfactory evaluation.

- Answer the fill-in-the-blank, mix and match, multiple choice, and true/false review questions after reading the chapter, with enough accuracy to obtain a satisfactory evaluation.

- Select the five-digit procedure code numbers, modifiers, and/or descriptors of each service, given a series of problems relating to various medical procedures and services and using the *Current Procedural Terminology* (CPT) code book, with enough accuracy to obtain a satisfactory evaluation.

- Abstract information from a clinical note to apply to coding.

- Calculate RBRVS.

STUDY OUTLINE

Understanding the Importance of Procedural Coding Skills
A Coding Specialist's Tools
Health Care Procedure Coding System
Level I: CPT Codes
Level II: HCPCS Codes
Current Procedural Terminology Content and Format
Category I Codes
Category II: Performance Measurement Codes
Category III: New and Emerging Technology Codes
Code Book Symbols
Unlisted Procedures
Evaluation and Management Services (99202-99499)
Office or Other Outpatient Services
Observation Care
Hospital Inpatient Services
Consultations
Emergency Department Services
Critical Care
Nursing Facilities, Prolonged Services, Case Management
Preventive Medicine
Prolonged Services and Standby
Other Evaluation and Management Codes
Anesthesia Services (00100-01999)
Surgery Guidelines
Coding from an Operative Report
Global Surgical Package

Never Event
Supplies
Integumentary System (10030-19499)
Musculoskeletal System (20005-29999)
Respiratory System (30000-32999)
Cardiovascular System (33010-37799)
Hemic and Lymphatic Systems (38100-38999)
Digestive System (40490-49999)
Urinary System (50100-53899)
Male Genital System (54000-55899)
Female Reproductive System (56405-58999)
Endocrine System (60000-60699)
Nervous System (61000-64999)
Eye and Auditory Systems (65091-69979)
Radiology (70010-79999)
Pathology and Laboratory (80047-89398)
Medicine Section (90281-99607)
Code Modifiers
Common Current Procedural Terminology Modifiers
HCPCS Level II Modifiers
Correct Coding Edits and Practices
National Correct Coding Initiative (NCCI)
Code Monitoring
Methods of Payment
Fee Schedule
Usual, Customary, and Reasonable
Relative Value Studies

ASSIGNMENT 13.1 REVIEW QUESTIONS

Part I Fill in the Blank

Review the objectives, key terms, and chapter information before completing the following review questions.

1. The coding system used for billing professional medical services and procedures is found in a book titled _____
_____ .

2. The Medicare program uses a system of coding composed of two levels, and this is called _____
_____ .

3. A medical service or procedure performed that differs in some way from the code description may be shown by using a CPT code with a/an _____ .

4. Explain the difference between HCPCS Level I and Level II code sets.

_____

_____

_____

5. Name the six sections of Category I in the CPT codebook published by the American Medical Association. (AMA)

   a. _____

   b. _____

   c. _____

   d. _____

   e. _____

   f. _____

6. Name five criteria for Medicare's definition of DME.

   a. _____

   b. _____

   c. _____

   d. _____

   e. _____

7. A surgical package includes:

_____

_____

_____

_____

8. A function of computer software that performs online checking of codes on an insurance claim to detect improper code submission is called a/an _____ .

9. A single code that describes two or more component codes bundled together as one unit is known as a/an _____
_____ .

10. Grouping related codes together is commonly referred to as _____.

11. Use of many procedural codes to identify procedures that may be described by one code is termed _____
    _____.

12. A code used on a claim that does not match the code system used by the third-party payer and is converted to the
    closest code rendering less payment is termed _____.

13. Intentional manipulation of procedural codes to generate increased reimbursement is called _____
    _____.

14. Give eight reasons for using modifiers on insurance claims.

    a. _____

    b. _____

    c. _____

    d. _____

    e. _____

    f. _____

    g. _____

    h. _____

15. What modifier is usually used when billing for an assistant surgeon who is not in a teaching hospital?
    _____

16. Explain when to use the -99 modifier code.

    _____

    _____

    _____

17. A *relative value scale* or *schedule* is a listing of procedure codes indicating the relative value of services performed,
    which is shown by _____.

18. Name three methods for basing payments adopted by insurance companies and by state and federal programs.

    a. _____

    b. _____

    c. _____

Part II Mix and Match

19. Match the symbols in the first column with the definitions in the second column. Write the correct letters on the
    blanks.

    _____ ►◄   a. New code

    _____ ●   b. Modifier -51 exempt

    _____ ↗   c. Add-on code

    _____ ⊘   d. New or revised text

    _____ +   e. Revised code

    _____ ▲   f. Reference material

162

20. Match the two-digit modifiers in the first column with the definitions in the second column. Write the correct letters on the blanks.

—— -23 a. Increased procedural service.

—— -22 b. Multiple procedures.

—— -25 c. Staged or related procedure.

—— -26 d. Decision for surgery.

—— -51 e. Significant, separately identifiable evaluation and management (E/M) service by the same physician on the same day of the procedure or other service.

—— -52 f. Unusual anesthesia.

—— -57 g. Reduced services.

—— -58 h. Professional component.

Part III Multiple Choice Questions

Choose the best answer.

21. The codes used to bill ambulance services, surgical supplies, and durable medical equipment are:
    a. CPT codes.
    b. CPT modifiers
    c. Level I HCPCS CPT codes.
    d. Level II HCPCS national codes.

22. A complex reimbursement system in which three fees are considered in calculating payment is known as:
    a. usual, customary, and reasonable (UCR).
    b. relative value studies (RVS).
    c. resource-based relative value scale (RBRVS).
    d. relative value unit (RVU).

23. Medicare defines the postoperative global periods as:
    a. 0, 25, 50, or 100 days.
    b. 0, 10, or 90 days.
    c. 0, 10, 20, or 50 days.
    d. 0, 20, 50, or 90 days.

24. To code numerous CPT codes to identify a procedure that can be described in a single comprehensive code is referred to as:
    a. unbundling.
    b. downcoding.
    c. bundling.
    d. upcoding.

25. When two surgeons work together as primary surgeons performing distinct parts of a procedure, and each doctor bills for performing his or her distinct part of the procedure, the CPT surgical code is listed with modifier:
    a. -62.
    b. -66.
    c. -80.
    d. -82.

Part IV True/False

Write "T" or "F" in the blank to indicate whether you think the statement is true or false.

_____26. Procedure coding is the translation of written descriptions of procedures and professional services into numeric designations (code numbers).

_____27. Category II codes describe clinical components that may be typically included in evaluation and management services or clinical services and do not have a relative value associated with them.

_____28. When multiple lacerations have been repaired using the same technique and are in the same anatomic category, each repair should be assigned a separate code when billing an insurance claim.

_____29. When listing a sterile tray for an in-office surgical procedure, the tray is bundled with the procedure, unless other supplies are needed in addition to those usually used.

_____30. HCPCS Level II modifiers always consist of two numeric characters.

In this chapter, the points awarded for assignments that require procedure codes are 1 point for each correct digit.

ASSIGNMENT 13.2 INTRODUCTION TO CPT AND CODING EVALUATION AND MANAGEMENT SERVICES

Performance Objective

Task: Locate the correct information and/or procedure code for each question and/or case scenario.

Conditions: Use a pen or a pencil and the CPT codebook.

Standards: Time: —————— minutes

                     Accuracy: —————

                     (Note: The time element and accuracy criteria may be given by your instructor.)

1. To become acquainted with the sections of the CPT codebook, match the code number in the left column with the appropriate description in the right column by writing the letters in the blanks. Locate each code number in the CPT codebook. As you progress through the assignment, the problems get more difficult and complex.

   99231 _____ a.   Chest x ray.

   59400 _____ b.   Anesthesia for procedures on cervical spine and cord.

   71045 _____ c.   Subsequent hospital care.

   00600 _____ d.   Supplies and materials.

   85025 _____ e.   Routine OB care, antepartum and postpartum.

   99070 _____ f.   CBC.

2. Name the section of the CPT where each of the following codes is located.

E/M	Radiology	Category I
Anesthesia	Pathology	Category II
Surgery	Medicine	

   a. 65091 _____

   b. 86038 _____

   c. 92596 _____

   d. 75984 _____

   e. 0042T _____

   f. 01320 _____

   g. 99324 _____

   h. 0503F _____

3. Evaluation and Management (E/M) codes are used by physicians to report a significant portion of their services. Remember, it is the physician's responsibility to assign E/M codes, and the exercises presented here are only for familiarization. The problems will acquaint you with the terminology for this section of the CPT codebook. Select the appropriate office visit codes using the elements identified:

a. A new patient office visit requiring a medically appropriate history and exam and low-level medical decision-making. The provider spends 40 minutes. _____

b. An established patient returns to the office for follow up to a straightforward medical problem. The provider spends 10 minutes. _____

c. A new patient office visit requiring a medically appropriate history and exam and straightforward medical decision-making. The provider spends 10 minutes. _____

d. An established patient visits the office for a new medical problem requiring moderate level medical decision-making and 30 minutes with the provider. _____

e. A new patient office visit requiring a medically appropriate history and exam with high level medical decision-making. The provider spends over an hour. _____

4. Evaluation and Management (E/M) codes **99202** to **99239** are used for services provided in the physician's office or in a hospital facility. Read the brief statement and then locate the code number in the *Current Procedural Terminology* codebook.

a. Office visit of a 20-year-old patient seen within the past 3 years for instruction in diabetes injection sites by RN (minimal problem). Patient not seen by physician at this brief visit. _____

b. Office visit of a 30-year-old new patient with allergic rhinitis. This case had a medical appropriate history & examination and straightforward decision-making. _____

c. Discussion of medication with the son of an 80-year-old patient with dementia on discharge from the observation unit. _____

d. Admission to hospital of 60-year-old established patient in acute respiratory distress with bronchitis. Comprehensive history & examination and medical decision-making of moderate complexity. _____

e. Hospital visit of a 4-year-old boy, now stable, who will be discharged the next day. This is a problem-focused interval history & examination and medical decision-making of low complexity. _____

f. New patient seen in the office for chest pain, congestive heart failure, and hypertension. The diagnosis required highly complex decision-making. _____

5. Evaluation and Management codes **99241** to **99255** are used for consultations provided in the physician's office or in an outpatient or inpatient hospital facility. A *consultation* is a service provided by a physician whose opinion about a case is requested by another physician. Read the brief statement and then locate the code number in the *Current Procedural Terminology* codebook.

a. Office consultation for a 30-year-old woman complaining of palpitations and chest pains. Her family physician described a mild systolic click. This is an expanded problem-focused history & examination and straightforward decision-making. _____

b. Subsequent inpatient consultation for a 54-year-old woman, who is now stable, admitted 2 days ago for a bleeding ulcer. This case requires a detailed history & examination and low-complexity decision-making. _____

c. Office consultation for a 14-year-old boy with poor grades in school and suspected alcohol abuse. This is a comprehensive history & examination and medical decision making of moderate complexity. _____

d. Subsequent inpatient consultation for a 50-year-old man who is diabetic and is suffering with fever, chills, gangrenous heel ulcer, rhonchi, and dyspnea (difficulty breathing), an unstable condition. The patient appears lethargic and tachypneic (rapid breathing). This case is a comprehensive history & examination with highly complex medical decision-making. _____

e. Initial emergency department (ED) consultation for a senior who presents with thyrotoxicosis, exophthalmos, cardiac arrhythmia, and congestive heart failure. This case is a comprehensive history & examination with highly complex medical decision-making. _____

f. Initial hospital consultation for a 30-year-old woman, post-abdominal surgery, who is exhibiting a fever. This case is an expanded problem-focused history & examination and straightforward medical decision-making. _____
_____

6. Evaluation and Management codes **99281** to **99499** are used for emergency department, critical care, nursing facility, rest home, custodial care, home, prolonged, physician standby, and preventive medicine services. Read the brief statement and then locate the code number in the *Current Procedural Terminology* code book.

a. First hour of critical care of a senior who, after major surgery, suffers a cardiac arrest from a pulmonary embolus. _____

b. A 40-year-old woman is admitted to the Obstetrical unit, and the primary care physician has requested the neonatologist to stand by for possible cesarean section and neonatal resuscitation. Code for a 1-hour standby. _____
_____

c. A child is seen in the ED with a fever, diarrhea, abdominal cramps, and vomiting. This case had an expanded problem-focused history & examination, and a moderately complex medical decision was made. _____

d. A patient is seen for an annual visit at a nursing facility for detailed history & comprehensive examination and low-complexity medical decision-making. _____

e. An initial visit is made to a domiciliary care facility for a developmentally disabled individual with a mild rash on hands and face. This case had an expanded problem-focused history & examination and low-complexity medical decision-making. _____

f. A 50-year-old man with a history of asthma comes into the office with acute bronchospasm and moderate respiratory distress. Office treatment is initiated. The case requires intermittent physician face-to-face time with the patient for 2 hours and prolonged services. Assume the appropriate E/M code has been assigned for this case. _____
_____

Performance Objective

Task: Locate the correct procedure and modifier, if necessary, for each question and/or case scenario.

Conditions: Use a pen or a pencil and CPT codebook.

Standards: Time: _____ minutes

                   Accuracy: _____

                   (Note: The time element and accuracy criteria may be given by your instructor.)

Directions: Anesthesia codes **00100** to **01999** may be used by anesthesiologists and physicians. Read the brief statement and then locate the Anesthesia Code in the *Current Procedural Terminology* codebook. Special modifiers **P1** through **P6** may be needed when coding for this section, as well as code numbers for cases that have difficult circumstances.

a. Cesarean delivery after neuraxial labor anesthesia, normal healthy patient.   _____   _____

b. Reduction mammoplasty of a woman with mild systemic disease.   _____

c. Total right hip replacement, 71-year-old patient, normal healthy patient.   _____   _____

d. Repair of cleft palate, newborn infant, normal healthy patient.   _____   _____

e. Transurethral resection of the prostate, normal healthy male.   _____

Performance Objective

Task: Locate the correct procedure code and modifier, if necessary, for each question and/or case scenario.

Conditions: Use a pen or a pencil and *Current Procedural Terminology* codebook.

Standards: Time: _____ minutes

               Accuracy: _____

               (Note: The time element and accuracy criteria may be given by your instructor.)

Directions: Surgery codes **10040** to **69979** are used for each anatomic part of the body. Read over each case carefully. Use the *Current Procedural Terminology* codebook to obtain the correct code number for each descriptor given. Full descriptors for services rendered have been omitted in some instances to give you practice in abstracting the correct descriptor from the available information. Indicate the correct two-digit modifier if necessary. The skill of critical thinking enters this section of the assignment, in that you may have to use your own judgment to code because the cases do not contain full details. Remember to use the index at the back of the CPT codebook.

Integumentary System 10040-19499

a. Removal of benign lesion from the back (1.0 cm) and left foot (0.5 cm)   _____

b. Drainage of deep breast abscess   _____

c. Laser destruction of two benign facial lesions   _____

Musculoskeletal System 20000-29909

Reminder: Be sure to read the "Application of casts and strapping" guidelines in your CPT codebook that appear before the 29000 codes.

d. Aspiration of fluid (arthrocentesis) from right knee joint; not infectious   _____

e. Deep tissue biopsy of left upper arm   _____

f. Fracture of the left tibia, closed treatment   _____

   Does the procedural code include application and removal of the first cast?   _____

   If done as an office procedure, may supplies be coded?   _____

   Does the procedural code include subsequent replacement of a cast for follow-up care? _____

   If not, list the code number for application of a walking short leg cast.   _____

Respiratory System 30000-32999

g. Parietal pleurectomy   _____

h. Removal of two nasal polyps, simple   _____

i. Diagnostic bronchoscopy with bronchial biopsy   _____

Cardiovascular System 33010-37799

j. Pacemaker insertion with transvenous electrode, atrial   _____

k. Thromboendarterectomy with patch graft, carotid artery   _____

l. Introduction of intracatheter and injection procedure for contrast venography   _____

169

Hemic/Lymphatic/Diaphragm 38100-39599

m. Partial splenectomy
_____

n. Excision, two deep cervical nodes
_____

Digestive System 40490-49999

o. Repair, esophageal/diaphragmatic hernia, transthoracic
_____

p. T & A, 12-year-old boy
_____

q. Endoscopic balloon dilation of esophagus
_____

Urinary System/Male and Female Genital 50010-55980

r. Marsupialization of urethral diverticulum from female patient
_____

s. Anastomosis of single ureter to bladder
_____

Laparoscopy/Peritoneoscopy/Hysteroscopy/Female Genital/Maternity 56300-59899

t. Routine OB care following a vaginal delivery, antepartum and postpartum care
_____

u. Therapeutic D & C, nonobstetric
_____

Nervous System (61000-64999)

v. Percutaneous needle biopsy of the spinal cord
_____

w. Carpal tunnel surgery (neuroplasty)
_____

Eye and Ocular Adnexa (65091-68899)

x. Enucleation of eye, with implant, muscles attached to implant
_____

y. Strabismus surgery, superior oblique muscle
_____

Auditory System (69000-69979

z. Cochlear device implantation
_____

aa. Bilateral, myringotomy including aspiration, requiring general anesthesia
_____

ASSIGNMENT 13.5 CODE PROBLEMS FOR RADIOLOGY AND PATHOLOGY

Performance Objective

Task: Locate the correct procedure code and modifier, if necessary, for each question and/or case scenario.

Conditions: Use a pen or a pencil and *Current Procedural Terminology* codebook.

Standards: Time: _____ minutes

              Accuracy: _____

              (Note: The time element and accuracy criteria may be given by your instructor.)

Radiologists, as well as other physicians in many specialties, perform these studies. A physician who interprets, dictates, and signs a report may not bill for the report separately because it is considered part of the radiology procedure.

Some medical practices perform basic laboratory tests under a waived test certificate that complies with the rules of the Clinical Laboratory Improvement Amendments (CLIA) of 1988, implemented in September 1992.

a. Upper GI x-ray study with films   _____

b. Ultrasound, pregnant uterus after first trimester, two gestations   _____ and _____

c. Routine urinalysis with microscopy, nonautomated   _____

d. Hemoglobin (Hgb), electrophoretic method   _____

Performance Objective

Task: Locate the correct procedure code and modifiers, if necessary, for each case scenario.

Conditions: Use a pen or a pencil and *Current Procedural Terminology* codebook.

Standards: Time: _____ minutes

                Accuracy: _____

                (Note: The time element and accuracy criteria may be given by your instructor.)

Directions: Find the correct procedure codes and modifiers, if necessary. This assignment will reinforce what you have already learned about procedural coding because code numbers for the case scenarios presented are located in all the sections of the CPT codebook. Also search for codes in the Medicine section, if necessary.

1. A new patient had five benign skin lesions on the right arm destroyed with surgical curettement. The patient was also evaluated and given a prescription for an upper respiratory infection. Complete the coding for the surgery.

Code Number   *Description*

a. _____   _____   Initial new patient visit with low level of medical decision making.

b. _____   _____   Destruction of five benign skin lesions rt arm.

2. Mrs. Stayman had four moles on her back. Dr. Davis excised the multiple nevi in one new-patient office visit. The information on the pathology report stated nonmalignant lesions measuring 2.2 cm, 1.5 cm, 1 cm, and 0.75 cm.

Code Number   *Description*

a. _____   Excision, benign lesion 2.2 cm.

b. _____   _____   Excision, benign lesion 1.5 cm.

c. _____   _____   Excision, benign lesion 1 cm.

d. _____   _____   Excision, benign lesion 0.75 cm.

3. Dr. Davis stated on his operative report that Mr. Allen was suffering from a complex, complicated nasal fracture. Dr. Davis debrided the wound because it was contaminated and performed an open reduction with internal fixation in a complex and complicated procedure.

Code Number   *Description*

_____   Open tx nasal fracture, complicated.

4. A registered nurse (RN), an established patient, age 40 years, sees the doctor for an annual physical. A Pap (Papanicolaou) smear is obtained and sent to an outside laboratory. The patient also has a furuncle on the right axilla at the time of the visit, which the doctor incises and drains (I & D).

Code Number   *Description*

a. _____   Periodic physical examination.

b. _____   Handling of specimen.

c. _____   I & D, furuncle, right axilla.

5. While making his rounds in the hospital during the noon hour, Dr. James sees a new patient in the ED for a laceration of the forehead, 5-cm long. The doctor does a workup for a possible concussion.

Code Number	Description
a. _____	Repair of laceration, simple, face.

The physician sees a patient in Problem 5 in his office as an infection has developed, and the needs his dressing changed. The patient is given a tetanus shot in his arm and sent home with an antibiotic for the infection

Code Number	Description
b. _____	Tet tox (tetanus toxoid) 0.5 mL.
c. _____	Administration intramuscular injection.

On day 11, the sutures are removed, and on day 12, a final dressing change is made, and the patient is discharged.

Code Number	Description
d. _____	Minimal service, OV (suture removal).
e. _____	Minimal service, OV (dressing change).

Note: Some fee schedules allow no follow-up days; Medicare fee schedule allows 10 follow-up days for the procedural code number for repair of laceration.

6. The physician sees 13-year-old Bobby Jones (established patient) for a Boy Scout physical. Bobby is in good health and well groomed. His troop is going for a 1-week camping trip in 12 days. The physician reviewed safety issues with Bobby, talked to him about school, and counseled him about not getting into drugs or alcohol. Bobby denied any problems with that or of being sexually active. He said that he plays baseball. He has no allergies. The physician performed a detailed examination. The physician completed information for scouting papers and cleared him for camping activity.

Code Number	Description
_____	Periodic preventive evaluation and management.

7. A new patient, David Ramsey, age 15 years, was seen by Dr. Menter for lapses of memory and frequent headaches. The doctor performed a complete history and exam with moderate complexity medical decision making. The doctor also performed an electroencephalogram (EEG) with extended monitoring for 60 minutes and spent 45 minutes working with the patient on psychophysiological therapy using biofeedback training. Dr. Astro Parkinson was called in as a consultant. Dr. Parkinson performed an expanded problem-focused history and exam with straightforward medical decision-making. All the test results were negative, and the patient was advised to come in for weekly psychotherapy.

Code Number	Description
Dr. Menter's bill:	
a. _____	OV, history & examination, moderate-complexity decision-making.
b. _____	EEG, extended monitoring (1 hour).
c. _____	Psychophysiological therapy using biofeedback training.
Dr. Parkinson's bill:	
d. _____	Consultation, expanded problem-focused history & examination, straightforward decision-making.

8. An established patient, age 70 years, requires repair of a bilateral initial inguinal hernia (reducible). The code for this initial procedure is

_____   _____.

Performance Objective

Task: Locate the correct HCPCS code and modifier, if necessary, for each medical drug, supply item, or service presented.

Conditions: Use a pen or a pencil and HCPCS code set.

Standards: Time: _____ minutes

                    Accuracy: _____

                    (Note: The time element and accuracy criteria may be given by your instructor.)

Directions: Match the HCPCS code in the first or second column with the description of the drug, supply item, or service presented in the third or fourth column. Write the correct letters on the blanks.

E1280	_____	a.	Vitamin B$_{12}$, 1000 mg
E0141	_____	b.	Injection, insulin per 5 units
J0290	_____	c.	Rigid walker, wheeled, without seat
J3420	_____	d.	Waiver of liability statement on file
J1815	_____	e.	Nonemergency transportation, taxi
P9010	_____	f.	Inj of calcitriol
J1212	_____	g.	Cervical occipital/mandibular support
J3370	_____	h.	Inj of lidocaine (Xylocaine)
E1092	_____	i.	Gloves, nonsterile
A4211	_____	j.	Supplies for self-administered drug injections
J0760	_____	k.	Blood (whole) for transfusion/unit
A9150	_____	l.	Heavy-duty wheelchair with detachable arms
J2001	_____	m.	Ampicillin inj, up to 500 mg
L0160	_____	n.	Dimethyl sulfoxide (DMSO) inj
L3100-RT	_____	o.	Urine strips
A4250	_____	p.	Vancomycin (Vancocin) inj
J2590	_____	q.	Oxytocin (Pitocin) inj
A4927	_____	r.	Wide, heavy-duty wheelchair with detachable arms and leg rests
A0100	_____	s.	Rt hallux valgus night splint
-GA	_____	t.	nonprescription drug

Performance Objective

Task: Locate the correct procedure code and modifier, if necessary, for each case scenario.

Conditions: Use a pen or a pencil and *Current Procedural Terminology* codebook.

Standards: Time: _____ minutes

               Accuracy: _____

               (Note: The time element and accuracy criteria may be given by your instructor.)

Directions: Find the correct procedure codes and modifiers, if necessary, for each case scenario.

1. The physician sees Horace Hart, a 60-year-old new patient, in the office for bronchial asthma, arteriosclerotic heart disease (ASHD), and hypertension. He performs an electrocardiogram (ECG) and urinalysis (UA) without microscopy and obtains x-rays. Comprehensive metabolic and lipid panels and a complete blood count (CBC) are done by an outside laboratory.

   Code Number   *Description*

   Physician's bill:

   a. _____   Initial OV, history & examination, high-complexity decision making.

   b. _____   ECG with interpret and report.

   c. _____   UA, routine, nonautomated.

   d. _____   Chest x-ray, two views.

   e. _____   Routine venipuncture for handling of specimen.

   f. _____   Handling of specimen.

   Laboratory's bill:

   g. _____   Comprehensive metabolic panel: albumin, bilirubin, calcium, carbon dioxide, chloride, creatinine, glucose, phosphatase (alkaline), potassium, protein, sodium, ALT, AST, and urea nitrogen.

   h. _____   Lipid panel.

   i. _____   CBC, completely automated with complete automated differential.

   If the doctor decides to have the chest x-rays interpreted by a radiologist, the procedural code billed by the radiologist would be _____.

2. Mr. Hart is seen again in the office on May 12. On May 25, he is seen at home at 2 AM with asthma exacerbation, possible myocardial infarct, and congestive heart failure. The doctor consulted with a thoracic cardiovascular surgeon by telephone. He also called to make arrangements for hospitalization. To complete the patient care, these services required 2 hours and 40 minutes of non-face-to-face time in addition to the time spent examining the patient during the house call.

   Code Number   *Description*

   a. _____   _____   May 12, OV, history & examination, straightforward decision-making.

   b. _____   _____   May 25, Home visit, detailed interval history & examination, high- complexity decision-making.

   c. _____   _____   Prolonged time.

3. On June 9, Horace Hart is seen again in the hospital. The thoracic cardiovascular surgeon who was telephoned the previous day was called in for consultation to formally examine the patient and says that surgery is necessary, which is scheduled the following day. The patient's physician sees the patient for his asthmatic condition and acts as assistant surgeon. The surgeon does the follow-up care and assumes care in the case.

Code Number

Description

Primary care physician/assistant surgeon's bill:

a. _____   Hospital visit, problem-focused history & examination, low-complexity decision making performed by PCP.

b. _____   _____   Pericardiotomy performed (PCP acting as assistant surgeon).

Thoracic cardiovascular surgeon's bill:

c. _____   _____   Consultation, comprehensive history & examination, moderate-complexity decision-making performed by surgeon.

d. _____   Pericardiotomy performed by surgeon.

ASSIGNMENT 13.9 CASE SCENARIO FOR CRITICAL THINKING

Performance Objective

Task: Locate the correct procedure code and modifier, if necessary, for each case scenario.

Conditions: Use a pen or a pencil and *Current Procedural Terminology* codebook.

Standards: Time: _____ minutes

               Accuracy: _____

               (Note: The time element and accuracy criteria may be given by your instructor.)

Directions: Read through this progress note on Roy A. Takashima. Abstract information from the note about the subjective symptoms, objective findings, and diagnoses. List the diagnostic and procedure codes you think this case would warrant.

Takashima, Roy A.
October 5, 20xx

   Patient presents with many things going on. First, he's had no difficulties after the feral cat bite, and the cat was normal on quarantine.
   He seemed to be recovering from the flu but is plagued with a persistent cough and pain down the center of his chest attributed to bronchitis without fever or grossly discolored phlegm.
   Physical examination shows expiratory rhonchi and gross exacerbation of his cough on forced expiration. Spirometry before and after bronchodilator was remarkably good; he is symptomatically improved with a Proventil inhaler, which he is given as a sample. I don't think other antibiotics would help.
   His reflux is under good control with proprietary antacids with a clear examination.
   He has several areas of seborrheic keratoses on his face and head that need attention.
   Finally, in follow-up, he needs a complete physical examination.

                                                              Ting Cho, MD

Diagnosis: Influenza and acute bronchitis

Subjective symptoms   _____

                       _____

Objective findings   _____

                       _____

                       _____

Diagnosis code   _____

                       _____

E/M code   _____

Spirometry code   _____

Performance Objective

Task: Calculate and insert the correct amounts for the Medicare scenario.

Conditions: Use a pen or a pencil, the description of the problem and the reference material listed in the problem.

Standards: Time: _____ minutes

                Accuracy: _____

                (Note: The time element and accuracy criteria may be given by your instructor.)

Problem: In the late 1980s, Medicare's Resource-Based Relative Value System (RBRVS) became the way payment was determined each year. However, since the early 1990s, annual fee schedules have been supplied by Medicare Administrative Contractors, so the RBRVS has become more useful in determining practice cost to convert patients to capitation in negotiations of managed care contracts. Because physicians may request determination of fees for certain procedures to discover actual cost and what compensation ratios should be, it is important to know how Medicare fees are determined. Each year, the *Federal Register* publishes geographic practice cost indices (GPCIs) by Medicare carrier and locality, as well as relative value units (RVUs) and related information. This assignment will give you some mathematical practice in using figures for annual conversion factors to determine fees for given procedures in various regions of the United States. Refer to , which are based on pages of the Figs. 13.1 and 13.2 *Federal Register and the CMS Final Rule for 2021.*

FORMULA:

(RVU physician work × GCPI physician work)

+ (RVU practice expense × GPCI practice expense)

+ (RVU malpractice cost × GCPI malpractice cost)

RVU TOTAL × CF = RBRVS

2021 conversion factor $32.4085

a. 47600: Removal of gallbladder. The medical practice is located in Phoenix, Arizona.

FORMULA:

(_____ × _____)

+ (_____ × _____)

+ (_____ × _____)

RVU TOTAL × CF = RBRVS

b. 47715: Excision of bile duct cyst. The medical practice is located in Arkansas.

FORMULA:

$$(\underline{\hspace{3cm}} \times \underline{\hspace{3cm}})$$

$$+ (\underline{\hspace{3cm}} \times \underline{\hspace{3cm}})$$

$$+ (\underline{\hspace{3cm}} \times \underline{\hspace{3cm}})$$

RVU TOTAL × CF = RBRVS

c. 48146: Pancreatectomy. The medical practice is located in Fresno, California.

FORMULA:

$$(\underline{\hspace{3cm}} \times \underline{\hspace{3cm}})$$

$$+ (\underline{\hspace{3cm}} \times \underline{\hspace{3cm}})$$

$$+ (\underline{\hspace{3cm}} \times \underline{\hspace{3cm}})$$

RVU TOTAL × CF = RBRVS

ADDENDUM D—GEOGRAPHIC PRACTICE COST INDICES BY MEDICARE CARRIER AND LOCALITY

Carrier number	Locality number	Locality name	Work	Practice expense	Mal-practice
510	5	Birmingham, AL	0.981	0.913	0.824
510	4	Mobile, AL	0.964	0.911	0.824
510	2	North Central AL	0.970	0.867	0.824
510	1	Northwest AL	0.985	0.869	0.824
510	6	Rest of AL	0.975	0.851	0.824
510	3	Southeast AL	0.972	0.869	0.824
1020	1	Alaska	1.106	1.255	1.042
1030	5	Flagstaff (city), AZ	0.983	0.911	1.255
1030	1	Phoenix, AZ	1.003	1.016	1.255
1030	7	Prescott (city), AZ	0.983	0.911	1.255
1030	99	Rest of Arizona	0.987	0.943	1.255
1030	2	Tucson (city), AZ	0.987	0.989	1.255
1030	8	Yuma (city), AZ	0.983	0.911	1.255
520	13	Arkansas	0.960	0.856	0.302
2050	26	Anaheim-Santa Ana, CA	1.046	1.220	1.370
542	14	Bakersfield, CA	1.028	1.050	1.370
542	11	Fresno/Madera, CA	1.006	1.009	1.370
542	13	Kings/Tulare, CA	0.999	1.001	1.370
2050	18	Los Angeles, CA (1st of 8)	1.060	1.196	1.370
2050	19	Los Angeles, CA (2nd of 8)	1.060	1.196	1.370

Fig. 13.1

ADDENDUM B—RELATIVE VALUE UNITS (RVUs) AND RELATED INFORMATION

HCPCS[1]	MOD	Status	Description	Work RVUs	Practice expense RVUs[2]	Mal-practice RVUs	Total	Global period	Update
47399	....	C	Liver surgery procedure	0.00	0.00	0.00	0.00	YYY	S
47400	....	A	Incision of liver duct	19.11	8.62	1.38	29.11	090	S
47420	....	A	Incision of bile duct	15.48	9.59	2.01	27.08	090	S
47425	....	A	Incision of bile duct	14.95	11.84	2.48	29.27	090	S
47440	....	A	Incision of bile duct	18.51	10.61	2.23	31.35	090	S
47460	....	A	Incision of bile duct sphincter	14.57	15.71	1.84	32.12	090	N
47480	....	A	Incision of gallbladder	8.14	7.68	1.61	17.43	090	S
47490	....	A	Incision of gallbladder	6.11	3.61	0.38	10.10	090	N
47500	....	A	Injection for liver x-rays	1.98	1.53	0.14	3.65	000	N
47505	....	A	Injection for liver x-rays	0.77	1.34	0.14	2.25	000	N
47510	....	A	Insert catheter, bile duct	7.47	2.90	0.25	10.62	090	N
47511	....	A	Insert bile duct drain	10.02	2.90	0.25	13.17	090	N
47525	....	A	Change bile duct catheter	5.47	1.61	0.16	7.24	010	N
47530	....	A	Revise, reinsert bile tube	5.47	1.53	0.19	7.19	090	N
47550	....	A	Bile duct endoscopy	3.05	1.58	0.35	4.98	000	S
47552	....	A	Biliary endoscopy, thru skin	6.11	1.38	0.21	7.70	000	S
47553	....	A	Biliary endoscopy, thru skin	6.42	3.84	0.63	10.89	000	N
47554	....	A	Biliary endoscopy, thru skin	9.16	3.97	0.68	13.81	000	S
47555	....	A	Biliary endoscopy, thru skin	7.64	2.66	0.30	10.60	000	N
47556	....	A	Biliary endoscopy, thru skin	8.66	2.66	0.30	11.62	000	N
47600	....	A	Removal of gallbladder	10.80	7.61	1.60	20.01	090	S
47605	....	A	Removal of gallbladder	11.66	8.23	1.77	21.66	090	S
47610	....	A	Removal of gallbladder	14.01	9.47	2.02	25.50	090	S
47612	....	A	Removal of gallbladder	14.91	14.39	3.08	32.38	090	S
47620	....	A	Removal of gallbladder	15.97	11.35	2.39	29.71	090	S
47630	....	A	Removal of bile duct stone	8.40	3.79	0.40	12.59	090	N
47700	....	A	Exploration of bile ducts	13.90	7.71	1.60	23.21	090	S
47701	....	A	Bile duct revision	26.87	8.30	1.92	37.09	090	S
47710	....	A	Excision of bile duct tumor	18.64	12.19	2.49	33.32	090	S
47715	....	A	Excision of bile duct cyst	14.66	8.31	1.73	24.70	090	S
47716	....	A	Fusion of bile duct cyst	12.67	6.63	1.55	20.85	090	S
47720	....	A	Fuse gallbladder and bowel	12.03	9.26	1.95	23.34	090	S
47721	....	A	Fuse upper gi structures	14.57	11.55	2.50	28.62	090	S
47740	....	A	Fuse gallbladder and bowel	14.08	10.32	2.16	26.56	090	S
47760	....	A	Fuse bile ducts and bowel	20.15	11.74	2.56	34.45	090	S
47765	....	A	Fuse liver ducts and bowel	19.25	14.77	3.00	37.02	090	S
47780	....	A	Fuse bile ducts and bowel	20.60	10.22	2.70	33.61	090	S
47800	....	A	Reconstruction of bile ducts	17.91	13.37	2.46	33.74	090	S
47801	....	A	Placement, bile duct support	11.41	5.54	0.82	17.77	090	S
47802	....	A	Fuse liver duct and intestine	16.19	10.38	1.77	28.34	090	S
47999	....	C	Bile tract surgery procedure	0.00	0.00	0.00	0.00	YYY	S
48000	....	A	Drainage of abdomen	13.25	7.13	1.42	21.80	090	S
48001	....	A	Placement of drain, pancreas	15.71	8.22	1.91	25.84	090	S
48005	....	A	Resect/debride pancreas	17.77	9.29	2.16	29.22	090	S
48020	....	A	Removal of pancreatic stone	13.12	6.86	1.59	21.57	090	S
48100	....	A	Biopsy of pancreas	10.30	4.26	0.80	15.36	090	S
48102	....	A	Needle biopsy, pancreas	4.48	2.44	0.25	7.17	010	N
48120	....	A	Removal of pancreas lesion	12.93	9.83	2.09	24.85	090	S
48140	....	A	Partial removal of pancreas	18.47	13.44	2.86	34.77	090	S
48145	....	A	Partial removal of pancreas	19.30	15.88	3.20	38.38	090	S
48146	....	A	Pancreatectomy	21.97	16.67	1.94	40.58	090	S
48148	....	A	Removal of pancreatic duct	14.57	8.32	1.70	24.59	090	S
48150	....	A	Partial removal of pancreas	34.55	22.79	4.80	62.14	090	S
48151	....	D	Partial removal of pancreas	0.00	0.00	0.00	0.00	090	O
48152	....	A	Pancreatectomy	31.33	22.79	4.80	58.92	090	S
48153	....	A	Pancreatectomy	34.55	22.79	4.80	62.14	090	S
48154	....	A	Pancreatectomy	31.33	22.79	4.80	58.92	090	S
48155	....	A	Removal of pancreas	19.65	20.63	4.31	44.59	090	S
48160	....	N	Pancreas removal, transplant	0.00	0.00	0.00	0.00	XXX	O
48180	....	A	Fuse pancreas and bowel	21.11	12.74	2.66	36.51	090	S
48400	....	A	Injection, intraoperative	1.97	1.04	0.24	3.25	ZZZ	S
48500	....	A	Surgery of pancreas cyst	12.17	8.62	1.68	22.47	090	S
48510	....	A	Drain pancreatic pseudocyst	11.34	7.62	1.46	20.42	090	S
48520	....	A	Fuse pancreas cyst and bowel	13.11	11.43	2.46	27.00	090	S
48540	....	A	Fuse pancreas cyst and bowel	15.95	12.80	2.68	31.43	090	S
48545	....	A	Pancreatorrhaphy	14.81	7.75	1.81	24.37	090	S
48547	....	A	Duodenal exclusion	21.42	11.20	2.61	35.23	090	S

[1] All numeric CPT HCPCS Copyright 1993 American Medical Association.
[2] *Indicates reduction of Practice Expense RVUs as a result of OBRA 1993.

Fig. 13.2

14 The Paper Claim: CMS-1500

Linda M. Smith

KEY TERMS

Your instructor may wish to select some words pertinent to this chapter for a test. For definitions of the terms, further study, and/or reference, the words, phrases, and abbreviations may be found in the glossary at the end of the Textbook. *Key terms for this chapter follow.*

Administrative Simplification Compliance Act	National Provider Identifier
clean claim	National Uniform Claim Committee
deleted claim	optical character recognition
dirty claim	paper claim
durable medical equipment number	pending claim
electronic claim	physically clean claim
employer identification number	purchased service provider
facility provider number	rejected claim
group National Provider Identifier (group NPI)	Social Security number
Health Insurance Claim Form (CMS-1500)	state license number
incomplete claim	suspended claim
intelligent character recognition	taxonomy code
invalid claim	

KEY ABBREVIATIONS

See how many abbreviations and acronyms you can translate and then use this as a handy reference list. Definitions for the key abbreviations are located near the back of the Textbook *in the glossary.*

ASCA _____	LMP _____
CMS-1500 _____	MSP _____
DME _____	NA, N/A _____
DNA _____	NPI _____
EIN _____	NUCC _____
EMG _____	OCR _____
EPSDT _____	SOF _____
ICR _____	SSN _____

PERFORMANCE OBJECTIVES

The student will be able to:

- Define and spell the key terms and key abbreviations for this chapter, given the information from the *Textbook* glossary, within a reasonable time period and with enough accuracy to obtain a satisfactory evaluation.

- After reading the chapter, answer the fill-in-the-blank, mix and match, multiple choice, and true/false review questions, with enough accuracy to obtain a satisfactory evaluation.

- Given the patients' medical chart notes and blank insurance claim forms, complete each CMS-1500 Health Insurance Claim Form for billing, within a reasonable time period and with enough accuracy to obtain a satisfactory evaluation.

STUDY OUTLINE

Part I Fill in the Blank

Review the objectives, key terms, chapter information, glossary definitions of key terms, and figures before completing the following review questions.

1. What legislation required all claims sent to the Medicare program be submitted electronically, effective October 16, 2003?

    _____

2. State the name of the health insurance claim form that was required for health care professionals and suppliers to use effective April 1, 2014. _____

3. What is the name of the organization that developed the CMS-1500 claim form? _____ _____

    _____

4. What is a pended claim?

    _____

5. How many days will it take to process a Medicare claim that is submitted electronically?

    _____

6. If a claim form is submitted with errors, what is it referred to as?

    _____

7. What is *dual coverage*?

    _____

8. The insurance company with the first responsibility for payment of a bill for medical services is known as the

    _____

9. The CMS-1500 claim form allows for reporting of a maximum of _____ diagnosis codes per claim form.

10. What internet resource can be used to find physician provider numbers?

    _____

11. For electronic submission of claims, what allows the physician's name to be printed in the signature block where it would normally be signed?

    _____

12. When preparing a claim that is to be optically scanned, birth dates are keyed in with how many digits?

    _____

13. If circumstances make it impossible to obtain a signature each time a paper claim is submitted, the patient's signature may be obtained and maintained in the patient's medical record. The claim block should be completed with _____ or _____, thus indicating the signature is on file.

Part II Mix and Match

14. Match the types of claims listed in the right column with their descriptions and fill in the blanks with the appropriate letters.

_____ Claim missing required information	a. Clean claim
_____ Phrase used when a claim is held back from payment	b. Paper claim
_____ Claim that is submitted and then optically scanned by the insurance carrier and converted to electronic form	c. Invalid claim
_____ Claim that needs manual processing because of errors or to solve a problem	d. Dirty claim
_____ Claim that needs clarification and answers to some questions	e. Electronic claim
_____ Claim that is canceled or voided if the incorrect claim form is used or itemized charges are not provided	f. Pending claim
_____ Claim that is paperless	g. Rejected claim
_____ Claim that is submitted within the time limit and correctly completed	h. Incomplete claim
_____ Medicare claim that contains information that is complete and necessary but is illogical or incorrect	i. Deleted claim

15. Match the types of numbers listed in the right column with their descriptions and fill in the blanks with the appropriate letters.

_____ A number issued by the federal government to each individual for personal use	a. State license number
_____ A Medicare lifetime provider number	b. Employer identification number
_____ A number listed on a claim when submitting insurance claims to insurance companies under a group name	c. Social Security number
_____ A number that a health care provider must obtain to practice in a state	d. Group national provider number
_____ A number used when billing for supplies and equipment	e. National Provider Identifier
_____ A number issued to a hospital	f. Durable medical equipment number
_____ An individual health care provider's federal tax identification number issued by the Internal Revenue Service	g. Facility provider number

PART III MULTIPLE CHOICE

Choose the best answer.

16. The basic paper claim form currently used by health care professionals and suppliers to bill insurance carriers for services provided to patients is the:
    a. UB-04 claim form.
    b. CMS-1500 claim form.
    c. Attending physician's statement.
    d. COMB-1.

17. What is the exception to the Administrative Simplification Compliance Act's (ASCA's) requirement for service providers to send claims to Medicare electronically?
    a. Chiropractors.
    b. Providers who have more than 25 full-time employees.
    c. Providers with fewer than 10 full-time employees.
    d. Any provider who requests a financial hardship.

18. Under ASCA, plans other than Medicare:
    a. may allow submission of claims on paper.
    b. will never allow submission of claims on paper.
    c. only allow submission of claims on paper.
    d. must follow the claims submission guidance of the American Medical Association (AMA).

19. The National Uniform Claim Committee (NUCC) is made up of which of the following?
    a. AMA representatives.
    b. Centers for Medicare and Medicaid Services (CMS) representatives.
    c. Providers.
    d. All of the above.

186

Chapter **14** **The Paper Claim: CMS-1500**

20. The most recently revised version of the 1500 Health Insurance Claim Form developed in 2012 accommodates:
    a. the change in the names of the government agency from Health Care Finance Administration to Centers for Medicare and Medicaid Services (CMS).
    b. requirements for allowing optical scanning of the claim.
    c. changes needed for implementation of the ICD-10 coding system.
    d. changes to the *Current Procedural Terminology* (CPT) coding system.

21. If a patient has dual coverage:
    a. insurance information for the primary carrier should be obtained.
    b. insurance information for both the primary and the secondary carrier should be obtained.
    c. insurance information for the secondary carrier can be obtained after the primary insurance carrier processes the claim.
    d. the primary carrier has insurance information for the secondary carrier and will automatically forward the claim to the secondary carrier if necessary.

22. Health Insurance Portability and Accountability Act (HIPAA) laws require that the provider rendering the service be identified on the claim form by:
    a. reporting of the correct provider number.
    b. reporting of the correct International Classification of Diseases (ICD)-10 code.
    c. reporting of the correct CPT code.
    d. reporting of the correct facility code.

23. The Omnibus Budget Reconciliation Act (OBRA) requires Medicare administrative contractors to:
    a. deny all claims received after 1 year from date of service.
    b. pay all clean claims that are submitted within 1 year from date of service.
    c. investigate all clean claims not paid on time.
    d. pay interest on all clean claims not paid on time.

24. A claim that is investigated on a postpayment basis that is found to be "not due" will require:
    a. resubmission of a claim.
    b. manual review of the claim.
    c. refund of the monies paid.
    d. additional medical records.

25. If there is a balance remaining on a patient's account after the patient's primary insurance has paid, and the patient has secondary coverage, the billing specialist should:

a. send a bill to the patient for the remaining balance.
    b. send a claim form to the secondary insurance for the remaining balance.
    c. send a claim form to the secondary insurance with a copy of the explanation of benefits from the primary carrier.
    d. monitor the claim to determine whether the patient has sent a claim to the secondary carrier.

26. The maximum number of diagnostic codes that can be submitted on the CMS-1500 claim form is:
    a. four.
    b. six.
    c. eight.
    d. twelve.

27. National Provider Identifier (NPI) numbers are used to report:
    a. referring physicians.
    b. ordering physicians.
    c. performing physicians.
    d. all of the above.

28. NPI numbers are assigned:
    a. each time a health care provider contracts with a new payer.
    b. annually, per health care provider.
    c. once in a lifetime, per health care provider.
    d. each time the provider moves to another state.

29. To correct a claim that has been denied because of an invalid procedure code, the billing specialist should:
    a. check the patient registration form to ensure all data were reported accurately.
    b. confirm the code in the CPT manual to ensure it is valid for the date of service.
    c. confirm the code in the ICD-10 manual to ensure it is valid for the date of service.
    d. confirm the provider's NPI number to make sure it was reported accurately.

30. To correct a claim that was denied because more than six lines were entered on the claim, the billing specialist should:
    a. readjust the printer, so all claim lines fit on the form, reprint, and send.
    b. reenter data with the appropriate code range for the dates of service and bill on one line.
    c. bill six claim lines on one claim and complete an additional paper claim for the additional claim lines.
    d. write off the additional claim lines that have been denied.

PART IV TRUE/FALSE

Write "T" or "F" in the blank to indicate whether you think the statement is true or false.

_____ 31. The insurance billing specialist does not need to know how to complete a paper claim because most claims are submitted electronically.

_____ 32. Physicians who experience downtimes of internet services that are out of their control for more than two days may submit claims to Medicare on paper.

_____ 33. The goal of the NUCC is to provide a warehouse for providers to purchase CMS-1500 claim forms.

_____ 34. Effective June 1, 2013, providers were required to use only the CMS-1500 claim form for processing.

_____ 35. Use of the standardized CMS-1500 claim form has simplified processing of paper claims.

_____ 36. Quantities of the CMS-1500 claim form can be purchased through CMS or downloaded from the CMS website and used for submission.

_____ 37. Interest rates that apply to the Prompt Payment Interest Rate can be located on the Treasury's Financial Fiscal Service page.

_____ 38. Medicare claims that require further investigation before being processed are referred to as "other" claims.

_____ 39. A diagnosis should never be submitted without supporting documentation in the medical record.

_____ 40. Claims for dates of services in two different years may be submitted on the same claim form.

_____ 41. Services that are inclusive in the global surgical package that have no charge associated with them should not be submitted on the CMS-1500 claim form.

_____ 42. Proofreading claims before submission can prevent denials and delay of claim processing.

_____ 43. When submitting supplemental documentation for processing of a claim, the patient's name and date of service need only be on the front of a two-sided document.

_____ 44. Handwriting is permitted on optically scanned paper claims.

_____ 45. Use the abbreviation "DNA" when information is not applicable.

ASSIGNMENT 14.2 COMPLETE A HEALTH INSURANCE CLAIM FORM FOR A PRIVATE CASE

Performance Objective

Task: Complete a health insurance claim form

Conditions: Use Merry M. McLean's patient record, one health insurance claim form, a computer or a pen.

Standards: Claim Productivity Measurement

                Time: _____ minutes

                Accuracy: _____

                (Note: The time element and accuracy criteria may be given by your instructor.)

Directions:

1. Complete the Health Insurance Claim Form, using NUCC guidelines, and send the form to the Prudential Insurance Company for Mrs. Merry M. McLean by referring to the patient record. Date the claim June 15 of the current year. Record on the financial account record/statement when you have billed the insurance company.

2. A Performance Evaluation Checklist may be reproduced from the "Instruction Guide to the Workbook" in a section before Chapter 1 if your instructor wishes you to submit it to assist with scoring and comments.

After the instructor has returned your work to you, either make the necessary corrections and place your work in a three-ring notebook for future reference, or, if you received a high score, place it in your portfolio for reference when applying for a job.

COLLEGE CLINIC
4567 Broad Avenue, Woodland Hills, XY 12345-0001
(555)-486-9002
Fax: (555) 487-8976
NPI: 3664021CC
Federal Tax ID#: XX12210XX

PATIENT INFORMATION:

Name:	Merry M. McLean
Address:	4919 Dolphin Way
	Woodland Hills, XY 12345
Telephone:	(555) 486-1859
Date of Birth:	02/02/1948
Social Security:	459-XX-9989
Occupation:	SECRETARY
Employer:	Porter Company
	5490 Wilshire Blvd.
	Merck, XY 12346
Status:	Married
Spouse:	Harry L. McLean

INSURANCE INFORMATION:

Primary:	Prudential Insurance
	5621 Wilshire Blvd.
	Merck, XY 12346
	(555) 664-9023
Policy Number:	459-XX-9989
Group Number:	8832
Subscriber:	Harry L. McLean
Secondary:	None

DIAGNOSIS INFORMATION

1. N32.0	Vesicle fistula, not otherwise specified	5.	
2. R32	Urinary incontinence, unspecified	6.	
3.		7.	
4.		8.	

PROCEDURE INFORMATION

Description	Date	Code	Charge
1. Office visit, new patient	05/06/20XX	99203	120.00
2. Urinalysis	05/06/20XX	81000	10.00
3. Cystoscopy	05/10/20XX	52000	230.00
4. Initial hospital care	05/16/20XX	99221	110.00
5. Repair vesicovaginal fistula	05/17/20XX	51900	910.00
6. Hospital visit	05/18/20XX	99024	N/C
7. Hospital visit	05/19/20XX	99024	N/C
8. Hospital visit	05/20/20XX	99024	N/C
9. Hospital visit	05/21/20XX	99024	N/C
10. Discharge	05/22/20XX	99024	N/C
11. Follow-up office visit	06/05/20XX	99024	N/C

NOTES: Referred by: Emdee Fine, MD, 5000 Wilshire Blvd., Merck, XY 12346
               NPI: 73027175XX
       Treating MD: Gene Ulibarri, MD
               NPI: 25678831XX
     Place of service: College Clinic for 5/6–5/10, 6/5
               College Hospital for 5/16–5/22 (Inpatient)
               4500 Broad Avenue, Woodland Hills, XY 12345
               NPI: X950731067
               Patient hospitalized 5/16/20xx-5/22/20xx

ASSIGNMENT 14.3 COMPLETE ONE HEALTH INSURANCE CLAIM FORM FOR A PRIVATE CASE

Performance Objective

Task: Complete one health insurance claim form.

Conditions: Use Walter J. Stone's E/M patient record, one health insurance claim form, a computer or a pen.

Standards: Claim Productivity Measurement

                 Time: _____ minutes

                 Accuracy: _____

                 (Note: The time element and accuracy criteria may be given by your instructor.)

Directions: You will be billing for all services listed on the patient's progress notes for Dr. Clarence Cutler.

1. Complete one Health Insurance Claim Form, addressing it to Travelers Insurance Company for Mr. Walter J. Stone by referring to patient record. Date the claim May 5 of the current year. Use NUCC guidelines.

2. A Performance Evaluation Checklist may be reproduced from the "Instruction Guide to the Workbook" that appears in a section before Chapter 1 if your instructor wishes you to submit it to assist with scoring and comments.

   After the instructor has returned your work to you, either make the necessary corrections and place your work in a three-ring notebook for future reference or, if you received a high score, place it in your portfolio for reference when applying for a job.

COLLEGE CLINIC
4567 Broad Avenue, Woodland Hills, XY 12345-0001
(555)-486-9002
Fax: (555) 487-8976
NPI: 3664021CC
Federal Tax ID#: XX12210XX

PATIENT INFORMATION:		INSURANCE INFORMATION:	
Name:	Walter J. Stone	Primary:	Travelers Insurance
Address:	2008 Converse Street		5460 Olympic Blvd.
	Woodland Hills, XY 12345		Woodland Hills, XY
Telephone:	(555) 345-0776		12345
Date of Birth:	03/14/1949	Policy Number:	456-XX-9989
Social Security:	456-XX-9989	Group Number:	6754
Occupation:	ADVERTISING AGENT	Subscriber:	Walter J. Stone
Employer:	RV Black and Associates	Secondary:	None
	1267 Broad Street		
	Woodland Hills, XY 12345		
Status:	Widowed		
Spouse:			

DIAGNOSIS INFORMATION

1. K25.0   Acute gastric ulcer with hemorrhage.

2. K80.18   Calculus of gallbladder and bile duct with cholecystitis, unspecified, without obstruction.

3. K92.2   Gastrointestinal hemorrhage, unspecified.

4. I10   Essential hypertension, benign.

PROCEDURE INFORMATION

Description	Date	Code	Charge
1. Initial hospital care	05/03/20XX	99222	150.00
2. Cholecystectomy	05/04/20XX	47600	1160.00
3. Endoscopy	05/04/20XX	43255-51 59	710.00

NOTES: Referred by: Gaston Input, MD, College Hospital
                            NPI: 32783127XX
             Treating MD: Clarence Cutler, MD
                            NPI: 43050047XX
             Place of service: College Hospital (Inpatient)
                            4500 Broad Avenue, Woodland Hills, XY 12345
                            NPI: X950731067
                            Patient hospitalized 5/3/20xx – 5/5/20xx

ASSIGNMENT 14.4 LOCATE ERRORS ON A COMPLETED HEALTH INSURANCE CLAIM FORM

Performance Objective

Task: Locate errors on a completed health insurance claim form and post the information to the patient's ledger card.

Conditions: Use Tom N. Parkinson's completed insurance claim (Fig. 14.1), one health insurance claim form, a computer or a pen.

         Standards:Time: _____ minutes

         Accuracy: _____

         (Note: The time element and accuracy criteria may be given by your instructor.)

Guidance: To alleviate frustration and ease the process of completing a claim form for the first time, you will be editing a claim and then taking the correct information and inserting it on a blank CMS-1500 form. Refer to Chapter 14 in the Textbook for block-by-block private payer instructions for completing the CMS-1500 insurance claim form.

Directions: Study the completed claim form (Fig. 14.1) and search for missing or incorrect information. If possible, verify all information. Highlight or circle in red all incorrect or missing information. Insert the correct information on the claim form. Now transfer all the data to a blank CMS-1500 claim form. If mandatory information is missing, insert the word "NEED" in the corresponding block of the claim form.

    A Performance Evaluation Checklist may be reproduced from the "Instruction Guide to the Workbook" that appears in a section before Chapter 1 if your instructor wishes you to submit it to assist with scoring and comments.

Optional: List, in block-by-block order, the reasons why the claim may either be rejected or delayed according to the errors found.

General Directions for Claim Form Completion

Assume that the Health Insurance Claim Form CMS-1500 is printed in red ink for processing by optical character recognition (OCR) or intelligent character recognition (ICR). Complete the form using NUCC guidelines and send it to the proper insurance carrier. Refer to Chapter 14 in the Textbook for block instructions. Claim form templates have been completed to use as visual examples for placement of data; they may be found at the end of Chapter 14 in the Textbook. Screened areas on each form do not apply to the insurance program example shown and should be left blank.

    All physicians in College Clinic accept assignment of benefits for all types of insurance that you will be billing for; indicate this by checking "yes" in Block 27. For each claim completed, be sure to insert your initials at the lower left corner of the claim form.

HEALTH INSURANCE CLAIM FORM

APPROVED BY NATIONAL UNIFOR MCLAIM COMMITTEE (NUCC) 02/12

| | PICA | | | | | | | PICA | |

1. MEDICARE ☐ (Medicare#)	MEDICAID ☐ (Medicaid#)	TRICARE ☐ (ID#DoD#)	CHAMPVA ☐ (Member ID#)	GROUP HEALTH PLAN ☒ (ID#)	FECA BLK LUNG ☐ (ID#)	OTHER ☐ (ID#)

1a. INSURED'S I.D. NUMBER (For Program in Item 1)
PX4278A

2. PATIENT'S NAME (Last Name, First Name, Middle Initial)
Parkinson, Tom, N

3. PATIENT'S BIRTH DATE   SEX
MM 04 | DD 06 | YY 1993   M ☒   F ☐

4. INSURED'S NAME (Last Name, First Name, Middle Initial)
Parkinson, Jamie, B

5. PATIENT'S ADDRESS (No., Street)
4510 South A Street

6. PATIENT RELATIONSHIP TO INSURED
Self ☐ Spouse ☐ Child ☒ Other ☐

7. INSURED'S ADDRESS (No., Street)
4510 South A Street

CITY   Woodland Hills   STATE XY

8. RESERVED FOR NUCC USE

CITY   Woodland Hills   STATE XY

ZIP CODE 12345-0000   TELEPHONE (Include Area Code) (555) 7421560

ZIP CODE 12345-0000   TELEPHONE (Include Area Code) (555) 7421560

9. OTHER INSURED'S NAME (Last Name, First Name, Middle Initial)

10. IS PATIENT'S CONDITION RELATED TO:

11. INSURED'S POLICY GROUP OR FECA NUMBER

a. OTHER INSURED'S POLICY OR GROUP NUMBER

a. EMPLOYMENT? (Current or Previous)
☐ YES ☒ NO

a. INSURED'S DATE OF BIRTH
MM | DD | YY   SEX M ☐ F ☐

b. RESERVED FOR NUCC USE

b. AUTO ACCIDENT?   PLACE (State)
☐ YES ☒ NO

b. OTHER CLAIM ID (Designated by NUCC)

c. RESERVED FOR NUCC USE

c. OTHER ACCIDENT?
☐ YES ☒ NO

c. INSURANCE PLAN NAME OR PROGRAM NAME

d. INSURANCE PLAN NAME OR PROGRAM NAME

10d. CLAIM CODES (Designated by NUCC)

d. IS THERE ANOTHER HEALTH BENEFIT PLAN?
☐ YES ☒ NO If yes, complete items 9, 9a, and 9d.

READ BACK OF FORM BEFORE COMPLETING & SIGNING THIS FORM.

12. PATIENT'S OR AUTHORIZED PERSON'S SIGNATUREI authorize the release of any medical or other information necessary to process this claim. I also request payment of government benefits either to myself or to the party who accepts assignment below.

SIGNED _____ DATE _____

13. INSURED'S OR AUTHORIZED PERSON'S SIGNATURE I authorize payment of medical benefits to the undersigned physician or supplier for services described below.

SIGNED _____

14. DATE OF CURRENT: ILLNESS, INJURY, or PREGNANCY(LMP)
MM | DD | YY   QUAL.

15. OTHER DATE
QUAL.   MM | DD | YY

16. DATES PATIENT UNABLE TO WORK IN CURRENT OCCUPATION
FROM MM | DD | YY   TO MM | DD | YY

17. NAME OF REFERRING PROVIDER OR OTHER SOURCE
17a.
17b. NPI

18. HOSPITALIZATION DATES RELATED TO CURRENT SERVICES
FROM MM | DD | YY   TO MM | DD | YY

19. ADDITIONAL CLAIM INFORMATION (Designated by NUCC)

20. OUTSIDE LAB?   ☐ YES ☒ NO $ CHARGES

21. DIAGNOSIS OR NATURE OF ILLNESS OR INJURY Relate A-L to service line below (24E)   ICD Ind. 0

A. |____   B. |____   C. |____   D. |____
E. |____   F. |____   G. |____   H. |____
I. |____   J. |____   K. |____   L. |____

22. RESUBMISSION CODE   ORIGINAL REF. NO.

23. PRIOR AUTHORIZATION NUMBER

24. A. DATE(S) OF SERVICE From / To	B. PLACE OF SERVICE	C. EMG	D. PROCEDURES, SERVICES, OR SUPPLIES (Explain Unusual Circumstances) CPT/HCPCS	MODIFIER	E. DIAGNOSIS POINTER	F. $ CHARGES	G. DAYS OR UNITS	H. EPSDT Family Plan	I. ID. QUAL.	J. RENDERING PROVIDER ID. #
1 07 14 20XX			99242			80 24	1		NPI	
2 07 14 20XX			71020		A	38 96	1		NPI	4627889700
3									NPI	
4									NPI	
5									NPI	
6									NPI	

25. FEDERAL TAX I.D. NUMBER   SSN ☐ EIN ☐
7034597

26. PATIENT'S ACCOUNT NO.

27. ACCEPT ASSIGNMENT? (For govt. claims, see back)
☒ YES ☐ NO

28. TOTAL CHARGE
$ 119 20

29. AMOUNT PAID
$

30. Rsvd for NUCC Use
$

31. SIGNATURE OF PHYSICIAN OR SUPPLIER INCLUDING DEGREES OR CREDENTIALS (I certify that the statements on the reverse apply to this bill and are made a part thereof.)
Gerald Practon   071420XX
SIGNED Gerald Practon   DATE

32. SERVICE FACILITY LOCATION INFORMATION
a. NPI   b.

33. BILLING PROVIDER INFO & PH # (555) 4869002
College Clinic
4567 Broad Avenue
Woodland Hills XY 12345-0001
a. 3664021CC   b.

NUCC Instruction Manual available at: www.nucc.org   PLEASE PRINT OR TYPE   OMB APPROVAL PENDING

CARRIER

PATIENT AND INSURED INFORMATION

PHYSICIAN OR SUPPLIER INFORMATION

Fig. 14.1

ASSIGNMENT 14.5 COMPLETE A CLAIM FORM FOR A MEDICARE/MEDICAID CASE

Performance Objective

Task: Complete a CMS-1500 claim form for a Medicare/Medicaid case.

Conditions: Use Helen P. Nolan's patient record, one health insurance claim form, a pen or a pencil.

Standards: Claim Productivity Measurement

Time: _____ minutes

Accuracy: _____

(Note: The time element and accuracy criteria may be given by your instructor.)

Directions:

1. Complete the CMS-1500 claim form, using NUCC guidelines for a Medicare/Medicaid case. If your instructor wants you to direct it to your local Medicare fiscal intermediary, obtain the name and address by going to the internet. Refer to Mrs. Helen P. Nolan's patient record for information. Date the claim May 31 of the current year.

2. Refer to Chapter 14 of the textbook for instructions on how to complete the CMS-1500 claim form.

3. A Performance Evaluation Checklist may be reproduced from the "Instruction Guide to the Workbook" that appears in a section before Chapter 1 if your instructor wishes you to submit it to assist with scoring and comments.

   After the instructor has returned your work to you, either make the necessary corrections and place your work in a three-ring notebook for future reference or, if you received a high score, place it in your portfolio for reference when applying for a job.

COLLEGE CLINIC

4567 Broad Avenue, Woodland Hills, XY 12345-0001

(555)-486-9002

Fax: (555) 487-8976

NPI: 3664021CC

Federal Tax ID#: XX12210XX

PATIENT INFORMATION:

Name:	Helen P. Nolan	
Address:	2588 Cedar Street	
	Woodland Hills, XY 12345-0001	
Telephone:	(555) 660-9878	
Date of Birth:	05/10/37	
Social Security:	732-XX-1573	
Occupation:	HOMEMAKER	
Employer:		
Status:	Widowed	
Spouse:		

INSURANCE INFORMATION:

Primary:	Medicare
Policy Number:	632XX3209D
Group Number:	
Subscriber:	
Secondary:	Medicaid
Policy Number:	1960235894901XX
Group Number:	

DIAGNOSIS INFORMATION

1. I84.131   Internal and external bleeding hemorrhoids.

2. K60.5   Anorectal fistula.

3.

4.

PROCEDURE INFORMATION

Description	Date	Code	Charge
1. Office visit, new patient	05/01/20XX	99203-25	120.00
2. Diagnostic proctoscopy	05/01/20XX	46614	160.00
3. Hemorrhoidectomy with fistulectomy	05/08/20XX	46258	510.00

NOTES: Referred by: James B. Jeffers, MD, 100 S. Broadway, Woodland Hills, XY 12345

NPI: 12345069XX

Treating MD: Rex Rumsey, MD

NPI: 19999047XX

Place of service: 5/1 College Clinic

5/8 College Hospital

4500 Broad Avenue, Woodland Hills, XY 12345

NPI: X950731067

Hospitalized from 5/8/20xx to 5/11/20xx (Inpatient)

ASSIGNMENT 14.6 COMPLETE A CLAIM FORM FOR A MEDICARE CASE

Performance Objective

Task: Complete a CMS-1500 claim form for a Medicare case.

Conditions: Use Elsa M. Mooney's patient record, one health insurance claim form, a pen or a pencil.

Standards: Claim Productivity Measurement

Time: _____ minutes

Accuracy: _____

(Note: The time element and accuracy criteria may be given by your instructor.)

Directions:

1. Complete the CMS-1500 claim form, using National Uniform Claim Committee (NUCC) guidelines for a Medicare case. If your instructor wants you to direct it to your local fiscal intermediary, obtain the name and address by going to the internet. Refer to Mrs. Elsa M. Mooney's patient record for information. Date the claim December 21 of the current year. Dr. Cardi is a participating physician who is accepting assignment.

2. Refer to Chapter 14 of the textbook for instructions on how to complete this claim form and a Medicare template.

3. A Performance Evaluation Checklist may be reproduced from the "Instruction Guide to the Workbook" that appears in a section before Chapter 1 if your instructor wishes you to submit it to assist with scoring and comments.

   After the instructor has returned your work to you, either make the necessary corrections and place your work in a three-ring notebook for future reference or, if you received a high score, place it in your portfolio for reference when applying for a job.

COLLEGE CLINIC
4567 Broad Avenue, Woodland Hills, XY 12345-0001
(555)-486-9002
Fax: (555) 487-8976
NPI: 3664021CC
Federal Tax ID#: XX12210XX

PATIENT INFORMATION:		INSURANCE INFORMATION:	
Name:	Elsa M. Mooney	Primary:	Medicare
Address:	5750 Canyon Road	Policy Number:	321XX2653A
	Woodland Hills, XY 12345	Group Number:	
Telephone:	(555) 452-4968	Subscriber:	
Date of Birth:	02/06/1930	Secondary:	none
Social Security:	321-XX-2653	Policy Number:	
Occupation:	RETIRED SECRETARY	Group Number:	
Employer:		Subscriber:	
Status:	Widowed		
Spouse:			

DIAGNOSIS INFORMATION

1. I25.119   Atherosclerotic heart disease of native coronary artery with unspecified angina pectoris

2.

3.

4.

PROCEDURE INFORMATION

Description	Date	Code	Charge
1. Initial office visit, new pt	12/15/20XX	99203	120.00
2. ECG with interpret & report	12/15/20XX	93000	20.00

NOTES: Referred by: George Gentle, MD, 1000 N. Main St., Woodland Hills, XY 12345
NPI: 40213102XX
Treating MD: Perry Cardi, MD
NPI: 67805027XX
Place of service: College Clinic
4500 Broad Avenue, Woodland Hills, XY 12345

ASSIGNMENT 14.7 COMPLETE A CLAIM FORM FOR A MEDICAID CASE

Performance Objective

Task: Complete a CMS-1500 claim form.

Conditions: Use Rose Clarkson's patient record, one health insurance claim form, a pen or a pencil.

Standards: Claim Productivity Measurement

Time: _____ minutes

Accuracy: _____

(Note: The time element and accuracy criteria may be given by your instructor.)

Directions:

1. Using National Uniform Claim Committee (NUCC) guidelines, complete the Health Insurance Claim Form and direct it to Medicaid for Rose Clarkson by referring to her patient record. Date the claim September 6 of the current year. If your instructor wants you to insert the name and address of your Medicaid fiscal agent on the claim, obtain the address by going to the internet.

2. Refer to Chapter 14 in the *Textbook* for instructions on how to complete this claim form and a Medicaid template.

3. A Performance Evaluation Checklist may be reproduced from the "Instruction Guide to the Workbook" in the section before Chapter 1 if your instructor wishes you to submit it to assist with scoring and comments.

After the instructor has returned your work to you, either make the necessary corrections and place your work in a three-ring notebook for future reference or, if you received a high score, place it in your portfolio for reference when applying for a job.

COLLEGE CLINIC
4567 Broad Avenue, Woodland Hills, XY 12345-0001
(555)-486-9002
Fax: (555) 487-8976
NPI: 3664021CC
Federal Tax ID#: XX12210XX

PATIENT INFORMATION:		INSURANCE INFORMATION:	
Name:	Rose Clarkson	Primary:	Medicaid
Address:	3408 Jackson Street	Policy Number:	CC99756329346X
	Hempstead, XY 11551-0300	Group Number:	
Telephone:	(555) 487-2209	Subscriber:	
Date of Birth:	03/09/1954	Secondary:	none
Social Security:	030-XX-9543	Policy Number:	
Occupation:	UNEMPLOYED	Group Number:	
Employer:		Subscriber:	
Status:			
Spouse:			

DIAGNOSIS INFORMATION

1. I50.9   Congestive heart failure

2. I34.1   Nonrheumatic mitral valve prolapse

3.

4.

PROCEDURE INFORMATION

Description	Date	Code	Charge
1. Initial office visit, new pt	09/04/20XX	99203	120.00
2. 12 lead ECG	09/04/20XX	93000	20.00
3. Echocardiogram with Doppler	09/04/20XX	99306	210.00
4. Chest x-ray	09/04/20XX	71045	30.00

NOTES: Referred by: James Jackson, MD, 100 N. Main St., Hempstead, XY 11551
                         NPI: 72011337XX
            Treating MD: Perry Cardi, MD
                         NPI: 67805027XX
        Place of service: College Clinic
                         4500 Broad Avenue, Woodland Hills, XY 12345
                         NPI: X950731067

ASSIGNMENT 14.8 COMPLETE A CLAIM FORM FOR A MEDICAID CASE

Performance Objective

Task: Complete a CMS-1500 claim form for a Medicaid case

Conditions: Use Stephen M. Drake's patient record, one health insurance claim form, a pen or a pencil.

Standards: Claim Productivity Measurement

               Time: _____ minutes

               Accuracy: _____

               (Note: The time element and accuracy criteria may be given by your instructor.)

Directions:

1. Using NUCC guidelines, complete the Health Insurance Claim Form and direct it to Medicaid for Stephen M. Drake by referring to his patient record. Date the claim May 26 of the current year. If your instructor wants you to insert the name and address of your Medicaid fiscal agent on the claim, obtain it by going to the internet. Do not list services not charged for (N/C) on the claim form. Remember that the physician must always sign all forms on Medicaid cases; stamped signatures are not allowed.

2. Refer to Chapter 14 in the Textbook for instructions on how to complete this claim form and a Medicaid template.

3. A Performance Evaluation Checklist may be reproduced from the "Instruction Guide to the Workbook" that appears in the section before Chapter 1 if your instructor wishes you to submit it to assist with scoring and comments.

    After the instructor has returned your work to you, either make the necessary corrections and place your work in a three-ring notebook for future reference or, if you received a high score, place it in your portfolio for reference when applying for a job.

COLLEGE CLINIC
4567 Broad Avenue, Woodland Hills, XY 12345-0001
(555)-486-9002
Fax: (555) 487-8976
NPI: 3664021CC
Federal Tax ID#: XX12210XX

PATIENT INFORMATION:		INSURANCE INFORMATION:	
Name:	Stephen M. Drake	Primary:	Medicaid
Address:	2317 Charnwood Avenue	Policy Number:	197152403316X
	Woodland Hills, XY 12345	Group Number:	
Telephone:	(555) 277-5831	Subscriber:	
Date of Birth:	04/03/1991	Secondary:	none
Social Security:	566-XX-0081	Policy Number:	
Occupation:	STUDENT	Group Number:	
Employer:		Subscriber:	
Status:			
Spouse:			

DIAGNOSIS INFORMATION

1. J03.90	Acute tonsillitis, unspecified.
2. J35.03	Chronic tonsillitis and adenoiditis.
3. J02.0	Streptococcal sore throat.
4.	

PROCEDURE INFORMATION

Description	Date	Code	Charge
1. Initial office visit, new pt	05/01/20XX	99203	120.00
2. Strep culture	05/01/20XX	87081	10.00
3. Injection, antibiotic	05/01/20XX	96372	20.00
4. Bicillin	05/01/20XX	J0540	10.00
5. Follow-up office visit	05/08/20XX	99212-57	50.00
6. Remove tonsils and adenoids	05/09/20XX	42821	330.00
7. Post-op office visit	05/17/20XX	99024	N/C

NOTES: Referred by: James Jeffers, MD, 100 S. Broadway, Hempstead, XY 12345
                          NPI: 12345069XX
              Treating MD: Gerald Practon, MD
                          NPI: 46278897XX
        Place of service: College Clinic for 5/1–5/8, 5/17
                          College Hospital for 5/9 (Outpatient)
                          4500 Broad Avenue, Woodland Hills, XY 12345
                          NPI: X950731067

ASSIGNMENT 14.9 COMPLETE A CLAIM FORM FOR A TRICARE STANDARD CASE

Performance Objective

Task: Complete a CMS-1500 claim form for a TRICARE Standard case.

Conditions: Use Rosa M. Sandoval's patient record, one health insurance claim form, a pen or a pencil.

Standards: Claim Productivity Measurement

                   Time: _____ minutes

                   Accuracy: _____

                   (Note: The time element and accuracy criteria may be given by your instructor.)

Directions:

1. Using National Uniform Claim Committee (NUCC) guidelines, complete the CMS-1500 claim form. Refer to Miss Rosa M. Sandoval's patient record for information. Date the claim May 31 of the current year. Dr. Atrics is not accepting assignment on this TRICARE Standard case but is completing the claim for the patient's convenience.

2. Refer to Chapter 14 (Fig. 14.8) of the Textbook for instructions on how to complete this claim form and to view a TRICARE template.

3. A Performance Evaluation Checklist may be reproduced from the "Instruction Guide to the Workbook" chapter if your instructor wishes you to submit it to assist with scoring and comments.

    After the instructor has returned your work to you, either make the necessary corrections and place your work in a three-ring notebook for future reference or, if you received a high score, place it in your portfolio for reference when applying for a job.

COLLEGE CLINIC
4567 Broad Avenue, Woodland Hills, XY 12345-0001
(555)-486-9002
Fax: (555) 487-8976
NPI: 3664021CC
Federal Tax ID#: XX12210XX

PATIENT INFORMATION:

Name:	Rosa M. Sandoval
Address:	209 Maple St
	Woodland Hills, XY 12345
Telephone:	(555) 456-3322
Date of Birth:	11/01/1991
Social Security:	994-XX-1164
Guarantor:	Herman J. Sandoval (Father)

INSURANCE INFORMATION:

Primary:	Tricare
	PO Box 1234
	West End, YZ 01222
Policy Number:	886-XX-0999
Group Number:	
Subscriber:	Herman J. Sandoval
	(DOB 2/10/70)
Secondary:	none
Policy Number:	
Group Number:	
Subscriber:	

DIAGNOSIS INFORMATION

1. H66.001   Acute suppurative otitis media without spontaneous rupture of ear drum, right ear.

2. H66.3x1   Chronic suppurative otitis media, NOS, right ear.

3.

4.

PROCEDURE INFORMATION

Description	Date	Code	Charge
1. Initial office visit, new pt	05/01/20XX	99202-25	90.00
2. Myringotomy	05/01/20XX	69420-RT	130.00
3. Post-op visit	05/03/20XX	99024	N/C
4. Post-op visit	05/08/20XX	99024	N/C

NOTES: Referred by: mother
            Treating MD: Pedro Atrics, MD
                    NPI: 137640017XX
        Place of service: College Clinic
                    4500 Broad Avenue, Woodland Hills, XY 12345
                    NPI: 3664021CC

ASSIGNMENT 14.10 COMPLETE A CLAIM FORM FOR A TRICARE EXTRA CASE

Performance Objective

Task: Complete a CMS-1500 claim form for a TRICARE Extra case.

Conditions: Use Darlene B. Drew's patient record, one health insurance claim form, a pen or a pencil.

Standards: Claim Productivity Measurement

Time: _____ minutes

Accuracy: _____

(Note: The time element and accuracy criteria may be given by your instructor.)

Directions:

1. Using NUCC guidelines, complete the CMS-1500 claim form. Refer to Mrs. Darlene B. Drew's patient record for information and post to the financial statement. Date the claim February 3 of the current year. The physician has been approved to treat the patient at College Hospital. Dr. Ulibarri is accepting assignment on this TRICARE Extra case.

2. Refer to Chapter 14 of the Textbook for instructions on how to complete this claim form and to view a TRICARE template.

3. A Performance Evaluation Checklist may be reproduced from the "Instruction Guide to the Workbook" shown in the section before Chapter 1 if your instructor wishes you to submit it to assist with scoring and comments.

After the instructor has returned your work to you, either make the necessary corrections and place your work in a three-ring notebook for future reference or, if you received a high score, place it in your portfolio for reference when applying for a job.

COLLEGE CLINIC

4567 Broad Avenue, Woodland Hills, XY 12345-0001

(555)-486-9002

Fax: (555) 487-8976

NPI: 3664021CC

Federal Tax ID#: XX12210XX

PATIENT INFORMATION:

Name:	Darlene B. Drew
Address:	720 Ganley Street
	Woodland Hills, XY 12345
Telephone:	(555) 466-1002
Date of Birth:	12/22/1941
Social Security:	450-XX-3762
Occupation:	SEAMSTRESS
Employer:	J. B. Talon Company
	2111 Ventura Blvd.
	Merck, XY 12346
Status:	Married
Spouse:	Harry M. Drew

INSURANCE INFORMATION:

Primary:	Tricare
	PO Box 1234
	West End, YZ 01222
Policy Number:	67531
Effective date:	1/1/1980
Subscriber:	Harry M. Drew
	Service# 221XX0711
	DOB 4/15/1937
Secondary:	none

DIAGNOSIS INFORMATION

1. N34.0   Abscess of urethral gland

2. B96.5   Pseudomonas (aeruginosa)

3.

4.

PROCEDURE INFORMATION

Description	Date	Code	Charge
1. Initial office visit, new pt	01/13/20XX	99203-25	120.00
2. Urinalysis	01/13/20XX	81000	10.00
3. Drainage of Skene's gland abscess	01/13/20XX	53060	210.00
4. Handling/transport culture specimen	01/13/20XX	99000	10.00
5. Office visit	01/18/20XX	99212	50.00
6. Excision of Skene's gland	01/24/20XX	53270-58	230.00
7. Post-op visit	01/27/20XX	99024	n/c

NOTES: Referred by: James B. Jeffers, MD, 100 S. Broadway, Woodland Hills, XY 12345
                    NPI: 12345069XX
            Treating MD: Gene Ulibarri, MD
                    NPI: 25678831XX
        Place of service: College Clinic for 1/13–18, 1/27
                    College Hospital for 1/24 (Outpatient)
                    4500 Broad Avenue, Woodland Hills, XY 12345
                    NPI: X950731067

Performance Objectives

Task: Complete a CMS-1500 claim form for a workers' compensation case.

Conditions: Use Glen M. Hiranuma's patient record, a CMS-1500 claim form, a pen or a pencil.

Standards: Claim Productivity Measurement

                    Time: _____ minutes

                    Accuracy: _____

                    (Note: The time element and accuracy criteria may be given by your instructor.)

Directions:

1. Using National Uniform Claim Committee (NUCC) guidelines, complete a CMS-1500 claim form and direct it to the proper workers' compensation carrier. Refer to Mr. Glen M. Hiranuma's patient record for information. As a result of this work-related injury, the patient was unable to work on 5/22 through the returning date of 6/5. Date the claim May 24 of the current year.

2. Refer to Chapter 14 of the Textbook for instructions on how to complete this claim form and to view a workers' compensation template.

3. A Performance Evaluation Checklist may be reproduced from the "Instruction Guide to the Workbook" that appears in the section before Chapter 1 if your instructor wishes you to submit it to assist with scoring and comments.

After the instructor has returned your work to you, either make the necessary corrections and place your work in a three-ring notebook for future reference or, if you received a high score, place it in your portfolio for reference when applying for a job.

COLLEGE CLINIC
4567 Broad Avenue, Woodland Hills, XY 12345-0001
(555)-486-9002
Fax: (555) 487-8976
NPI: 3664021CC
Federal Tax ID#: XX12210XX

PATIENT INFORMATION:		INSURANCE INFORMATION:	
Name:	Glen M. Hiranuma	Primary:	State Insurance Fund
Address:	4372 Hanley Avenue		14156 Magnolia Blvd.
	Woodland Hills, XY 12345		Torres, XY 12349
Telephone:	(555) 467-3383	Policy Number:	016-2432-211
Date of Birth:	12/24/1955	Date of Injury:	05/22/20XX
Social Security:	558-XX-9960	Subscriber:	
Occupation:	HOUSE PAINTER	Secondary:	none
Employer:	Pittsburgh Paint Company	Policy Number:	
	3725 Bonfield Avenue	Group Number:	
	Woodland Hills, XY 12345	Subscriber:	
Status:	Married		
Spouse:	Esme M. Hiranuma		

DIAGNOSIS INFORMATION

1. S06.0x1A   Concussion with loss of consciousness of 30 minutes or less.

2. S43.92xA   Unspecified sprain of left shoulder girdle.

3. S70.212A   Abrasion of left hip.

4. S80.812A   Abrasion left lower leg.

5. W11.xxxA   Fall on and from ladder, initial encounter.

PROCEDURE INFORMATION

Description	Date	Code	Charge
1. Hospital admit	05/22/20XX	99222	150.00
2. WC Report	05/22/20XX	99080	10.00
3. Discharge	05/23/20XX	99238	80.00

NOTES: Referred by: Pittsburgh Pain Company
          Treating MD: Gerald Practon, MD
          NPI: 46278897XX
          Place of service: College Hospital (Inpatient)
          4500 Broad Avenue, Woodland Hills, XY 12345
          NPI: X950731067
          Patient unable to work from 5/22/20xx to 06/05/20xx

ASSIGNMENT 14.12 COMPLETE A CLAIM FORM FOR A WORKERS' COMPENSATION CASE

Performance Objective

Task: Complete a CMS-1500 claim form for a workers' compensation case.

Conditions: Use Carlos A. Giovanni's patient record, a CMS-1500 claim form, a pen or a pencil.

Standards: Claim Productivity Measurement

Time: _____ minutes

Accuracy: _____

(Note: The time element and accuracy criteria may be given by your instructor.)

Directions:

1. Using NUCC guidelines, complete a CMS-1500 claim form for November dates of service and direct it to the correct workers' compensation carrier for this workers' compensation claim. Refer to Mr. Carlos A. Giovanni's patient record for information to record on the claim. Date the claim November 30 of the current year.

2. Refer to Chapter 14 of the textbook for instructions on how to complete this claim form and to view a workers' compensation template.

3. A Performance Evaluation Checklist may be reproduced from the "Instruction Guide to the Workbook" that appears in a section before Chapter 1 if your instructor wishes you to submit it to assist with scoring and comments.

After the instructor has returned your work to you, either make the necessary corrections and place your work in a three-ring notebook for future reference or, if you received a high score, place it in your portfolio for reference when applying for a job.

COLLEGE CLINIC
4567 Broad Avenue, Woodland Hills, XY 12345-0001
(555)-486-9002
Fax: (555) 487-8976
NPI: 3664021CC
Federal Tax ID#: XX12210XX

PATIENT INFORMATION:

Name:	Carlos A. Giovanni
Address:	89 Beaumont Court
	Woodland Hills, XY 12345
Telephone:	(555) 677-3485
Date of Birth:	10/24/1945
Social Security:	556-XX-9699
Occupation:	TV REPAIRMAN
Employer:	Giant Television Company
	8764 Ocean Avenue
	Woodland Hills, XY 12345
Status:	Married
Spouse:	Maria Giovanni

INSURANCE INFORMATION:

Primary:	State Compensation Ins Fund
	600 S. Lafayette Park Place
	Ehrlich, XY 12350
Policy Number:	57780
Date of Injury:	11/11/20XX
Subscriber:	
Secondary:	none
Policy Number:	
Group Number:	
Subscriber:	

DIAGNOSIS INFORMATION

1. S02.91xA   Fracture of skull and facial bones, initial encounter for closed fracture.

2. S06.0x1A   Concussion with loss of consciousness of 30 minutes or less.

3. W13.xxxA   Fall from, out of or through building or structure.

PROCEDURE INFORMATION

Description	Date	Code	Charge
1. Hospital admit	11/11/20XX	99223-57	220.00
2. WC Report	11/11/20XX	99080	10.00
3. Craniotomy	11/12/20XX	61314	1930.00
4. Hospital visits	11/13-29/20XX	99024	N/C
5. Discharge	11/30/20XX	99024	N/C
6. Office visit	12/07/20XX	99024	N/C
7. Office visit	12/21/20XX	99024	N/C
8. Office visit	12/29/20XX	99024	N/C

NOTES: Referred by: Giant Television Company
            Treating MD: Astro Parkinson, MD
                NPI: 46789377XX
        Place of service: College Clinic for 12/7–12/29
                College Hospital for 11/11–11/30 (Inpatient)
                4500 Broad Avenue, Woodland Hills, XY 12345
                NPI: X950731067
                Patient unable to work from 11/12/20xx–01/14/20xx

15 The Electronic Claim

Linda M. Smith

KEY TERMS

Your instructor may wish to select some words pertinent to this chapter for a test. For definitions of the terms, further study, and/or reference, the words, phrases, and abbreviations may be found in the glossary at the end of the Textbook. *Key terms for this chapter follow.*

Accredited Standards Committee X12 (ASCX12)
Accredited Standards Committee X12 Version 5010
Administrative Simplification Enforcement Tool
American National Standards Institute
application service provider
ASC X12 Version 5010
audit trail
batch
business associate agreement
cable modem
carrier-direct system
claim attachments
clearinghouse
code sets
covered entity
data elements

digital subscriber line
direct data entry
electronic data interchange
electronic funds transfer
electronic remittance advice
encoder
encryption
HIPAA Transaction and Code Set Rule
National Standard Format
real time
standard transactions
syntax error
T-1
taxonomy codes
trading partner

KEY ABBREVIATIONS

See how many abbreviations and acronyms you can translate, and then use this as a handy reference list. Definitions for the key abbreviations are located near the back of the Textbook *in the glossary.*

ANSI _____

ASC X12 _____

ASET _____

ASP _____

ATM _____

DDE _____

DHHS _____

DSL _____

EDI _____

EFT _____

EHR _____

EMC _____

EOMB _____

ERA _____

HPID _____

IRS _____

MAC _____

NDC _____

NSF _____

TCS rule _____

PERFORMANCE OBJECTIVES

The student will be able to:

- Define and spell the key terms and key abbreviations for this chapter, given the information from the textbook glossary, within a reasonable time period and with enough accuracy to obtain a satisfactory evaluation.

- After reading the chapter, answer the fill-in-the-blank, multiple choice, and true/false review questions with enough accuracy to obtain a satisfactory evaluation.

- Input data into the element for place of service codes for 837P electronic claims submission.

- Indicate the patient's relationship to the insured by using the individual relationship code numbers for 837P electronic claims submission.

- Select the correct taxonomy codes for the specialists for submission of 837P electronic claims submission.

STUDY OUTLINE

The Electronic Claim
Electronic Data Interchange
Accounts Receivable Management System
Application Service Providers (ASP)
Transmission of Electronic Claims
Advantages of Electronic Claim Submission
Transaction and Code Set Regulations: Streamlining Electronic Data Interchange
Transaction and Code Set Standards
Data Requirements
Required and Situational
Electronic Standard HIPAA 837P
Accredited Standards CommitteeX12 Version 5010
Claim Attachments Standards
Standard Unique Identifiers
Standard Unique Employer Identifier
Standard Unique Health Care Provider Identifier

Standard Unique Health Plan Identifier
Standard Unique Patient Identifier
Building the Electronic Claim
Keying Insurance Data for Claim Transmission
Encoder
Signature Requirements
Clean Electronic Claims Submission
Follow-Up of Electronic Claims Processing
Interactive Transactions
Electronic Remittance Advice
Electronic Funds Transfer
Transmission Reports
Electronic Processing Problems
Solutions to Electronic Processing Problems
Billing and Account Management Schedule
Administrative Simplification Enforcement Tool

ASSIGNMENT 15.1 REVIEW QUESTIONS

Part I Fill in the Blank

Review the objectives, key terms, glossary definitions of key terms, chapter information, and figures before completing the following review questions.

1. Exchange of data in a standardized format through computer systems is a technology known as _____.

2. The act of converting computerized data into a code so that unauthorized users are unable to read it is a security system known as _____.

3. If a health care organization does not have an on-site accounts receivable management system, they can contract with a business that will supply software application and services for use over the internet. The business is referred to as a/an _____.

4. A private company that will receive information from the health care organization, translate it into a standard format and send claims to insurance carriers is a _____.

5. Payment to the provider of service of an electronically submitted insurance claim may be received in approximately _____.

6. A chronological record of submitted data built by an electronic transmission that allows the data to be traced to the source of the place of origin is a/an _____.

7. Refer to Table 15.1 in the *textbook* to list benefits of using Health Insurance Portability and Accountability Act (HIPAA) standard transactions and code sets:
   a. _____
   b. _____
   c. _____
   d. _____
   e. _____
   f. _____

8. Refer to Table 15.2 in the *textbook* to name the standard code sets used for the following:
   a. Physician services _____
   b. Diseases and injuries _____
   c. Pharmaceuticals and biologics _____

9. The family practice taxonomy code is _____.

10. The American National Standards Institute formed the _____, which developed the electronic data exchange standards.

11. Refer to Table 15.3 in the *textbook* to complete these statements.
   a. The staff at College Clinic submit professional health care claims for each of their providers and must use the industry standard electronic format called _____ to transmit them electronically.
   b. The billing department at College Hospital must use the industry standard electronic format called _____ to transmit health care claims electronically.
   c. The Medicare fiscal intermediary (insurance carrier) uses the industry standard electronic format called _____ to transmit payment information to the College Clinic and College Hospital.
   d. It has been three weeks since Gordon Marshall's health care claim was transmitted to the XYZ insurance company, and you wish to inquire about the status of the claim. The industry standard electronic format that must be used to transmit this inquiry is called _____.
   e. Dr. Practon's insurance billing specialist must use the industry standard electronic format called _____ to obtain information about Beatrice Garcia's health policy benefits and coverage from the insurance plan.

12. Refer to Table 15.4 in the textbook to name the levels for data collected to construct and submit an electronic claim.
   a. _____

b. _____

c. _____

d. _____

e. _____

f. _____

13. HIPAA electronic standards for claim submission were upgraded to Version _____, and all providers, payers, and clearinghouses were required to use it effective January 1, 2012.

14. The Claims Attachments Standards have not yet been adopted; however, it was mandated for compliance as of _____, as required under the Affordable Care Act.

15. The _____ is an all numeric 10-character number assigned to each provider and required for all transactions with health plans effective May 23, 2007.

16. Although a standard unique patient identifier is supported by HIPAA and the ACA, efforts to implement a system have been protested by public interest groups and considered to be a/an _____ threat.

17. To look for and correct all errors before the health claim is transmitted to the insurance carrier, you _____ or _____.

18. List different types of information that a software code editor can identify during the edit and error process:
_____
_____
_____

19. Add-on software to a practice management system that can reduce the time it takes to build or review a claim before batching is known as a/an _____.

20. Many insurance companies, such as Medicare, provide instant access to information about pending claims through online _____.

21. An electronic funds transfer (EFT) agreement may allow for health plans to _____ overpayments from a provider's bank account.

22. A transmission report generated to track the claims process, which shows how many claims were originally received by the payer, and how many claims were automatically rejected _____.

23. A transmission report used to identify which claims are not included in processing and require the insurance billing specialist to correct and refile them _____.

24. Under the 5010 guidelines, EINs or Social security numbers cannot be used as primary identifiers for healthcare providers; only a/an _____ can be used.

25. Under HIPAA transaction standard Accredited Standards Committee (ASC) X12 Version 5010, a _____ digit ZIP code is required to report service facility locations.

26. The _____ is an electronic tool that enables organizations to file a complaint against a noncompliant covered entity that is negatively affecting the efficient processing of claims.

Part II Multiple Choice

Choose the best answer.

27. Electronic claims are submitted by means of:
    a. the US Postal Service.
    b. fax transmission.
    c. phone transmission.
    d. electronic data interchange (EDI).

28. Today, most claims are submitted by means of:
    a. the US Postal Service.
    b. fax transmission.
    c. phone transmission.
    d. EDI.

29. The online error-edit process allows providers to:
    a. correct claim errors before transmission of the claim.
    b. decrease labor costs by freeing staff to do other duties.
    c. reduce postage fees and trips to the post office.
    d. reduce storage of claims.

30. Under HIPAA, data elements that are used uniformly to document why patients are seen (diagnosis) and what is done to them during their encounter (procedure) are known as:
    a. medical code sets.
    b. information elements.
    c. transaction and code set (TCS) standards.
    d. National Standard Format (NSF).

31. The standard transaction that replaces the paper CMS-1500 claim form and more than 400 versions of the electronic NSF is called the:
    a. 270.
    b. 837I.
    c. 837P.
    d. 837D.

32. The next version of the electronic claims submission that will be proposed for consideration once lessons are learned from implementation of Version 5010 will be:
    a. Version 5011.
    b. Version 5012.
    c. Version 6001.
    d. Version 7030.

33. A standard unique number that will be assigned to identify individual health plans under the Affordable Care Act is referred to as a/an:
    a. employer identification number (EIN).
    b. electronic remittance advice (ERA).
    c. health plan identifier (HPID).
    d. National Provider Identifier (NPI).

34. Uniform patient identifiers:
    a. were required on all claims effective May 23, 2007.
    b. were required on all claims effective October 1, 2012.
    c. were required on all claims effective October 1, 2014.
    d. are not yet required, and the proposal is on hold for implementation of the standard.

35. An authorization and assignment of benefits signature for a patient who was treated in the hospital but has never been to the provider's office:
    a. should be obtained by the provider when he or she sees the patient in the hospital.
    b. must be mailed to the patient for signature before submission of a claim.
    c. can be obtained from the patient at his or her first office visit.
    d. is not required; the authorization obtained by the hospital applies to that provider's claim filing.

36. A paperless computerized system that enables payments to be transferred automatically to a physician's bank account by a third-party payer may be done via:
    a. electronic savings account.
    b. ERA.
    c. EFT.
    d. EDI.

37. An electronic Medicare remittance advice that takes the place of a paper Medicare explanation of benefits (EOB) is referred to as:
    a. American National Standards Institute (ANSI) 277.
    b. ANSI 820.
    c. ANSI 830.
    d. ANSI 835.

38. A method for submitting claims electronically by keying information into the payer system for processing is accomplished through use of:
    a. a clearinghouse.
    b. carrier direct entry.
    c. an application service provider.
    d. digital subscriber line (DSL).

39. A report that is generated by a payer and sent to the provider to show how many claims were received as electronic claims and how many of the claims were automatically rejected and will not be processed is called a:
    a. send-and-receive file report.
    b. scrubber report.
    c. transaction transmission summary.
    d. rejection analysis report.

40. The HIPAA transaction standard ASC X12 Version 5010 requires that anesthesia services be reported:
    a. per day.
    b. per unit.
    c. per second.
    d. per minute.

Part III True/False

Write "T" or "F" in the blank to indicate whether you think the statement is true or false.

_____ 41. Like paper claims, electronic claims require the performing physician's signature.

_____ 42. Claims can be submitted to various insurance payers in a single-batch electronic transmission.

_____ 43. Under HIPAA, insurance payers can require health care providers to use the payer's own version of local code sets.

_____ 44. As *International Classification of Diseases* (ICD) and *Current Procedural Terminology* (CPT) codes are deleted and become obsolete, they should immediately be removed from the practice's computer system.

_____ 45. Under HIPAA's TCS standards, there are 15 different "relationship to patient" indicators that can be assigned to a claim.

_____ 46. HIPAA's electronic standard transactions are identified by a four-digit number that precedes "ASC X12N."

_____ 47. Implementation of ICD-10 resulted in the upgrade to HIPAA transaction standard ASC X12 Version 6020.

_____ 48. HIPAA requires that the NPI number be used to identify employers rather than inputting the actual name of the company when submitting claims.

_____ 49. When transmitting electronic claims, inaccuracies that violate the HIPAA standard transaction format are known as *syntax errors*.

_____ 50. Failure to implement the HIPAA TCS rule, can result in civil monetary penalties.

ASSIGNMENT 15.2 INPUT DATA INTO ELEMENT FOR PLACE OF SERVICE CODES FOR 837P ELECTRONIC CLAIMS SUBMISSIONS

Performance Objective

Task: Insert the correct place of service code for each location description where the medical professional service was rendered.

Conditions: Place of service codes reference (Fig. 15.1), list of places where medical care was rendered, and a pen or a pencil.

Standards: Time: _____ minutes

                Accuracy: _____

                (Note: The time element and accuracy criteria may be given by your instructor.)

Directions: When submitting the 837P electronic claim, place of service codes must be entered. Refer to the place of service codes reference list and insert the correct code for each place of service for the following locations.

a. Inpatient psychiatric facility   _____

b. Physician's office   _____

c. Outpatient hospital   _____

d. Intermediate nursing facility   _____

e. Independent clinic   _____

f. Independent laboratory   _____

g. Birthing center   _____

h. End-stage renal disease treatment facility

i. Inpatient hospital   _____

j. Hospice   _____

PLACE OF SERVICE CODES	
Codes	**Place of Service**
01	Pharmacy
00-02	Unassigned
03	School
04	Homeless shelter
05	Indian health service free-standing facility
06	Indian health service provider-based facility
07	Tribal 638 free-standing facility
08	Tribal 638 provider-based facility
09	Prison/correctional facility
10	Unassigned
11	Doctor's office
12	Patient's home
13	Assisted living facility
14	Group home
15	Mobile unit
16	Temporary lodging
17-19	Unassigned
20	Urgent care facility
21	Inpatient hospital
22	Outpatient hospital or urgent care center
23	Emergency department—hospital
24	Ambulatory surgical center
25	Birthing center
26	Military treatment facility/uniformed service treatment facility
27-30	Unassigned
31	Skilled nursing facility (swing bed visits)
32	Nursing facility (intermediate/long-term care facilities)
33	Custodial care facility (domiciliary or rest home services)
34	Hospice (domiciliary or rest home services)
35-40	Unassigned
41	Ambulance—land
42	Ambulance—air or water
43-48	Unassigned
49	Independent clinic
50	Federally qualified health center
51	Inpatient psychiatric facility
52	Psychiatric facility—partial hospitalization
53	Community mental health care (outpatient, twenty-four-hours-a-day services, admission screening, consultation, and educational services)
54	Intermediate care facility/mentally retarded
55	Residential substance abuse treatment facility
56	Psychiatric residential treatment center
57	Nonresidential substance abuse treatment facility
58-59	Unassigned
60	Mass immunization center
61	Comprehensive inpatient rehabilitation facility
62	Comprehensive outpatient rehabilitation facility
63-64	Unassigned
65	End-stage renal disease treatment facility
66-70	Unassigned
71	State or local public health clinic
72	Rural health clinic
73-80	Unassigned
81	Independent laboratory
82-98	Unassigned
99	Other unlisted facility

Fig. 15.1

ASSIGNMENT 15.3 SELECT THE CORRECT INDIVIDUAL RELATIONSHIP CODE NUMBER FOR 837P ELECTRONIC CLAIMS SUBMISSION

Performance Objective

Task: Insert the correct individual relationship code for the patient's relationship to the insured.

Conditions: Individual relationship code number reference (Fig. 15.2), list of individuals or entities, and a pen or a pencil.

Standards: Time: _____ minutes

                 Accuracy: _____

                 (Note: The time element and accuracy criteria may be given by your instructor.)

Directions: Refer to the individual relationship code number list, choose the correct code for the patient's relationship to the insured for the following persons, and insert it on the lines.

a. Mother   _____

b. Spouse   _____

c. Child   _____

d. Father   _____

e. Stepdaughter   _____

f. Emancipated minor   _____

g. Adopted child   _____

h. Handicapped dependent   _____

i. Stepson   _____

j. Sponsored dependent   _____

Individual Relationship Code	
Code	**Relationship**
01	Spouse
04	Grandfather or grandmother
05	Grandson or granddaughter
07	Nephew or niece
09	Adopted child
10	Foster child
15	Ward
17	Stepson or stepdaughter
19	Child
20	Employee
21	Unknown
22	Handicapped dependent
23	Sponsored dependent
24	Dependent of a minor dependent
29	Significant other
32	Mother
33	Father
34	Other adult
36	Emancipated minor
39	Organ donor
40	Cadaver donor
41	Injured plaintiff
43	Child where insured has no financial responsibility
53	Life partner
G8	Other relationship

Fig. 15.2

ASSIGNMENT 15.4 SELECT THE CORRECT TAXONOMY CODES FOR MEDICAL SPECIALISTS FOR 837P ELECTRONIC CLAIMS SUBMISSION

Performance Objective

Task: Choose the correct taxonomy code for each specialist for submission of 837P electronic claims by referring to the Health Care Provider Taxonomy code list.

Conditions: Health Care Provider Taxonomy code list (Fig. 15.3), list of providers of service, and a pen or a pencil.

Standards: Time: _____ minutes

Accuracy: _____

(Note: The time element and accuracy criteria may be given by your instructor.)

Directions: Refer to the Health Care Provider Taxonomy code list, choose the correct code for each of the following specialists, and insert the code numbers on the lines.

a. Raymond Skeleton, MD, orthopedist   _____

b. Gaston Input, MD, gastroenterologist   _____

c. Vera Cutis, MD, dermatologist   _____

d. Gene Ulibarri, MD, urologist   _____

e. Bertha Caesar, MD, obstetrician/gynecologist   _____

f. Gerald Practon, MD, general practitioner   _____

g. Pedro Atrics, MD, pediatrician   _____

h. Astro Parkinson, MD, neurosurgeon   _____

i. Brady Coccidioides, MD, pulmonary disease   _____

j. Max Gluteus, RPT, physical therapist   _____

College Clinic Staff		
Health Care Provider Taxonomy Codes		
Name	**Specialty**	**Taxonomy Code**
Concha Antrum, MD	Otolaryngologist	207Y00000X
Pedro Atrics, MD	Pediatrician	208000000X
Bertha Caesar, MD	Obstetrician/Gynecologist	207V00000X
Perry Cardi, MD	Cardiologist	207RC0000X
Brady Coccidioides, MD	Pulmonary disease	207RP1001X
Vera Cutis, MD	Dermatologist	207N00000X
Clarence Cutler, MD	General surgeon	208600000X
Dennis Drill, DDS	Dentist	122300000X
Max Gluteus, RPT	Physical therapist	208100000X
Cosmo Graff, MD	Plastic surgeon	208200000X
Malvern Grumose, MD	Pathologist	207ZP0105X
Gaston Input, MD	Gastroenterologist	207RG0100X
Adam Langerhans, MD	Endocrinologist	207RE0101X
Cornell Lenser, MD	Ophthalmologist	207W00000X
Michael Menter, MD	Psychiatrist	2084P0800X
Arthur O. Dont, DDS	Orthodontist	1223X0400X
Astro Parkinson, MD	Neurosurgeon	207T00000X
Nick Pedro, MD	Podiatrist	213E00000X
Gerald Practon, MD	General practitioner	208D00000X
Walter Radon, MD	Radiologist	2085R0202X
Rex Rumsey, MD	Proctologist	208C00000X
Sensitive E. Scott, MD	Anesthesiologist	207L00000X
Raymond Skeleton, MD	Orthopedist	207X00000X
Gene Ulibarri, MD	Urologist	208800000X

Fig. 15.3

16 Receiving Payments and Insurance Problem Solving

Linda M. Smith

KEY TERMS

Your instructor may wish to select some words pertinent to this chapter for a test. For definitions of the terms, further study, and/or reference, the words, phrases, and abbreviations may be found in the glossary at the end of the textbook. Key terms for this chapter follow.

adjudication
Administrative Law Judge
aging report
appeal
claim denial management
delinquent claim
denied claim
determination
explanation of benefits
inquiry
insurance payment poster
insurance payment posting
lost claim
medical necessity

overpayment
peer review
Qualified Independent Contractor
reassess
rebill (resubmit)
reimbursement
rejected claim
remittance advice
revenue cycle management
review
state insurance commissioner
suspended claim
suspense
tracer

KEY ABBREVIATIONS

See how many abbreviations and acronyms you can translate, and then use this as a handy reference list. Definitions for the key abbreviations are located near the back of the textbook in the glossary.

ALJ _____

CMS _____

EOB _____

HIPAA _____

NPI _____

QIC _____

RA _____

RCM _____

PERFORMANCE OBJECTIVES

The student will be able to:

- Define and spell the key terms and key abbreviations for this chapter, given the information from the textbook glossary, within a reasonable time period and with enough accuracy to obtain a satisfactory evaluation.

- After reading the chapter, answer the fill-in-the-blank, multiple choice, and true/false review questions with enough accuracy to obtain a satisfactory evaluation.

- Review an aging report to determine the method of follow-up needed to zero out all patient accounts.

- Locate the errors on each claim, given three returned insurance claims, within a reasonable time period and with enough accuracy to obtain a satisfactory evaluation.

- File an appeal by composing and printing a letter with envelope, within a reasonable time period and with enough accuracy to obtain a satisfactory evaluation.

STUDY OUTLINE

Revenue Cycle Management
Response From a Submitted Claim
Claim Policy Guidelines
    Insured
    Contracts and Fee Schedules
    Reimbursement Time Frames
Explanation of Benefits
    Components of an Explanation of Benefits
    Interpreting an Explanation of Benefits
    Posting an Explanation of Benefits
    Secondary Insurance
    Explanation of Benefits Management
Claim Management Techniques
    Insurance Claims Register
    Purging Paid Files

    Aging Reports
Claim Inquiries
    Problem Claims
    Rebilling
Review and Appeal Process
    Filing an Appeal
State Insurance Commissioner
    Types of Problems
    State Insurance Department Inquries
Claim Denial Management
    Claim Denial Identification
    Claim Denial Review and Appeal
    Categorizing Claim Denials
    Measuring Claim Denials
    Developing Strategies to Prevent Future Denials

Part I Fill in the Blank

Review the objectives, key terms, and chapter information before completing the following review questions.

1. The process in the health care organization uses to track services provided from registration and appointment scheduling to the final payment for services is referred to as _____.

2. Once a claim has been successfully submitted to the insurance carrier, the next step in the revenue cycle is for the insurance billing specialist to _____ the claim until a response is received from the responsible party and the service has been paid in full.

3. Who dictates the guidelines for claims submission, such as which services are covered, the reimbursement rates, and time limits for claim submission and payment?

   _____   _____

4. Time limits for filing claims promptly can be found in the _____ or the _____.

5. What is the purpose of prompt payment laws?

   _____

6. After an insurance claim is processed by the insurance carrier (paid, suspended, rejected, or denied), a document known as a/an _____ is sent to the patient and to the provider of professional medical services.

7. A claim that is processed by a third-party payer but is held in an indeterminate state is referred to as a _____ claim.

8. Claims paid with no errors are designated as _____.

9. Claims that are not paid within 30–45 days of the service date are referred to as _____ claims.

10. A _____ claim is a submitted claim that does not follow specific third-party payer instructions or contains technical errors.

11. A service is considered _____ if it is provided in accordance with the generally accepted standards of medical practice and is clinically appropriate.

12. State the solution if a claim for routine foot care has been denied as a noncovered service.

   _____

   _____

   _____

13. State the solution if a claim has been denied because the professional service rendered was for an injury that is being considered as compensable under workers' compensation.

   _____

   _____

   _____

14. When an insurance carrier changes the code submitted to one of lesser value and it reduces the reimbursement amount, it is referred to as _____.

15. When an insurance carrier reimburses a service at an amount over and above the amount due, it is referred to as an _____.

16. Patient accounts with a balance should be billed on a _____ basis.

17. A/an _____ is a request for a review and reconsideration of a claim that has been underpaid, incorrectly paid, or denied by an insurance company.

18. A/an _____ is an evaluation of a denied claim performed by a group of unbiased practicing physicians or other health care professionals to judge the effectiveness and efficiency of professional care rendered and to determine if payment can be made.

19. Name the five levels for appealing a Medicare claim.

    a. _____

    b. _____

    c. _____

    d. _____

    e. _____

20. A/an _____ is an independent contractor who conducts reconsiderations for Medicare claims going through the appeals process.

21. To pursue judicial review of a Medicare claim in federal district court, the amount of the case must meet the minimum dollar amount of _____ in 2020.

22. A TRICARE expedited appeal must be filed within _____ of the receipt of the initial denial.

23. A TRICARE nonexpedited appeal must be filed within _____ of the receipt of the initial denial.

24. _____ are public officials who regulate the Insurance Industry in their state.

25. Effective claim denial management starts with _____ the reason for denials.

Part II Multiple Choice

Choose the best answer.

26. When reviewing an aging report to determine which unpaid claims require that an inquiry for claims status be made by the insurance billing specialist, claims should qualify for review at:
    a. 10–15 days old
    b. 15–30 days old
    c. 30–45 days old
    d. 45–60 days old

27. When an electronic claim is transmitted for several services and one service is rejected for incomplete information, the solution is to:
    a. resubmit a paper claim with the needed data for the rejected services only.
    b. submit a corrected claim for appeal.
    c. review the rejection code, correct the field and resubmit the electronic claim.
    d. write it off; it will never be paid.

28. A request for payment to a third-party payer asking for a review of an insurance claim that has been denied is referred to as a/an:
    a. review.
    b. appeal.
    c. request.
    d. demand.

29. When overpayments are identified, the Office of Inspector General (OIG) strongly advises that:
    a. service providers hold it for 30 days to make sure it was not due them.
    b. service providers place in a hold account until the insurance carrier requests it.
    c. service providers return the overpayment within 180 days of receipt of payment.
    d. service providers return the overpayment promptly when the insurance poster identifies it.

30. The steps in claim denial management are:
    a. Identify, Appeal, Categorize, Measure, Strategize.
    b. Appeal, Identify, Categorize, Strategize, Measure.
    c. Strategize, Categorize, Measure, Identify, Appeal.
    d. Identify, Measure, Categorize, Appeal, Strategize.

Part III True/False

Write "T" or "F" in the blank to indicate whether you think the statement is true or false.

_____ 31. An insurance billing specialist's primary goal is to assist in management of the revenue cycle.

_____ 32. A patient's insurance card specifies the detailed benefits and coverages.

_____ 33. All health insurance companies are obligated to reimburse health care organizations promptly for services rendered.

_____ 34. The elements within a remittance advice (RA) document and an explanation of benefits (EOB) document are different.

_____ 35. There is a standard format for EOB forms that all carriers are expected to follow.

_____ 36. Due to issues concerning timely filing, it is wise to be aggressive on claims that are outstanding for more than 30–45 days.

_____ 37. Information collected at the front desk does not impact denials.

_____ 38. One of the criteria for a service to be considered medically necessary is that the service must be in accordance with the generally accepted standards of medical practice.

_____ 39. If any insurance carrier has downcoded a claim, thereby reducing reimbursement, there is no other recourse than to write off the balance.

_____ 40. If a claim has not been paid within a reasonable amount of time, the most effective follow-up method is to simply rebill the claim.

ASSIGNMENT 16.2 USING AN AGING REPORT FOR FOLLOW-UP

Performance Objective

Task: Use the aging report in Fig. 16.1 to complete follow-up.

Conditions: Refer to the aging report (see Fig. 16.1) and use a pen or a computer.

Standards: Time: _____ minutes

               Accuracy: _____

               (Note: The time element and accuracy criteria may be given by your instructor.)

Directions: Review the aging report in Fig. 16.1 and consider the following scenario:

The Happy Day Primary Care Office is reviewing their aging report to follow up on outstanding payments. The office charges Aetna $260 for initial office visits and $145 for established patient office visits. Electronic claims that are filed to Aetna are reimbursed within to the office within 30 days of initial electronic claim submission. Answer the following questions.

1. Who were the three patients who were most recently billed?

   _____

   _____

   _____

2. Do phone calls to Aetna need to be made for patients that are in the 0–30 days categories? Why or why not?

   _____

   _____

3. Which two patients have balances that are different from typical office visit charges submitted to Aetna?

   _____

   _____

4. What would account for the difference in the balance from the original total charges submitted to Aetna?

   _____

   _____

5. Would it be appropriate to send the patients in categories beyond 60 days to a collection agency? Why or why not?

   _____

   _____

AETNA

Patient Name	Acct #	Primary Insurance	Secondary Insurance	0–30 days	31–60 days	61–90 days	91–120 days	Over 120 days	Total Balance
Bassett, Eleanor	75846	AETNA		$145.00	$0.00	$0.00	$0.00	$0.00	$145.00
Herron, John	83029	AETNA		$0.00	$42.41	$0.00	$0.00	$0.00	$42.41
Holt, Maxine	64739	AETNA	BLUE SHIELD	$145.00	$0.00	$0.00	$0.00	$0.00	$145.00
Kellog, Keenan	24537	AETNA		$0.00	$0.00	$145.00	$0.00	$0.00	$145.00
Lincoln, Frank	85940	AETNA		$0.00	$15.00	$0.00	$0.00	$0.00	$15.00
Markham, Melanie	14263	AETNA	MEDICARE	$0.00	$0.00	$0.00	$260.00	$0.00	$260.00
McDonald, Lydia	56374	AETNA		$260.00	$0.00	$0.00	$0.00	$0.00	$260.00
McLean, Mary	24395	AETNA		$0.00	$0.00	$0.00	$0.00	$260.00	$260.00
				$550.00	$57.41	$145.00	$260.00	$260.00	$1,272.41

Fig. 16.1

ASSIGNMENT 16.3 POST TO A FINANCIAL ACCOUNTING RECORD (LEDGER) FROM AN EXPLANATION OF BENEFITS (EOB) DOCUMENT

Performance Objective

Task: Post data from an EOB document to a patient's financial accounting record (ledger).

Conditions: Use a blank financial accounting record (ledger) (Fig. 16.2), an EOB document (Fig. 16.3), and a pen or a computer.

Standards: Time: _____ minutes

                Accuracy: _____

                (Note: The time element and accuracy criteria may be given by your instructor.)

Background: Most payments in the medical office are posted in the same practice management billing software that the electronic claims are submitted from. However, to develop the skills and understanding for payment posting, a paper financial accounting ledger has been provided.

Directions: Post in ink the payment received and preferred provider organization (PPO) adjustment to a patient's financial accounting record (ledger) (see Fig. 16.2) by referring to an EOB document (see Fig. 16.3).

After the instructor has returned your work to you, either make the necessary corrections and place your work in a three-ring notebook for future reference or, if you received a high score, place it in your portfolio for reference when applying for a job.

1. Locate patient's financial accounting record (ledger) and EOB.

2. Ledger lines 3 and 4: Insert date of service (DOS), reference (CPT code number, check number, or dates of service for posting adjustments or when insurance was billed), description of the transaction, charge amounts, payments, adjustments, and running current balance. The posting date is the actual date the transaction is recorded. If the DOS differs from the posting date, list the DOS in the reference or description column.

Chapter **16 Receiving Payments and Insurance Problem Solving**

Acct No. ___9-3___

STATEMENT
Financial Account
COLLEGE CLINIC
4567 Broad Avenue
Woodland Hills, XY 12345-0001
Tel. 555-486-9002
Fax No. 555-487-8976

Mr. Jabe Bortolussi
989 Moorpark Road
Woodland Hills, XY 12345

Phone No. (H) __(555) 230-8870__   (W) __(555) 349-6689__   Birth date _____04-07-71_____

Primary Insurance Co. _____ABC Insurance Company_____   Policy/Group No. __4206/010__

DATE	REFERENCE	DESCRIPTION	CHARGES		CREDITS PYMNTS.		ADJ.		BALANCE	
					BALANCE FORWARD ⟶					
6-3-xx	99204	E/M NP Level 4	180	00					180	00
6-3-xx	94010	Spirometry	40	00					220	00

PLEASE PAY LAST AMOUNT IN BALANCE COLUMN ⟹

THIS IS A COPY OF YOUR FINANCIAL ACCOUNT AS IT APPEARS ON OUR RECORDS

Fig. 16.2

ABC Insurance Company
P.O. Box 4300
Woodland Hills, XY 12345-0001

Claim No.:	1-00-16987087-00-zmm
Group Name:	COLLEGE CLINIC
Group No.:	010
Employee:	JABE V. BORTOLUSSI
Patient:	JABE V. BORTOLUSSI
SSN:	554-XX-8876
Plan No.:	4206
Prepared by:	M. SMITH
Prepared on:	07/04/20XX

GERALD PRACTON MD
4567 BROAD AVENUE
WOODLAND HILLS XY 12345

Patient Responsibility	
Amount not covered:	00
Co-pay amount:	00
Deductible:	00
Co-insurance:	64.61
Patient's total responsibility:	64.61
Other insurance payment:	00

EXPLANATION OF BENEFITS

Treatment Dates	Service Code	CPT Code	Charge Amount	Not Covered	Reason Code	PPO Discount	Covered Amount	Deductible Amount	Co-pay Amount	Paid At	Payment Amount
06/03/xx	200	99204	180.00	00	48	20.00	160.00	00	00	80%	128.00
06/03/xx	540	94010	40.00	00	48	00	40.00	00	00	80%	32.00
		TOTAL	220.00	00		20.00	200.00	00	00		160.00

Other Insurance Credits or Adjustments   00

Total Payment Amount   160.00

Reason Code
48 CON DISCOUNT/PT NOT RESPONSIBLE

CPT Code
99204 OFFICE/OUTPT VISIT E&M NEW MOD-HI SEVERIT
94375 RESPIRATORY FLOW VOLUM LOOP
94060 BRONCHOSPSM EVAL SPIROM PRE & POST BRON
94664 AEROSOL/VAPOR INHALA; INIT DEMO & EVAL
94760 NONINVASIVE EAR/PULSE OXIMETRY-02 SAT

Participant GERALD PRACTON MD	Date 07-04-xx
Patient JABE V. BORTOLUSSI	ID Number 554-XX-8876

Plan Number 4206	Patient Number	Office No. 010

GC 1234567890

160.00

PAY TO THE ORDER OF

COLLEGE CLINIC
4567 BROAD AVENUE
WOODLAND HILLS XY 12345

J M Smith
ABC Insurance Company

Fig. 16.3

ASSIGNMENT 16.4 LOCATE ERRORS ON A RETURNED INSURANCE CLAIM

Performance Objective

Task: Highlight the blocks on the insurance claim form where errors are discovered.

Conditions: Use an insurance claim form (Fig. 16.4) and a highlighter or a red pen.

Standards: Time: _____ minutes

                Accuracy: _____

                (Note: The time element and accuracy criteria may be given by your instructor.)

Directions: An insurance claim (see Fig. 16.4) was returned by the Prudential Insurance Company. Highlight or circle in red all blocks on the claim form where errors are discovered.

Option 1: Retype the claim and either insert the correction, if data are available to fix the error, or insert the word "NEED" in the block of the claim form.

Option 2: On a separate sheet of paper, list the blocks from 1 to 33 and state where errors occur. A Performance Evaluation Checklist may be reproduced from the "Instruction Guide to the Workbook" chapter if your instructor wishes you to submit it to assist with scoring and comments.

After the instructor has returned your work to you, either make the necessary corrections and place your work in a three-ring notebook for future reference or, if you received a high score, place it in your portfolio for reference when applying for a job.

HEALTH INSURANCE CLAIM FORM

APPROVED BY NATIONAL UNIFOR MCLAIM COMMITTEE (NUCC) 02/12

Prudential Insurance Company
500 South Bend Street
Woodland Hills XY 12345-0001

| | PICA | | | | | | | PICA | |

1. MEDICARE (Medicare#) **MEDICAID** (Medicaid#) **TRICARE** (ID#DoD#) **CHAMPVA** (Member ID#) **GROUP HEALTH PLAN** (ID#) **FECA BLK LUNG** (ID#) **OTHER** [X] (ID#)

1a. INSURED'S I.D. NUMBER (For Program in Item 1)

2. PATIENT'S NAME (Last Name, First Name, Middle Initial)
Johnson, Emily B.

3. PATIENT'S BIRTH DATE MM 02 DD 12 YY 1903 **SEX** M [ ] F [ ]

4. INSURED'S NAME (Last Name, First Name, Middle Initial)
Johnson, Erron T.

5. PATIENT'S ADDRESS (No., Street)
4391 Everett Street

6. PATIENT RELATIONSHIP TO INSURED
Self [ ] Spouse [X] Child [ ] Other [ ]

7. INSURED'S ADDRESS (No., Street)
Same

CITY Woodland Hills **STATE** XY

8. RESERVED FOR NUCC USE

CITY **STATE**

ZIP CODE 123450001 **TELEPHONE** (Include Area Code) ( )

ZIP CODE **TELEPHONE** (Include Area Code) ( )

9. OTHER INSURED'S NAME (Last Name, First Name, Middle Initial)

10. IS PATIENT'S CONDITION RELATED TO:

11. INSURED'S POLICY GROUP OR FECA NUMBER

a. OTHER INSURED'S POLICY OR GROUP NUMBER

a. EMPLOYMENT? (Current or Previous) YES [ ] NO [ ]

a. INSURED'S DATE OF BIRTH MM DD YY **SEX** M [ ] F [ ]

b. RESERVED FOR NUCC USE

b. AUTO ACCIDENT? YES [ ] NO [ ] **PLACE** (State)

b. OTHER CLAIM ID (Designated by NUCC)

c. RESERVED FOR NUCC USE

c. OTHER ACCIDENT? YES [ ] NO [ ]

c. INSURANCE PLAN NAME OR PROGRAM NAME

d. INSURANCE PLAN NAME OR PROGRAM NAME

10d. CLAIM CODES (Designated by NUCC)

d. IS THERE ANOTHER HEALTH BENEFIT PLAN? YES [ ] NO [X] If yes, complete items 9, 9a, and 9d.

READ BACK OF FORM BEFORE COMPLETING & SIGNING THIS FORM.
12. PATIENT'S OR AUTHORIZED PERSON'S SIGNATURE I authorize the release of any medical or other information necessary to process this claim. I also request payment of government benefits either to myself or to the party who accepts assignment below.
SIGNED *Emily B. Johnson* DATE 1/4/2020

13. INSURED'S OR AUTHORIZED PERSON'S SIGNATURE I authorize payment of medical benefits to the undersigned physician or supplier for services described below.
SIGNED *Emily B. Johnson*

14. DATE OF CURRENT: ILLNESS, INJURY, or PREGNANCY(LMP) MM DD YY QUAL.

15. OTHER DATE QUAL. MM DD YY

16. DATES PATIENT UNABLE TO WORK IN CURRENT OCCUPATION FROM MM DD YY TO MM DD YY

17. NAME OF REFERRING PROVIDER OR OTHER SOURCE
17a.
17b. NPI 67805027XX

18. HOSPITALIZATION DATES RELATED TO CURRENT SERVICES FROM MM DD YY TO MM DD YY

19. ADDITIONAL CLAIM INFORMATION (Designated by NUCC)

20. OUTSIDE LAB? YES [ ] NO [X] $ CHARGES

21. DIAGNOSIS OR NATURE OF ILLNESS OR INJURY Relate A-L to service line below (24E) ICD Ind. 0

A. B. C. D.
E. F. G. H.
I. J. K. L.

22. RESUBMISSION CODE ORIGINAL REF. NO.

23. PRIOR AUTHORIZATION NUMBER

24. A. DATE(S) OF SERVICE From MM DD YY	To MM DD YY	B. PLACE OF SERVICE	C. EMG	D. PROCEDURES, SERVICES, OR SUPPLIES (Explain Unusual Circumstances) CPT/HCPCS	MODIFIER	E. DIAGNOSIS POINTER	F. $ CHARGES	G. DAYS OR UNITS	H. EPSDT Family Plan	I. ID. QUAL.	J. RENDERING PROVIDER ID. #
1 01 04 20XX		11		99213		A	90 00	1		NPI	705687717XX
2 01 04 20XX		11		99213		A	90 00			NPI	
3										NPI	
4										NPI	
5										NPI	
6										NPI	

25. FEDERAL TAX I.D. NUMBER 7180561XX SSN [ ] EIN [ ]

26. PATIENT'S ACCOUNT NO. 237819

27. ACCEPT ASSIGNMENT? (For govt. claims, see back) YES [X] NO [ ]

28. TOTAL CHARGE $ 180 00

29. AMOUNT PAID $ 0 00

30. Rsvd for NUCC Use $

31. SIGNATURE OF PHYSICIAN OR SUPPLIER INCLUDING DEGREES OR CREDENTIALS (I certify that the statements on the reverse apply to this bill and are made a part thereof.)
SIGNED *Vera Cutis, MD* DATE 01/06/20XX

32. SERVICE FACILITY LOCATION INFORMATION
a. NPI b.

33. BILLING PROVIDER INFO & PH # (555) 4869002
College Clinic
4567 Broad Avenue
Woodland Hills XY 123450001
a. 3664021CC b.

NUCC Instruction Manual available at: www.nucc.org *PLEASE PRINT OR TYPE* OMB APPROVAL PENDING

Fig. 16.4

Performance Objective

Task: Highlight the blocks on the insurance claim form where errors are discovered.

Conditions: Use an insurance claim form (Fig. 16.5) and a highlighter or a red pen.

Standards: Time: _____ minutes

                    Accuracy: _____

                    (Note: The time element and accuracy criteria may be given by your instructor.)

Directions: An insurance claim was returned by the Healthtech Insurance Company. Highlight or circle in red all blocks on the claim form where errors are discovered.

Option 1: Retype the claim and either insert the correction if data are available to fix the error or insert the word "NEED" in the block of the claim form.

Option 2: On a separate sheet of paper, list the blocks from 1 to 33 and state where errors occur. A Performance Evaluation Checklist may be reproduced from the "Instruction Guide to the Workbook" that appears in the section before Chapter 1 if your instructor wishes you to submit it to assist with scoring and comments.

After the instructor has returned your work to you, either make the necessary corrections and place your work in a three-ring notebook for future reference or, if you received a high score, place it in your portfolio for reference when applying for a job.

HEALTH INSURANCE CLAIM FORM

APPROVED BY NATIONAL UNIFOR MCLAIM COMMITTEE (NUCC) 02/12

Healthtech Insurance Company
4821 West Lake Avenue
Woodland Hills XY 12345-0001

CARRIER

| | PICA | | | | | | | | PICA | |

1. MEDICARE (Medicare#) ☐ MEDICAID (Medicaid#) ☒ TRICARE (ID#DoD#) ☒ CHAMPVA (Member ID#) ☐ GROUP HEALTH PLAN (ID#) ☐ FECA BLK LUNG (ID#) ☐ OTHER (ID#) ☒

1a. INSURED'S I.D. NUMBER (For Program in Item 1)
433129870ANC

2. PATIENT'S NAME (Last Name, First Name, Middle Initial)
Dugan, Charles C

3. PATIENT'S BIRTH DATE MM 12 | DD 24 | YY 1968 **SEX** M ☒ F ☐

4. INSURED'S NAME (Last Name, First Name, Middle Initial)
Same

5. PATIENT'S ADDRESS (No., Street)
5900 Elm Street

6. PATIENT RELATIONSHIP TO INSURED Self ☒ Spouse ☐ Child ☐ Other ☐

7. INSURED'S ADDRESS (No., Street)
Same

CITY Woodland Hills **STATE** XY

8. RESERVED FOR NUCC USE

CITY **STATE**

ZIP CODE 123450001 **TELEPHONE** (Include Area Code) (555) 5593300

ZIP CODE **TELEPHONE** (Include Area Code) ( )

9. OTHER INSURED'S NAME (Last Name, First Name, Middle Initial)

10. IS PATIENT'S CONDITION RELATED TO:

11. INSURED'S POLICY GROUP OR FECA NUMBER

a. OTHER INSURED'S POLICY OR GROUP NUMBER

a. EMPLOYMENT? (Current or Previous) YES ☐ NO ☒

a. INSURED'S DATE OF BIRTH MM | DD | YY **SEX** M ☐ F ☐

b. RESERVED FOR NUCC USE

b. AUTO ACCIDENT? YES ☐ NO ☒ PLACE (State)

b. OTHER CLAIM ID (Designated by NUCC)

c. RESERVED FOR NUCC USE

c. OTHER ACCIDENT? YES ☐ NO ☒

c. INSURANCE PLAN NAME OR PROGRAM NAME

d. INSURANCE PLAN NAME OR PROGRAM NAME

10d. CLAIM CODES (Designated by NUCC)

d. IS THERE ANOTHER HEALTH BENEFIT PLAN? YES ☐ NO ☐ If yes, complete items 9, 9a, and 9d.

READ BACK OF FORM BEFORE COMPLETING & SIGNING THIS FORM.
12. PATIENT'S OR AUTHORIZED PERSON'S SIGNATURE I authorize the release of any medical or other information necessary to process this claim. I also request payment of government benefits either to myself or to the party who accepts assignment below.

SIGNED _____ DATE _____

13. INSURED'S OR AUTHORIZED PERSON'S SIGNATURE I authorize payment of medical benefits to the undersigned physician or supplier for services described below.

SIGNED _____

PATIENT AND INSURED INFORMATION

14. DATE OF CURRENT: ILLNESS, INJURY, or PREGNANCY(LMP) MM | DD | YY QUAL.

15. OTHER DATE QUAL. MM | DD | YY

16. DATES PATIENT UNABLE TO WORK IN CURRENT OCCUPATION FROM MM | DD | YY TO MM | DD | YY

17. NAME OF REFERRING PROVIDER OR OTHER SOURCE

17a.
17b. NPI 67805027XX

18. HOSPITALIZATION DATES RELATED TO CURRENT SERVICES FROM MM | DD | YY TO MM | DD | YY

19. ADDITIONAL CLAIM INFORMATION (Designated by NUCC)

20. OUTSIDE LAB? YES ☐ NO ☒ $ CHARGES

21. DIAGNOSIS OR NATURE OF ILLNESS OR INJURY Relate A-L to service line below (24E) ICD Ind. 0

A. S51.801   B. _____   C. _____   D. _____
E. _____   F. _____   G. _____   H. _____
I. _____   J. _____   K. _____   L. _____

22. RESUBMISSION CODE ORIGINAL REF. NO.

23. PRIOR AUTHORIZATION NUMBER

24. A. DATE(S) OF SERVICE						B. PLACE OF SERVICE	C. EMG	D. PROCEDURES, SERVICES, OR SUPPLIES (Explain Unusual Circumstances) CPT/HCPCS MODIFIER	E. DIAGNOSIS POINTER	F. $ CHARGES	G. DAYS OR UNITS	H. EPSDT Family Plan	I. ID. QUAL.	J. RENDERING PROVIDER ID. #
From MM 09	DD 55	YY 20XX	To MM	DD	YY	11		99203	A	120 00	1		NPI	46278897XX
09	55	20XX				11		12001	A	100 00			NPI	46278897XX
													NPI	
													NPI	
													NPI	
													NPI	

25. FEDERAL TAX I.D. NUMBER 7034597XX SSN ☐ EIN ☒

26. PATIENT'S ACCOUNT NO. 238293

27. ACCEPT ASSIGNMENT? (For govt. claims, see back) YES ☒ NO ☐

28. TOTAL CHARGE $

29. AMOUNT PAID $

30. Rsvd for NUCC Use $

31. SIGNATURE OF PHYSICIAN OR SUPPLIER INCLUDING DEGREES OR CREDENTIALS (I certify that the statements on the reverse apply to this bill and are made a part thereof.)
SIGNED Gerald Practon, MD DATE 09/30/20XX

32. SERVICE FACILITY LOCATION INFORMATION
College Hospital
4500 Broad Avenue
Woodland Hills XY 123450001
a. 937310XX   b.

33. BILLING PROVIDER INFO & PH # (555) 4869002
College Clinic
4567 Broad Avenue
Woodland Hills XY 123450001
a. 3664021CC   b.

PHYSICIAN OR SUPPLIER INFORMATION

NUCC Instruction Manual available at: www.nucc.org   *PLEASE PRINT OR TYPE*   OMB APPROVAL PENDING

Fig. 16.5

ASSIGNMENT 16.6 LOCATE ERRORS ON A RETURNED INSURANCE CLAIM

Performance Objective

Task: Highlight the blocks on the insurance claim form where errors are discovered.

Conditions: Use an insurance claim form (Fig. 16.6) and a highlighter or a red pen.

Standards: Time: _____ minutes

                Accuracy: _____

                (Note: The time element and accuracy criteria may be given by your instructor.)

Directions: An insurance claim (see Fig. 16.6) was returned by an insurance plan. Highlight or circle in red all blocks on the claim form where errors are discovered.

Option 1: Retype the claim and either insert the correction if data are available to fix the error or insert the word "NEED" in the block of the claim form.

Option 2: On a separate sheet of paper, list the blocks from 1 to 33 and state where errors occur. A Performance Evaluation Checklist may be reproduced from the "Instruction Guide to the Workbook" that appears in the section before Chapter 1 if your instructor wishes you to submit it to assist with scoring and comments.

After the instructor has returned your work to you, either make the necessary corrections and place your work in a three-ring notebook for future reference or, if you received a high score, place it in your portfolio for reference when applying for a job.

HEALTH INSURANCE CLAIM FORM

APPROVED BY NATIONAL UNIFOR MCLAIM COMMITTEE (NUCC) 02/12

American Insurance Company
509 Main Street
Woodland Hills XY 12345-0001

CARRIER

	PICA		PICA	

1. MEDICARE ☐ (Medicare#) MEDICAID ☐ (Medicaid#) TRICARE ☐ (ID#DoD#) CHAMPVA ☐ (Member ID#) GROUP HEALTH PLAN ☐ (ID#) FECA BLK LUNG ☐ (ID#) OTHER ☒ (ID#)

1a. INSURED'S I.D. NUMBER   (For Program in Item 1)

2. PATIENT'S NAME (Last Name, First Name, Middle Initial)
Mary T Avery

3. PATIENT'S BIRTH DATE
MM 05 DD 07 YY 1980   SEX M ☐ F ☐

4. INSURED'S NAME (Last Name, First Name, Middle Initial)
Same

5. PATIENT'S ADDRESS (No., Street)
4309 Main Street

6. PATIENT RELATIONSHIP TO INSURED
Self ☒ Spouse ☐ Child ☐ Other ☐

7. INSURED'S ADDRESS (No., Street)

CITY Woodland Hills   STATE XY

8. RESERVED FOR NUCC USE

CITY   STATE

ZIP CODE 123450001   TELEPHONE (Include Area Code) (555) 4509899

ZIP CODE   TELEPHONE (Include Area Code) ( )

9. OTHER INSURED'S NAME (Last Namo, Firot Name, Middle Initial)

10. IS PATIENT'S CONDITION RELATED TO:

11. INSURED'S POLICY GROUP OR FECA NUMBER

a. OTHER INSURED'S POLICY OR GROUP NUMBER

a. EMPLOYMENT? (Current or Previous) ☐ YES ☒ NO

a. INSURED'S DATE OF BIRTH MM DD YY   SEX M ☐ F ☐

b. RESERVED FOR NUCC USE

b. AUTO ACCIDENT? ☐ YES ☒ NO   PLACE (State)

b. OTHER CLAIM ID (Designated by NUCC)

c. RESERVED FOR NUCC USE

c. OTHER ACCIDENT? ☐ YES ☒ NO

c. INSURANCE PLAN NAME OR PROGRAM NAME

d. INSURANCE PLAN NAME OR PROGRAM NAME

10d. CLAIM CODES (Designated by NUCC)

d. IS THERE ANOTHER HEALTH BENEFIT PLAN? ☐ YES ☐ NO   *If yes,* complete items 9, 9a, and 9d.

READ BACK OF FORM BEFORE COMPLETING & SIGNING THIS FORM.

12. PATIENT'S OR AUTHORIZED PERSON'S SIGNATUREI authorize the release of any medical or other information necessary to process this claim. I also request payment of government benefits either to myself or to the party who accepts assignment below.
SIGNED Mary T. Avery   DATE 11/20/2007

13. INSURED'S OR AUTHORIZED PERSON'S SIGNATURE I authorize payment of medical benefits to the undersigned physician or supplier for services described below.
SIGNED Mary T. Avery

PATIENT AND INSURED INFORMATION

14. DATE OF CURRENT: ILLNESS, INJURY, or PREGNANCY(LMP) MM DD YY   QUAL.

15. OTHER DATE QUAL.   MM DD YY

16. DATES PATIENT UNABLE TO WORK IN CURRENT OCCUPATION
FROM 11 09 20XX   TO 11 30 20XX

17. NAME OF REFERRING PROVIDER OR OTHER SOURCE
Gerald Practon MD
17a.
17b. NPI

18. HOSPITALIZATION DATES RELATED TO CURRENT SERVICES
FROM 11 11 20XX   TO 11 12 20XX

19. ADDITIONAL CLAIM INFORMATION (Designated by NUCC)

20. OUTSIDE LAB? ☐ YES ☒ NO $ CHARGES

21. DIAGNOSIS OR NATURE OF ILLNESS OR INJURY Relate A-L to service line below (24E)   ICD Ind. 0
A. J03.90 B. C. D.
E. F. G. H.
I. J. K. L.

22. RESUBMISSION CODE   ORIGINAL REF. NO.

23. PRIOR AUTHORIZATION NUMBER

24. A. DATE(S) OF SERVICE From MM DD YY	To MM DD YY	B. PLACE OF SERVICE	C. EMG	D. PROCEDURES, SERVICES, OR SUPPLIES (Explain Unusual Circumstances) CPT/HCPCS	MODIFIER	E. DIAGNOSIS POINTER	F. $ CHARGES	G. DAYS OR UNITS	H. EPSDT Family Plan	I. ID. QUAL.	J. RENDERING PROVIDER ID. #
1	11 10 20XX		11		99203		A	120 00	1		NPI	43050047XX
2	11 11 20XX		21		42821		A	330 00			NPI	43050047XX
3	11 22 20XX		21		99231		A	50 00			NPI	
4											NPI	
5											NPI	
6											NPI	

25. FEDERAL TAX I.D. NUMBER 715737291XX SSN ☐ EIN ☒

26. PATIENT'S ACCOUNT NO. 456273

27. ACCEPT ASSIGNMENT? (For govt. claims, see back) ☐ YES ☐ NO

28. TOTAL CHARGE $

29. AMOUNT PAID $

30. Rsvd for NUCC Use $

31. SIGNATURE OF PHYSICIAN OR SUPPLIER INCLUDING DEGREES OR CREDENTIALS (I certify that the statements on the reverse apply to this bill and are made a part thereof.)
SIGNED   DATE 11/15/20XX

32. SERVICE FACILITY LOCATION INFORMATION
College Hospital
4500 Broad Avenue
Woodland Hills XY 123450001
a. X950731067 b.

33. BILLING PROVIDER INFO & PH # (555) 4869002
College Clinic
4567 Broad Avenue
Woodland Hills XY 123450001
a. 3664021CC b.

PHYSICIAN OR SUPPLIER INFORMATION

NUCC Instruction Manual available at: www.nucc.org   *PLEASE PRINT OR TYPE*   OMB APPROVAL PENDING

Fig. 16.6

Performance Objective

Task: Compose, format, key, proofread, and print a letter of appeal, and attach to this document photocopies of information to substantiate reimbursement requested.

Conditions: Computer, printer, letterhead paper, envelope, attachments, thesaurus, English dictionary, medical dictionary, and a pen or a pencil.

Standards: Time: _____ minutes

               Accuracy: _____

               (Note: The time element and accuracy criteria may be given by your instructor.)

Scenario: After retyping and resubmitting Mary T. Avery's insurance claim in Assignment 16.6 (see Fig. 16.6), the insurance company sends an EOB/RA (health insurance claim number 123098) with a check in the amount of $200.00 to the College Clinic for payment of the claim. Dr. Cutler wishes an appeal to be made for an increase of the payment for the surgical procedure (CPT 42821). Only $100.00 of the $330.00 charge was approved for payment of the surgical procedure. The provider is asking for a review of the claim. (Note: This patient's marital status is single, and the insured's identification number is T45098.)

Directions: Use the retyped claim to Assignment 16.6 for Mary T. Avery. Follow these basic step-by-step procedures.

1. Compose, format, key, proofread, and print a letter.

2. Include the beneficiary's name, health insurance claim number, dates of service in question, and items or services in question with the name, address, and signature of the provider.

3. Compose a letter with an introduction that stresses the medical practice's qualifications, the physician's commitment to complying with regulations and providing appropriate services, and the importance of the practice to the payer's panel of physicians or specialists.

4. Provide a detailed account of the necessity of the treatment given and its relationship to the patient's problems and chief complaint. You might cross-reference the medical record and emphasize parts of it that the reviewer may have missed.

5. Explain the reason why the provider does not agree with the payment. Use a blank sheet, labeling it "Explanation of Benefits," because you do not have this printed document to attach.

6. Abstract excerpts from the coding resource book if necessary.

7. Direct the correspondence to Mr. Donald Pearson, a claims adjuster at the American Insurance Company, 509 Main Street, Woodland Hills, XY 12345.

8. Address an envelope for the letter.

9. Retain copies of all data sent for the physician's files.

17 Collection Strategies

Linda M. Smith

KEY TERMS

Your instructor may wish to select some words pertinent to this chapter for a test. For definitions of the terms, further study, and/or reference, the words, phrases, and abbreviations may be found in the glossary at the end of the textbook. Key terms for this chapter follow.

accounts receivable
age analysis
automatic stay
balance
bankruptcy
bonding
cash flow
collateral
collection ratio
credit
credit card
creditor
cycle billing
debit card
debt
debtor
discount
dun messages

embezzlement
estate administrator
estate executor
fee schedule
financial accounting record
garnishment
itemized statement
lien
netback
no charge
nonexempt assets
professional courtesy
secured debt
skip
statute of limitations
unsecured debt
write-off

KEY ABBREVIATIONS

See how many abbreviations and acronyms you can translate and then use this as a handy reference list. Definitions for the key abbreviations are located near the back of the textbook in the glossary.

A/R _____

ATM _____

e-check _____

FACT _____

FCBA _____

FCRA _____

FDCPA _____

FTC _____

N/A _____

NC _____

NSF _____

TILA _____

W2 _____

PERFORMANCE OBJECTIVES

The student will be able to:

- Define and spell the key terms and key abbreviations for this chapter, given the information from the *textbook* glossary, within a reasonable time period and with enough accuracy to obtain a satisfactory evaluation.

- After reading the chapter, answer the fill-in-the-blank, mix and match, multiple choice, and true/false review questions with enough accuracy to obtain a satisfactory evaluation.

- Select an appropriate dun message for a patient's bill, given a patient's ledger/statement, within a reasonable time period and with enough accuracy to obtain a satisfactory evaluation.

- Post a courtesy adjustment, given a patient's ledger/statement, within a reasonable time period and with enough accuracy to obtain a satisfactory evaluation.

- Post a patient's charges and payment to the patient's financial accounting record, within a reasonable time period and with enough accuracy to obtain a satisfactory evaluation.

- Compose a collection letter for a delinquent account, given letterhead stationery, within a reasonable time period and with enough accuracy to obtain a satisfactory evaluation.

- Complete a financial agreement, given a patient's ledger/statement, within a reasonable time period and with enough accuracy to obtain a satisfactory evaluation.

STUDY OUTLINE

Collection Strategies
 Accounts Receivable
Patient Education
 Patient Registration Form
Fees
 Fee Schedule
 Missed Appointments
 Fee Adjustments
 Discussing Fees
Collecting Fees
 Encounter Forms
 Patient Excuses for Nonpayments
 Credit and Debit Cards
 Payment by Check
 Payment Through Patient Portals
Self-Pay Billing
 Itemized Patient Statement
 Accounts Receivable and Age Analysis by Aging Report
 Dun Messages
 Electronic Media
 Computer Billing
 Billing Services
 Billing Guidelines

 Payment Plans
Credit and Collection Laws
 Statute of Limitations
The Collection Process
 Telephone Collection Procedures
 Collection Letters
 After-Insurance Collection
 Collection Agencies
 Small Claims Court
 Federal Wage Garnishment Laws
 Tracing a Skip
Special Collection Issues
 Bankruptcy
 Terminally Ill Patients
 Estate Claims
 Litigation
 Liens
 Patient Complaints
Collection Controls
 Bonding
 Embezzlement
 Precautions for financial protection

Part I Fill in the Blank

Review the objectives, key terms, chapter information, glossary definitions of key terms, and figures before completing the following review questions.

1. Third-party payers who generate a large percentage of reimbursement to health care organizations are composed of

   a. _____

   b. _____

   c. _____

   d. _____ .

2. The unpaid balance due from patients and third-party payers for professional services rendered is known as a/an

   _____ .

3. The days in accounts receivable for payment that is collected at the time of service is _____ days.

4. Write the formula for calculating a health care organization's collection ratio.

   _____

   _____

   _____

5. What is the collection rate if a total of $40,300 was collected for the month and the total of the accounts receivable is $50,670? _____

6. The Affordable Care Act allows young adults up to the age _____ to remain on their parent's health care plan.

7. A listing of accepted charges for specific medical services and procedures provided by a health care provider is a

   _____ .

8. The procedure of systematically arranging the accounts receivable, by age, from the date of service is called _____

   _____ .

9. Patient accounts that are open to charges made from time to time are referred to as

   _____ .

10. A court order attaching a debtor's property or wages to pay off a debt is known as _____

    _____ .

11. An individual who owes on an account and moves, leaving no forwarding address, is called a/an _____

    _____ .

12. What are the two kinds of bankruptcy petitions? _____ and _____ .

13. A straight petition in bankruptcy or absolute bankruptcy is also known as a/an _____ .

14. A wage earner's bankruptcy is sometimes referred to as a/an _____ .

15. State three bonding methods.

    a. _____

    b. _____

    c. _____

16. A system of billing accounts at spaced intervals during the month on the basis of a breakdown of accounts by alphabet, account number, insurance type, or date of service is known as _____ .

Part II Mix and Match

17. Match the credit and collection terms in the right column with the descriptions, and fill in the blank with the appropriate letter.

_____ Reductions of the normal fee based on a specific amount of money or a percentage of the charge

_____ Phrase to remind a patient about a delinquent account

_____ Item that permits bank customers to withdraw cash at any hour from an automated teller machine

_____ Individual owing money

_____ Claim on the property of another as security for a debt

_____ Individual record indicating charges, payments, adjustments, and balances owed for services rendered

_____ Detailed summary of all transactions of a creditor's account

_____ Person to whom money is owed

_____ Listing of accepted charges or established allowances for specific medical procedures

a. debtor

b. itemized statement

c. fee schedule

d. discounts

e. financial account record (ledger)

f. creditor

g. dun message

h. debit card

i. lien

18. Match the following federal acts with their descriptions, and fill in the blank with the appropriate letter.

_____ Law stating that a person has 60 days to complain about an error from the date that a statement is mailed

_____ Consumer protection act that applies to anyone who charges interest or agrees on payment of a bill in more than four installments, excluding a down payment

_____ Regulates collection practices of third-party debt collectors and attorneys who collect debts for others

_____ Federal law prohibiting discrimination in all areas of granting credit

_____ Regulates agencies that issue or use credit reports on consumers

a. Equal Credit Opportunity Act

b. Fair Credit Reporting Act

c. Fair Credit Billing Act

d. Truth in Lending Act

e. Fair Debt Collection Practices Act

Part III Multiple Choice

Choose the best answer.

19. Signing another person's name on a check to obtain money or pay off a debt without permission is called:
    a. embezzlement.
    b. stealing.
    c. garnishing.
    d. forgery.

20. When sending monthly statements to patients for balances due, the postal service can forward mail if the addressed envelopes contain the statement:
    a. "Please Forward."
    b. "Forwarding Service Requested."
    c. "Forwarding and Return Receipt Requested."
    d. "Send Forward."

21. When accepting a credit card as payment on an account, the proper guideline(s) to follow is/are to:
    a. ask for photo identification.
    b. accept a card only from the person whose name is on the card.

    c. get approval from the credit card company.
    d. all of the above.

22. Stealing money that has been entrusted in one's care is known as:
    a. embezzlement
    b. discounting
    c. forgery.
    d. bonding.

23. Insurance payment checks should be stamped in the endorsement area on the back "For Deposit Only," which is called a/an:
    a. conditional endorsement.
    b. qualified endorsement.
    c. special endorsement.
    d. restrictive endorsement.

Part IV True/False

Write "T" or "F" in the blank to indicate whether you think the statement is true or false.

_____ 24. Insurance companies and the federal government do not recommend waiving copayments to patients.

_____ 25. Regulation Z of the Truth in Lending Consumer Credit Cost Disclosure law applies if the patient is making three payments.

_____ 26. Most state collection laws allow telephone calls to the debtor between 8 AM and 9 PM.

_____ 27. When a patient has declared bankruptcy, it is permissible to continue to send monthly statements for a balance due.

_____ 28. A collection agency must follow all the laws stated in the Fair Debt Collection Practices Act.

Performance Objective

Task: Select an appropriate dun message and insert it on a patient's financial accounting record (ledger card).

Conditions: Use the patient's financial accounting record (Fig. 17.1), computer, and a printer.

Standards: Time: _____ minutes

                  Accuracy:_____

                  (Note: The time element and accuracy criteria may be given by your instructor.)

Background: Most patient account activities are recorded in the medical billing software. However, to develop the skills and understanding for payment posting, a paper financial accounting statement has been provided.

Directions: Read the scenario and refer to the patient's financial accounting record (see Fig. 17.1). Select appropriate dun messages for each month the patient has been billed.

Scenario: Carrie Jones was on vacation in June and July and did not pay on her account. It is August (current year).

June 1, 20XX, dun message _____

July 1, 20XX, dun message _____

August 1, 20XX, dun message _____

After the instructor has returned your work to you, either make the necessary corrections and place your work in a three-ring notebook for future reference or, if you received a high score, place it in your portfolio for reference when applying for a job.

STATEMENT
Financial Account
COLLEGE CLINIC
4567 Broad Avenue
Woodland Hills, XY 12345-0001
Tel. 555-486-9002
Fax No. 555-487-8976

Carrie Jones
15543 Dean Street
Woodland Hills, XY 12345

Phone No. (H) _____ (555) 439-8800 _____ (W) _____ (555) 550-8706 _____   Birth date _____ 05-14-72 _____

Primary Insurance Co. _____ Prudential Insurance Company _____   Policy/Group No. _____ 450998 _____

	REFERENCE	DESCRIPTION	CHARGES		CREDITS		BALANCE	
					PYMNTS.	ADJ.		
				BALANCE FORWARD ⟶				
4-16–xx	99215	Established patient visit; level 5					160	00
4-17–xx		Prudential billed (4-16-xx)						
5-27 xx		Rec'd insurance ck #435			30	00	130	00
6-1-xx		Billed pt					130	00
7-1-xx		Billed pt					130	00
8-1-xx		Billed pt					130	00

PLEASE PAY LAST AMOUNT IN BALANCE COLUMN ⬆

THIS IS A COPY OF YOUR FINANCIAL ACCOUNT AS IT APPEARS ON OUR RECORDS

Fig. 17.1

Performance Objective

Task: Post a courtesy adjustment to a patient's financial accounting record (ledger card).

Conditions: Use the patient's financial accounting record (Fig. 17.2) and a pen.

Standards: Time: _____ minutes

                  Accuracy: _____

                  (Note: The time element and accuracy criteria may be given by your instructor.)

Background: Most patient account activities are recorded in the medical billing software. However, to develop the skills and understanding for payment posting, a paper financial accounting statement has been provided.

Directions: Read the case scenario and refer to the patient's financial accounting record (see Fig. 17.2).

Scenario: Maria Smith recently lost her job and is raising two children as a single parent. It is September 1 (current year). A discussion with Dr. Gerald Practon leads to a decision to write off the balance of the current charges on the account but not the balance forward.

After the instructor has returned your work to you, either make the necessary corrections and place your work in a three-ring notebook for future reference or, if you received a high score, place it in your portfolio for reference when applying for a job.

Acct No. 10-3

STATEMENT
Financial Account
COLLEGE CLINIC
4567 Broad Avenue
Woodland Hills, XY 12345-0001
Tel. 555-486-9002
Fax No. 555-487-8976

Ms. Maria Smith
3737 Unser Road
Woodland Hills, XY 12345

Phone No. (H) (555) 430-8877   (W)   (555) 908-1233   Birth date 06-11-80

Primary Insurance Co.   Metropolitan Insurance Company   Policy/Group No.   4320870

	REFERENCE	DESCRIPTION	CHARGES		CREDITS PYMNTS.	ADJ.	BALANCE	
					BALANCE FORWARD ➡		20	00
5-19-xx	99214	Est. office visit	120	00			140	00
5-20-xx		Metropolitan billed (5-19-xx)						
6-20-xx		Rec'd ins ck #6778			25	00	115	00
7-1-xx		Pt billed					115	00
8-1-xx		Pt billed					115	00

PLEASE PAY LAST AMOUNT IN BALANCE COLUMN

THIS IS A COPY OF YOUR FINANCIAL ACCOUNT AS IT APPEARS ON OUR RECORDS

Fig. 17.2

Performance Objective

Task: Post a payment to a patient's financial accounting record (ledger card).

Conditions: Use the patient's financial accounting record (Fig. 17.3), and a pen.

Standards: Time: _____ minutes

                    Accuracy: _____

                    (Note: The time element and accuracy criteria may be given by your instructor.)

Background: Most patient account activities are recorded in the medical billing software. However, to develop the skills and understanding for payment posting, a paper financial accounting statement has been provided.

Directions: Read the case scenario; refer to the patient's financial accounting record (see Fig. 17.3). Post the charges for the services rendered and payment to the patient's financial accounting record.

Scenario:

Date of service: October 12 (current year)

Patient: Kenneth Brown; 8896 Aster Drive; Woodland Hills, XY, 12345

Patient Phone: 555-760-5211 (home) 555-987-3855 (work)

Date of birth: 1/15/82

Insurance: None

Service Provided: EKG (CPT 93000) Fee: $20.00

Service Provided: New patient visit level III (CPT 99203) Fee: $120.00

Patient paid by personal check: $50.00 (check #3421)

After the instructor has returned your work to you, either make the necessary corrections and place your work in a three-ring notebook for future reference or, if you received a high score, place it in your portfolio for reference when applying for a job.

Acct No. 10-4

STATEMENT
Financial Account
COLLEGE CLINIC
4567 Broad Avenue
Woodland Hills, XY 12345-0001
Tel. 555-486-9002
Fax No. 555-487-8976

Mr. Kenneth Brown
8896 Aster Drive
Woodland Hills, XY 12345

Phone No. (H) (555) 760-5211   (W) (555) 987-3355   Birth date 01-15-82

Primary Insurance Co. none   Policy/Group No.

REFERENCE	DESCRIPTION	CHARGES	CREDITS		BALANCE
			PYMNTS.	ADJ.	
		BALANCE FORWARD ⟶			

PLEASE PAY LAST AMOUNT IN BALANCE COLUMN ⬆

THIS IS A COPY OF YOUR FINANCIAL ACCOUNT AS IT APPEARS ON OUR RECORDS

Fig. 17.3

ASSIGNMENT 17.5 COMPOSE A COLLECTION LETTER

Performance Objective

Task: Compose a letter for the physician's signature and post the entry on the patient's financial accounting record (ledger card).

Conditions: Use the patient's financial accounting record (Fig. 17.4), one sheet of letterhead paper (Fig. 17.5), a number 10 envelope, English dictionary, thesaurus, medical dictionary, computer, printer, and pen.

Standards: Time: _____ minutes

                 Accuracy: _____

                 (Note: The time element and accuracy criteria may be given by your instructor.)

Background: Most patient account activities are recorded in the medical billing software. However, to develop the skills and understanding for payment posting, a paper financial accounting statement has been provided.

Directions: Read the case scenario, refer to the patient's financial accounting record (see Fig. 17.4), and compose a collection letter, using your signature and requesting payment. Print on letterhead stationery in full block format (paragraphs to left margin). Include a paragraph stating that a copy of the delinquent statement is enclosed. Post an entry on the patient's financial accounting record.

Scenario: It is December 1 (current year), and you have sent Mr. Ron Kelsey two statements with no response. You have tried to reach him by telephone without success and have decided to send him a collection letter (see Fig. 17.5).

After the instructor has returned your work to you, either make the necessary corrections and place your work in a three-ring notebook for future reference or, if you received a high score, place it in your portfolio for reference when applying for a job.

Acct No. 17-5

STATEMENT
Financial Account
COLLEGE CLINIC
4567 Broad Avenue
Woodland Hills, XY 12345-0001
Tel. 555-486-9002
Fax No. 555-487-8976

Mr. Ron Kelsey
6321 Ocean Street
Woodland Hills, XY 12345

Phone No. (H) (555) 540-9800   (W) (555) 890-7766   Birth date 03-25-75

Primary Insurance Co. XYZ Insurance Company   Policy/Group No. 8503Y

	REFERENCE	DESCRIPTION	CHARGES		CREDITS PYMNTS.	ADJ.	BALANCE	
					BALANCE FORWARD →			
07-09-xx	99283	ER Visit; Level 3	80	00			80	00
07-10-xx		XYZ Insurance billed (3-9-xx)					80	00
09-20-xx		EOB rec'd pt has not met deductible					80	00
10-01-xx		Billed pt					80	00
11-01-xx		Billed pt					80	00

PLEASE PAY LAST AMOUNT IN BALANCE COLUMN ⬆

THIS IS A COPY OF YOUR FINANCIAL ACCOUNT AS IT APPEARS ON OUR RECORDS

Fig. 17.4

COLLEGE CLINIC
4567 Broad Avenue
Woodland Hills, XY 12345-0001
Tel. (555) 486-9002
FAX (555) 487-8976

Fig. 17.5

ASSIGNMENT 17.6 ACCEPTING CREDIT CARD PAYMENTS

Performance Objective

Task: Accept a credit card payment through various tools.

Conditions: Use a credit card terminal, credit card reader attachment, or secured online web portal for credit card payments and credit card receipts, and pen or pencil.

Standards: Time: _____ minutes

Accuracy: _____

(Note: The time element and accuracy criteria may be given by your instructor.)

Background: The medical office has many different tools to accept credit card payments, such as:

- *Credit card terminal payment:* These lightweight devices use an internet connection to complete the payment transaction. The terminal can scan the credit card data including the cardholder's name, credit card number, and expiration date, through a swipe. The terminal also can process credit card transactions in which the user manually enters credit card information; in this scenario, the transaction requires the credit card number, the expiration date, the card security code (CVV), and the patient's billing ZIP code. Both transactions, the swipe method and the manual method, cause the terminal to typically print out two receipts per transaction, one for the medical office and one for the patient. If the credit card is swiped, the patient signs the medical office receipt because it states their name in the transaction. When manually entering the credit card data, the receipt will not print the patient's name, so the medical assistant must document the patient's name, date of service, and/or medical record number on the receipt. Renting a credit card terminal can be costly, so smaller medical offices prefer to use other credit card accepting options.

- *Credit card reader payment:* A smaller medical office might choose a pay-for-use credit card that accepts software packages. The package includes a tablet or smartphone attachment device for scanning credit cards and a downloadable application. The application is user-friendly and is able to send the patient a receipt via email or by text message. There is a minimal fee per transaction ($0.25 to $0.30) and a percent charged based on the total amount.

- *Online credit card payment:* Some medical offices use an online merchant service to accept patient credit card payments. Through a secure web portal, patients can view their medical bills online and make payments by credit card or through a service such as PayPal. The transaction receipt is emailed to the patient and to the medical office. When the medical assistant receives the transaction via email, he or she updates the patient's account to reflect the current balance. There is a per-transaction cost for this service similar to other credit card acceptance applications.

Directions: Read each case scenario, review the accompanying figures, and answer the following questions:

A. Kevin Long is attending the College Clinic on May 26 (current year) for an office visit and needs to pay for his $30 copay. He presents a credit card for payment (Fig. 17.6A).

1. What should the medical assistant do to verify Kevin Long's identity before accepting the credit card for payment?

   _____

2. Which tool can be used to accept Kevin Long's payment?

   _____

3. Will the credit card receipt have Kevin's name printed? Why or why not?

   _____

4. Does the medical office credit card receipt require the patient's signature? Why or why not?

   _____

B. It is November 6 (current year), and you receive a phone call at the College Clinic. It is Kevin Long, who has an unpaid balance of $24.32, and it is up to you to discuss this delinquency with Mr. Long and come to an agreement on how the account can be paid. After discussion, Mr. Long decides to pay the total balance due by credit card, giving you his authorization (Fig. 17.6B).

1. Which tool can be used to accept Kevin Long's payment?

   _____

2. Will the credit card receipts have Kevin's name printed? Why or why not?

_____

3. What must a medical assistant do to the receipt if the patient's name is not printed?

_____

4. How can a credit card receipt be sent to the patient?

_____

C. Kevin Long received a statement from the College Clinic for an outstanding balance of $63.52 from a date of service December 12 (current year). He notices that the clinic allows him to log in to pay online. He visits the medical office's website and clicks the "Pay Your Bill" feature. The secure online web portal asks Kevin to complete a form requests his name, billing address, an email address, the credit card number, expiration date, and CVV (Fig. 17.6C). Prior to submitting the online form, Kevin notices the following statement: "By clicking this box, the user agrees to the terms of this transaction." Kevin checks the box and clicks submit to send his credit card payment electronically. A receipt for the transaction is emailed to Kevin.

1. Which tool can be used to accept Kevin Long's payment?

_____

2. Will the credit card receipt have Kevin's name printed? Why or why not?

_____

_____

3. How is the credit card receipt sent to the patient?

_____

4. What should the medical assistant do with the transaction email received?

_____

COLLEGE CLINIC
4567 Broad Avenue
Woodland Hills, XY 12345-0001

05/26/20XX	09:39:14
Merchant ID:	00000000262026XX
Terminal ID:	038802XX
0150302859XX	

CREDIT CARD

MC SALE

Name	Kevin Long
CARD#	XXXXXXXXX4021
INVOICE	009
Batch #:	00716
Approval Code:	4123P
Entry Method:	Swiped
SALE AMOUNT	**$30.00**

Kevin Long

_____
Customer Signature

MERCHANT COPY

Fig. 17.6

COLLEGE CLINIC
4567 Broad Avenue
Woodland Hills, XY 12345-0001

11/6 /20XX	**09:39:14**
Merchant ID:	**00000000262026XX**
Terminal ID:	**038802XX**
0150302859XX	

CREDIT CARD

MC SALE

CARD#	**XXXXXXXXX4021**
INVOICE	**009**
Batch#:	**00716**
Approval Code:	**4123P**
Entry Method:	**Manual Entry**
Mode:	**Online**
SALE AMOUNT	**$24.32**

Approved by patient over the phone.

_____
Customer Signature

MERCHANT COPY

11/6/20XX: Spoke with Kevin Long (MR 354689); he agreed to pay balance in full with a credit card over the phone. Payment for date of service 7/3/20XX. Balance paid in full.

Fig. 17.6, cont'd

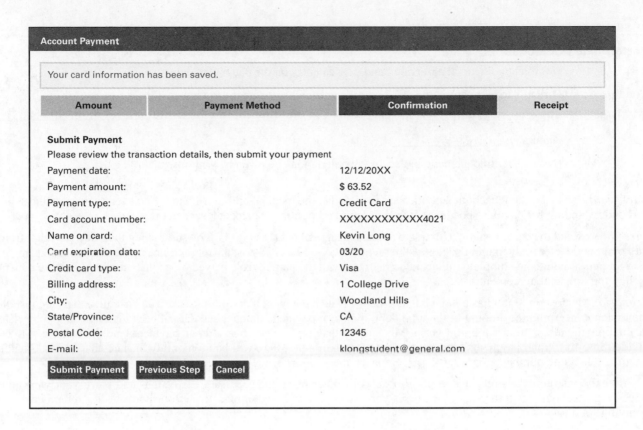

Account Payment

Your card information has been saved.

| Amount | Payment Method | Confirmation | Receipt |

Submit Payment

Please review the transaction details, then submit your payment

Payment date:	12/12/20XX
Payment amount:	$ 63.52
Payment type:	Credit Card
Card account number:	XXXXXXXXXXXX4021
Name on card:	Kevin Long
Card expiration date:	03/20
Credit card type:	Visa
Billing address:	1 College Drive
City:	Woodland Hills
State/Province:	CA
Postal Code:	12345
E-mail:	klongstudent@general.com

Submit Payment   Previous Step   Cancel

Fig. 17.6, cont'd

Performance Objective

Task: Complete a financial agreement and post an entry on the patient's ledger.

Conditions: Patient's ledger card is Fig. 17.7 and the financial agreement form is Fig. 17.8.

Standards: Time: _____ minutes

                   Accuracy: _____

                   (Note: The time element and accuracy criteria may be given by your instructor.)

Background: Most patient account activities are recorded in the medical billing software. However, to develop the skills and understanding for payment posting, a paper financial accounting statement has been provided.

Directions: Read the case scenario. Complete a financial agreement (see Fig. 17.8 by subtracting the down payment from the total debt. Refer to the patient's ledger/statement (see Fig. 17.7) and post an appropriate entry to the ledger/statement using a pen. Review the completed financial agreement with the patient (role played by another student). Ask the patient to sign the financial agreement.

Scenario: Mr. Joseph Small has a large balance due. Create a payment plan for this case. You have discussed the installment plan concerning the amount of the total debt, the down payment, amount and date of each installment, and the date of final payment. On June 1 (current year), Mr. Small is paying $500 cash as a down payment, and the balance is to be divided into five equal payments, due on the first of each month. There will be no monthly finance charge. Mr. Small's daytime telephone number is 555-760-5502. He is a patient of Dr. Brady Coccidioides.

After the instructor has returned your work to you, either make the necessary corrections and place your work in a three-ring notebook for future reference or, if you received a high score, place it in your portfolio for reference when applying for a job.

Acct No. 10-7

STATEMENT
Financial Account
COLLEGE CLINIC
4567 Broad Avenue
Woodland Hills, XY 12345-0001
Tel. 555-486-9002
Fax No. 555-487-8976

Mr. Joseph Small
655 Sherry Street
Woodland Hills, XY 12345

Phone No. (H) (555) 320-8801   (W) (555) 760-5502   Birth date 11-04-77

Primary Insurance Co. Blue Shield   Policy/Group No. 870-XX-4398

	REFERENCE	DESCRIPTION	CHARGES		CREDITS			BALANCE	
---	---	---	---	---	PYMNTS.		ADJ.		
					BALANCE FORWARD ➔				
04-19-xx	99215	OV Level 5	160	00				160	00
04-30-xx	99218	Adm hosp	110	00				270	00
04-30-xx	32440	Pneumonectomy, total	1690	00				1960	00
05-20-xx		Blue Shield billed (1-19 to 30-xx)							
05-15-xx		BS EOB Pt deductible $1000 rec'd ck #544			960	00		1000	00

PLEASE PAY LAST AMOUNT IN BALANCE COLUMN ⬑

THIS IS A COPY OF YOUR FINANCIAL ACCOUNT AS IT APPEARS ON OUR RECORDS

Fig. 17.7

College Clinic
4567 Broad Avenue
Woodland Hills, XY 12345-0001
Phone: 555/486-9002
Fax: 555/487-8976

FINANCIAL PAYMENT PLAN AGREEMENT

For medical professional services rendered to:

Patient Name_____ Account No. _____

Responsible Party _____

Address _____

_____

Telephones: Home _____

Mobile _____

Business _____

1. Cash price of total medical treatment	$	_____
2. Down payment (partial payment)	$	_____
3. Amount covered by insurance plan	$	_____
4. Unpaid balance due	$	_____
5. **ANNUAL PERCENTAGE RATE** (interest rate)		_____ %
6. **FINANCE CHARGE** ($ amt of cost to patient)	$	_____
7. Total amount of unpaid balance due		_____
8. Monthly payment amount	$	_____

TERMS:

1. ALL PAYMENTS ARE DUE ON OR BEFORE YOUR DUE DATE EACH MONTH.

2. The patient agrees to be fully responsible for the total payment of medical services performed in this office including any amounts not covered by any health insurance plan.

3. The patient has the right at any time to pay the unpaid balance due without penalty.

4. First payment due ____ / ____ / _____ and subsequent payments on the same day of each consecutive month until paid in full.

_____
Signature of Patient/Responsible Party   Date

_____
Physician's signature or Authorized representative   Date

Fig. 17.8

18 Introduction to Health Care Facilities and Ambulatory Surgery Centers

Cheryl Fassett

KEY TERMS

Your instructor may wish to select some words pertinent to this chapter for a test. For definitions of the terms, further study, and/or reference, the words, phrases, and abbreviations may be found in the glossary at the end of the Textbook. *Key terms for this chapter follow.*

72-hour rule
accreditation
Accreditation Association for Ambulatory
    Health Care
Accreditation Association of Hospitals/
    Health Systems
activities of daily living
acute care facility
admission review
against medical advice
Ambulance Fee Schedule
ambulatory care
ambulatory payment classifications
ambulatory surgery center
Ambulatory Surgical Center Quality Reporting
    Program
ambulatory surgery units
American College of Surgeons
American Hospital Association
American Medical Association
American Osteopathic Association
Ambulatory Surgery Center payment system
Capitation
case mix groups
chargemaster
clinic
Complication/Comorbidity
concurrent review
Consumer Assessment of Health Care Providers
    and Systems Outpatient and Ambulatory
    Surgery Survey
continued stay review
cost outlier
critical access hospital
discharge
discharge disposition
Discharge Not Final Billed
discounting
downcoding
DRG creep
Emergency Medical Treatment and Labor Act
Grouper
Healthcare Facilities Accreditation Program
health insurance prospective payment system code set

home health agency
Home Health Prospective Payment System
Hospice
Hospice Prospective Payment System
Hospital
hospital-acquired conditions
Hospital Acquired Condition Reduction Program
Hospital Standardization Program
Hospital Value-Based Purchasing Program
inpatient
Inpatient Only List
Inpatient Psychiatric Facility Prospective Payment System
Inpatient Prospective Payment System
Inpatient Rehabilitation Facility Patient Assessment
    Instrument
Inpatient Rehabilitation Facility Prospective Payment
    System
long-term care facility
Long-Term Care Hospital Prospective Payment System
major complications/comorbidities
major diagnostic categories
Medicare Severity Diagnosis-Related Groups
national unadjusted payment
never event
nonpatient
observation
osteopathic medicine
outpatient
outpatient code editor
Outpatient Prospective Payment System
packaging
pass throughs
patient dumping
per diem
preadmission
preadmission testing
preauthorization
present on admission
prospective payment system
Prospective reviews
Quality Improvement Organizations
rehabilitation impairment category
relative weight
Resident Assessment Instrument

retrospective review
revenue code
revenue cycle
skilled nursing facility
Skilled Nursing Facility Prospective Payment System
status (payment) indicator
swing bed

The Accreditation Association
The Joint Commission
Two Midnight Rule
Uniform Bill 04 (UB-04)
utilization management
upcoding

KEY ABBREVIATIONS

AAAHC _____

ACS _____

ADLs _____

AHA _____

AMA _____

AOA _____

APC _____

ASCQR _____

ASU _____

CAH _____

CCs _____

CMGs _____

DNFB _____

EMTALA _____

HACs _____

HACRP _____

HFAP _____

HHA _____

HH PPS _____

HIPPS _____

IPF PPS _____

IPPS _____

IRF PAI _____

IRF PPS _____

LTCH PPS _____

MCCs _____

MDCs _____

MS-DRGs _____

OAS CAHOP _____

OCE _____

OPPS _____

PAT _____

POA _____

PPS _____

QIO _____

RAI _____

RIC _____

SNF _____

SNF PPS _____

TJC _____

UB-04 _____

UM _____

VBP _____

PERFORMANCE OBJECTIVES

The student will be able to:

- Define and spell the key terms and key abbreviations for this chapter, given the information from the textbook glossary, within a reasonable time period and with enough accuracy to obtain a satisfactory evaluation.

- Answer the multiple choice and essay questions with enough accuracy to obtain a satisfactory evaluation.

- Determine if prior authorization is required on a health insurance policy.

- Calculate projected payments on MS-DRGs.

- Determine if an APC is subject to discounting based on status indicators.

- Locate and evaluate inpatient rehabilitation patient assessment instruments.

STUDY OUTLINE

History of Health Care Facilities
Types of Health Care Facilities
    Acute Care Facilities
    Critical Care Hospital
    Ambulatory Surgery Centers
    Clinics
    Skilled Nursing Facilities
    Long-Term Care Facilities
    Hospice
    Home Health Agencies
Regulation of Health Care Facilities
    Accreditation
    Emergency Medical Treatment and Labor Act
    Medicare Certification of Ambulatory Surgery Centers
Inpatient, Outpatient and Nonpatient Services
    Inpatient Only List
    72-hour rule
Revenue Cycle in Health Care Facilities
    Preadmission
    Patient Care
    Postdischarge

Reimbursement Methodologies
    Medicare Prospective Payment Systems
    Self-Pay
    Capitation
    Fee For Service
    Other Reimbursement Methodologies
Quality in Health Care Facilities
    Never Events
    Hospital Acquired Conditions
    Utilization Management
    Ambulatory Surgery Center Quality Reporting
    Hospital Value-Based Purchasing Program
    Consumer Assessment of Health Care Providers and Systems Outpatient and Ambulatory Surgery Survey
    Quality Improvement Organizations

Part I Multiple Choice

Choose the best answer.

1. The Joint Commission develops guidelines for hospitals and other health care facilities that address standards in which of the following areas?
   a. patient care
   b. infection control
   c. Medicare reimbursement
   d. both A and B

2. A small rural hospital established to provide care to assure Medicare beneficiaries have access to health care is called a _____?
   a. long-term care facility
   b. acute care facility
   c. critical access hospital
   d. ambulatory surgery center

3. What type of facility has seen significant growth over the last few decades due to reduced health care costs and technological advancement?
   a. skilled nursing facilities
   b. ambulatory surgery centers
   c. home health agencies
   d. acute care facilities

4. A voluntary assessment process that facilities use to assess their performance against national benchmarks and established standards of care is called _____.
   a. quality improvement organization
   b. accreditation
   c. prospective review
   d. certification

5. What organization developed the Health care Facilities Accreditation Program to evaluate osteopathic hospitals?
   a. TJC
   b. AMA
   c. AHA
   d. AOA

6. Patient dumping was addressed in which piece of legislation?
   a. EMTALA
   b. ACA
   c. HHA PPS
   d. COBRA

7. In the ASC exclusion list, CMS allows which of the following procedures to be done in an ASC?
   a. procedures involving major blood vessels
   b. procedures that are emergent in nature
   c. procedures that usually result in extensive blood loss
   d. procedures that do not typically involve an overnight stay

8. The Two-Midnight Rule is often used to determine which of the following?
   a. if a patient is considered to be an inpatient
   b. if the procedure can be done in an ASC
   c. if the patient is in observation
   d. if the procedure requires preauthorization

9. The rule used to determine if treatments related to an inpatient admission are bundled with the inpatient claim is known as _____.
   a. Two-Midnight Rule
   b. 72-hour Rule
   c. Birthday Rule
   d. Inpatient Only List

10. A list or database of all of the services, supplies and equipment provided by the hospital and the charges associated with them is called the _____.
    a. UB-04
    b. chargemaster
    c. preauthorization
    d. discharge summary

11. Which prospective payment system uses MS-DRGs?
    a. IPPS
    b. HHA PPS
    c. OPPS
    d. SNF PPS

12. The type of payment used by insurance carriers to control costs that are considered risky for the health care professional is:
    a. reimbursement
    b. coinsurance
    c. fee-for-service
    d. capitation

13. The _____ is the process of patient health and financial information moving into, through and out of the Ambulatory Surgery Center.
    a. revenue stream
    b. revenue cycle
    c. audit procedure
    d. managed care method

14. ASCs use _____ to bundle all supplies, medications, and other components of a service.
    a. packaging
    b. bundling
    c. bulk billing
    d. groupers

15. _____ payments were established by Congress to encourage facilities to use new technology.
   a. incentive
   b. bonus
   c. pass-through
   d. capitation

16. ASC claims are submitted to Medicare using a _____, while outpatient hospital claims are submitted on a _____.
   a. CMS-1500, UB-04
   b. UB-04, CMS-1500
   c. both use a UB-04
   d. both use a CMS-1500

17. What type of rate is the IPF PPS based on?
   a. capitation
   b. fee-for-service
   c. per diem
   d. bundled

18. Hospice services include which of the following?
   a. medical supplies
   b. grief counseling
   c. dietary management
   d. all of the above

19. A Never Event is defined as _____.
   a. when a patient does not show up for surgery
   b. an error in medical treatment that is preventable
   c. a procedure that is performed despite it not being authorized
   d. a procedure that is written off

20. _____ is performed to control costs and to ensure a patient's care is medically necessary.
   a. preauthorization
   b. quality improvement
   c. utilization management
   d. accreditation

21. Conditions flagged by CMS to indicate a potential quality issue are known as _____.
   a. hospital acquired conditions
   b. present on admission
   c. complication
   d. comorbidity

22. The Ambulance Fee Schedule requires that a service meet which of the following criteria?
   a. It must be medically necessary.
   b. The patient must have no other form of transportation.
   c. The patient must be covered by Medicare.
   d. Both A and C.

23. SNF PPS groups patients into the following categories.
   a. physical therapy, occupational therapy, speech therapy, nursing, non-therapy
   b. inpatient, outpatient, nonpatient
   c. long-term, short-term, residential living
   d. male, female, other

24. Discounting in the APC payment system can occur in which of the following scenarios?
   a. the patient applies for a discount due to financial hardship
   b. the surgery is cancelled after the patient is prepared for surgery
   c. two or more procedures are performed in the same operative session
   d. b and c

25. In the IPPS, hospitals can qualify for additional payment for which of the following?
   a. teaching medical residents
   b. use of approved technologies
   c. disproportionate number of indigent patients
   d. all of the above

Part II True/False

Write "T" or "F" in the blank to indicate whether you think the statement is true or false.

_____ 26. A patient may leave a hospital against medical advice.

_____ 27. A prospective payment system is a method of reimbursement in which Medicare payment is based on hospital-specific reasonable costs.

_____ 28. The DNFB report is a list of all facility claims that have not been billed to the insurance for payment.

_____ 29. The discharge disposition is documented in the health record to indicate if the patient is improving or terminal when discharged from the hospital.

_____ 30. It is mandatory for a facility to complete the accreditation process.

_____ 31. Hospice services may be provided at any facility or the patient's home.

_____ 32. ASCs can be freestanding or owned by a hospital.

_____ 33. Acute care facilities provide services only on an emergency basis.

_____ 34. CMS requires all ASCs to be certified.

_____ 35. Prospective payment systems were mandated under the Affordable Care Act.

_____ 36. When the cost of a patient's care is excessively large compared to a typical patient it is called a cost outlier.

_____ 37. In the OPPS, every patient is given a status indicator.

_____ 38. The average length of stay in a long-term care hospital must be 25 days or longer.

_____ 39. The IRF PAI measures areas such as mobility, dexterity, mood, thought process, speech, vision and hearing.

_____ 40. The IPF PPS uses the CPT code set to assign codes to claims.

Part III Matching

41. Match the type of service to the appropriate term.

_____ inpatient admission	a. resident assessment instrument
_____ ambulatory surgery center	b. case mix groups
_____ skilled nursing facility	c. ≥25 day stay
_____ long-term health care facility	d. Two-Midnight Rule
_____ hospice	e. HIPPS
_____ critical access hospital	f. APC
_____ inpatient psychiatric facility	g. ≤25 beds
_____ inpatient rehabilitation facility	h. end of life care plan
_____ home health	i. HHRGs

Part IV Fill in the Blank

42. Explain the difference between a complication and a comorbidity.

_____

_____

_____

43. What is the difference between grouper software and outpatient code editors?

_____

_____

_____

44. List six things that are included in an ASC payment?

_____

_____

_____

_____

_____

_____

45. Name three reasons why an LTCH payment may be reduced.

_____

_____

_____

46. Explain the difference between prospective, concurrent and retrospective reviews in utilization management.

_____

_____

_____

_____

47. What are some of the measures included in the ASCQR which could preclude an ASC from receiving full payment? List four.

_____

_____

_____

48. List six examples of never events.

_____

_____

_____

_____

_____

49. Name five payment methodologies besides prospective payment systems.

_____

_____

_____

_____

50. List five examples of facility licensing requirements in most states.

_____

_____

_____

_____

ASSIGNMENT 18.2 PREAUTHORIZATION

Research the internet and identify 10 procedures that frequently require preauthorization from the insurer before completion. Are the procedures covered only if they are done in a particular facility such as an Ambulatory Surgery Center? Are there other stipulations as to when the procedures may be covered or not covered?

ASSIGNMENT 18.3 CALCULATING MS-DRG

For each of the MS-DRGs identified, complete the table. Use the information in Fig. 18.1 below that reflects data extracted from the 2021 MS-DRG tables from the Centers for Medicare and Medicaid Services. The formula for calculating MS-DRG is outlined in the textbook.

Facility base rate is $4,022.00 and the add-on is $340.

MS-DRG	Relative Weight	Calculations
10		
61		
101		
206		
329		

Chapter **18 Introduction to Health Care Facilities and Ambulatory Surgery Centers**

MS-DRG	TABLE 5.—LIST OF MEDICARE SEVERITY DIAGNOSIS-RELATED GROUPS (MS-DRGS), RELATIVE WEIGHTING FACTORS,	Weights
	MS-DRG Title	
007	LUNG TRANSPLANT	11.5743
008	SIMULTANEOUS PANCREAS AND KIDNEY TRANSPLANT	5.4268
010	PANCREAS TRANSPLANT	3.6177
058	MULTIPLE SCLEROSIS AND CEREBELLAR ATAXIA WITH MCC	1.7367
059	MULTIPLE SCLEROSIS AND CEREBELLAR ATAXIA WITH CC	1.1265
060	MULTIPLE SCLEROSIS AND CEREBELLAR ATAXIA WITHOUT CC/MCC	0.9156
061	ISCHEMIC STROKE, PRECEREBRAL OCCLUSION OR TRANSIENT ISCHEMIA WITH THROMBOLYTIC AGENT WITH MCC	2.8882
062	ISCHEMIC STROKE, PRECEREBRAL OCCLUSION OR TRANSIENT ISCHEMIA WITH THROMBOLYTIC AGENT WITH CC	1.9872
099	NON-BACTERIAL INFECTION OF NERVOUS SYSTEM EXCEPT VIRAL MENINGITIS WITHOUT CC/MCC	1.3973
100	SEIZURES WITH MCC	1.8736
101	SEIZURES WITHOUT MCC	0.8870
102	HEADACHES WITH MCC	1.1517
204	RESPIRATORY SIGNS AND SYMPTOMS	0.7925
205	OTHER RESPIRATORY SYSTEM DIAGNOSES WITH MCC	1.6823
206	OTHER RESPIRATORY SYSTEM DIAGNOSES WITHOUT MCC	0.8842
207	RESPIRATORY SYSTEM DIAGNOSIS WITH VENTILATOR SUPPORT >96 HOURS	5.7264
208	RESPIRATORY SYSTEM DIAGNOSIS WITH VENTILATOR SUPPORT <=96 HOURS	2.5423
327	STOMACH, ESOPHAGEAL AND DUODENAL PROCEDURES WITH CC	2.6096
328	STOMACH, ESOPHAGEAL AND DUODENAL PROCEDURES WITHOUT CC/MCC	1.6655
329	MAJOR SMALL AND LARGE BOWEL PROCEDURES WITH MCC	4.8503
330	MAJOR SMALL AND LARGE BOWEL PROCEDURES WITH CC	2.5390
331	MAJOR SMALL AND LARGE BOWEL PROCEDURES WITHOUT CC/MCC	1.7101

Fig. 18.1

ASSIGNMENT 18.4 APC DISCOUNTING

Determine which of the following is subject to discounting.

The status indicator legend can be found at: https://med.noridianmedicare.com/web/jea/provider-types/opps/opps-payment-status-indicators

APC	Status Indicator	Subject to Discounting Yes/No
1	C	
2	S	
3	G	
4	T	

ASSIGNMENT 18.5 CRITIQUE OF THE INPATIENT REHABILITATION FACILITY-PATIENT ASSESSMENT INSTRUMENT (IRF-PAI)

Review the IRF-PAI document found at: https://www.cms.gov/Medicare/Medicare-Fee-for-Service-Payment/Inpatient RehabFacPPS/IRFPAI.html.

Critique the assessment instrument. Answer the following questions using the content from the book and the IRF-PAI to support your opinions.

1. What is the IRF-PAI used for?

2. Why do you think it is important to identify a patient's ethnicity?

3. Why do you think it is important to identify a patient's race?

4. Why do you think it is important to determine a patient's level of literacy?

5. What, if anything, on the assessment instrument surprised you?

19 Billing for Health Care Facilities

Cheryl Fassett

KEY TERMS

Your instructor may wish to select some words pertinent to this chapter for a test. For definitions of the terms, further study, and/or reference, the words, phrases, and abbreviations may be found in the glossary at the end of the Textbook. *Key terms for this chapter follow.*

Approach character
Body Part character
Body System character
Device character
First listed diagnosis
form locators
International Classification of Disease,
    Tenth Edition, Procedure Coding System

National Uniform Billing Committee
principal diagnosis
principal procedure
Qualifier character
reason for encounter
Root Operation character
Section character
Uniform Bill

KEY ABBREVIATIONS

See how many abbreviations and acronyms you can translate, and then use this as a handy reference list. Definitions for the key abbreviations are located near the back of the Textbook *in the glossary.*

CMS-1450 _____

FL _____

ICD-10-PCS _____

NPI _____

NUBC _____

POA _____

PPS _____

UB-04 _____

PERFORMANCE OBJECTIVES

The student will be able to:

- Define and spell the key terms and key abbreviations for this chapter, given the information from the *Textbook* glossary, within a reasonable time period and with enough accuracy to obtain a satisfactory evaluation.
- After reading the chapter, answer the fill-in-the-blank, mix and match, multiple choice, and true/false review

questions, with enough accuracy to obtain a satisfactory evaluation.
- Assign ICD-10-PCS codes to simple procedure descriptions.
- Abstract information from charge master to apply to UB-04.

STUDY OUTLINE

Introduction to Facilities Billing
Outpatient and Inpatient Diagnosis Coding Guidelines
    First Listed Diagnosis
    Principal Diagnosis
Introduction to Inpatient Facility Procedure Coding
    ICD-10-PCS Code Structure
    ICD-10-PCS Coding Manual
    ICD-10-PCS Official Guidelines

CMS 1450/Uniform Bill UB-04
    Section 1: Provider Information
    Section 2: Patient Information
    Section 3: Billing Information
    Section 4: Payer Information
    Section 5: Diagnostic Information

Part I Fill in the Blank

Review the objectives, key terms, glossary definitions of key terms, chapter information, and figures before completing the following review questions.

1. The first listed diagnosis is used for processing _____ claims, while the principal diagnosis is used for processing _____ claims.

2. If a patient is admitted as an inpatient due to a complication from an outpatient surgery, the diagnosis for the _____ should be listed as the principal diagnosis. If no complication is documented, assign the _____. If the patient is admitted for a reason unrelated to the surgery, assign the _____ as the principal diagnosis.

3. The _____ is the code set used to assign inpatient procedures.

4. ICD-10-PCS codes are _____ characters long.

5. List four types of devices identified by the device character.

   _____

   _____

   _____

   _____

6. What is the difference between an open, laparoscopic, or endoscopic procedure?

   _____

   _____

   _____

7. What are the three valid body part characters in the obstetric section?

   _____

   _____

   _____

8. In general, the terms upper and lower in the body part character descriptions refer to body parts located above or below the _____.

9. In a coronary artery bypass, the body part character indicates _____, while the qualifier specifies _____.

10. List the four root operations used when a procedure is performed on a device and not a body part.

    _____

    _____

11. Match the words or phrases used for ICD-10-PCS characters in the left column with the definitions in the right column. Write the correct letters in the blanks.

_____ Section	a.	objective of procedure
_____ Body System	b.	technique used to reach the site of the procedure
_____ Root Operation	c.	medical specialty
_____ Body Part	d.	other information such as the origin of transplant
_____ Approach	e.	area the procedure is performed on
_____ Device	f.	device left in place after the procedure
_____ Qualifier	g.	specific part of the body system procedure is performed on

12. Match the root operation in the left column to its definition in the right column. Write the appropriate letter in the blank.

_____ Alteration	a.	Completely closing an orifice or the opening of a tubular body part
_____ Bypass	b.	Pulling out or stripping out all or a portion of a body part by use of force
_____ Control	c.	Altering the route of passage of the contents of a tubular body part
_____ Creation	d.	Cutting into a body part, without draining fluids and/or gases from the body part, in order to separate or transect a body part
_____ Destruction	e.	Modifying the anatomic structure of a body part without affecting the function of the body part
_____ Detachment	f.	Putting in or on biological or synthetic material to form a new body part that to the extent possible replicates the anatomic structure or function of an absent body part
_____ Division	g.	Taking or cutting out solid matter from a body part
_____ Excision	h.	Freeing a body part from an abnormal physical constraint by cutting or by the use of force
_____ Extirpation	i.	Cutting out or off, without replacement, all of a body part
_____ Extraction	j.	Stopping, or attempting to stop, postprocedural or other acute bleeding
_____ Occlusion	k.	Taking out or off a device from a body part
_____ Release	l.	Cutting out or off, without replacement, a portion of a body part
_____ Removal	m.	Physical eradication of all or a portion of a body part by the direct use of energy force, or a destructive agent
_____ Resection	n.	Moving, without taking out, all or a portion of a body part to another location to take over the function of all or a portion of a body part
_____ Transfer	o.	Cutting off all or a portion of the upper or lower extremities

Part III Multiple Choice

Choose the best answer.

13. An open procedure performed with endoscopic assistance should be coded as
    a. open.
    b. endoscopic.
    c. laparoscopic.
    d. closed.

14. If a biopsy is followed by resection, the coding specialist should code the root operation
    a. excision.
    b. resection.
    c. biopsy.
    d. both biopsy and resection.

15. What organization is responsible for the design and distribution of the CMS-1450?
    a. CMS.
    b. AMA.
    c. NUBC.
    d. AHA.

16. The following types of services are always billed on a CMS-1450 (UB-04)
    a. professional services.
    b. all inpatient services.
    c. ambulatory surgery in an ASC.
    d. ED services.

17. What information is identified by the Type of Bill code on the UB-04?
    a. type of facility.
    b. type of care.
    c. sequence of bill.
    d. all of the above.

18. Procedures performed by force applied to the skin would be coded as
    a. open.
    b. percutaneous.
    c. external.
    d. endoscopic.

19. A procedure using a puncture to insert instrumentation through the skin to visualize the site of the procedure would be coded as
    a. percutaneous endoscopic.
    b. percutaneous.
    c. open.
    d. external.

20. In inpatient procedural coding, a device is coded when
    a. it is used to perform the procedure.
    b. it remains in the body after the procedure.
    c. it is used to visualize the site of the procedure.
    d. it is an external fixation device.

Part IV True/False

Write "T" or "F" in the blank to indicate whether you think the statement is true or false.

_____ 21. All facilities bill using the UB-04 form.

_____ 22. In the absence of a confirmed diagnosis, signs and symptoms may be coded in inpatient claims.

_____ 23. If two or more contrasting diagnoses are given on an inpatient record, only the first listed is coded.

_____ 24. The root operation E in the obstetrical section refers to the delivery of the newborn and is used in both vaginal deliveries and c-sections.

_____ 25. In ICD-10-PCS coding, procedural steps necessary to reach the site and close the site are coded separately.

_____ 26. If a procedure is discontinued before any root operation is performed, it should be coded as Inspection.

_____ 27. If multiple procedures are coded during the same episode, they are never coded separately. Only the most invasive procedure is coded.

_____ 28. Abnormal laboratory findings are always reported on inpatient claims.

CRITICAL THINKING ASSIGNMENTS

ASSIGNMENT 19.2 ASSIGNING CHARACTER 1 FOR SECTION (ICD-10-PCS)

Using Table 19.2 in the textbook, and the ICD-10-PCS, fill in the appropriate section that would be coded for Character 1 Section.

1. A patient with a tumor in the esophagus has an esophagectomy to remove it. _____

2. A patient has his PICC line flushed. _____

3. A patient has his cervical spine manipulated by a chiropractor. _____

4. A patient has amniocentesis for genetic testing. _____

5. A patient has an MRI of the brain. _____

6. A patient has a hearing aid assessment for a cochlear implant. _____

7. A patient has pulmonary function testing. _____

8. A patient has high does Iridium treatment for cancer. _____

9. A patient is on a ventilator in ICU. _____

10. A patient is admitted for a psychiatric evaluation. _____

Using Table 19.3 in the textbook, and the ICD-10-PCS, fill in the appropriate root operation that would be used to code the following procedures.

1. diagnostic dilatation and curettage   _____

2. wedge biopsy of right breast   _____

3. sigmoid colectomy   _____

4. thrombectomy   _____

5. lithotripsy of kidney stones   _____

6. corneal transplant   _____

7. closed reduction of right tibial fracture   _____

8. total knee arthroplasty   _____

9. breast augmentation   _____

10. tubal ligation   _____

Using the ICD-10-PCS, and Procedure 19.1 in the textbook, code the following procedures.

1. A patient has a mitral valve replacement with a synthetic valve. The surgeon uses an open technique.

    _____

2. A patient has an open splenectomy. _____

3. A colonoscopy is discontinued due to poor prep. _____

4. A patient has an extraperitoneal c-section at full-term. _____

5. A patient in the ICU is on a respirator for a week. _____

6. A child has a CT of the brain with and without low osmolar contrast. _____

7. A patient receives cognitive behavioral therapy for alcohol addiction. _____

8. A patient with a possible fungal infection has a toenail biopsy performed. _____

9. An elderly patient receives a left total knee arthroplasty. The surgeon inserts a unicondylar medial synthetic prosthesis. _____

10. A cancer patient receives percutaneous infusion of chemotherapy through central vein catheter.

    _____

11. A patient in the cardiac unit receives an external EKG. _____

12. After suffering a stroke, a patient receives Aphasia (speech) assessment by the speech therapist.

    _____

13. A patient has a triple coronary artery bypass, using patient's own left internal mammary artery. This is done with an open approach. _____

14. A patient requires an application of dressing to the right hand. _____

15. A patient with neck pain receives mechanically assisted chiropractic treatment of cervical spine.

    _____

16. A patient has a bilateral breast augmentation with silicone implants. _____

17. A patient receives a high dose radiation brachytherapy of bladder using Iridium 192. _____

18. A pregnant patient has a MRI of fetal spine with contrast. _____

19. A patient has a right and a left percutaneous cardiac catheterization for sampling and pressure.

    _____

20. A young boy needs an open reduction with internal fixation of his left radius after falling off his bike.

    _____

Using workbook Fig. 19.1 and information in the textbook, answer the following questions regarding the UB-04.

1. Match the following fields on the UB-04 to the description of the data they should contain. Be careful as some of the answers include more than one FL.

FL 50 -51(A-C)	FL12	FL 63 (A-C)	FL 61-62
FL 10	FL42	FL 77	FL 72
FL 74	FL44	FL 1	FL 69
FL 17	FL46	FL 18-28	FL 43
FL 3 (a-b)	FL 53	FL 4	FL 8-9

   a. _____ description of services that link to the revenue code

   b. _____ revenue codes based on type of service or item

   c. _____ number of days, quantity of items or dose of medication for each revenue code

   d. _____ patient's name and address

   e. _____ type of bill code

   f. _____ insured's group name and number

   g. _____ discharge status such as home, SNF, or expired

   h. _____ admitting diagnosis code

   i. _____ patient identifiers such as account number and medical record number

   j. _____ operating physician name and identifier

   k. _____ payer names and identification numbers

   l. _____ treatment authorization codes

   m. _____ condition codes that may affect processing of the claim

   n. _____ principal procedure code and date

   o. _____ external cause of injury code and the present on admission indicator

   p. _____ admission date

   q. _____ patient date of birth

   r. _____ HCPCS codes or accommodation rates

   s. _____ assignment of benefits authorization indicator

   t. _____ billing provider name, address and telephone number

2. Based on information in workbook Fig. 19.1, workbook Fig. 19.2, and the textbook, answer the following questions.

   a. What is the Type of Bill code that would be entered in FL 4 if the UB-04 encompassed the patient's entire inpatient admission? _____

   b. Did the patient complete paperwork allowing the insurance companies to pay the hospital directly? _____ Where would this be indicated on the UB-04? _____

   c. On the final page of the UB-04, what line would list the total charges and what revenue code would be listed? _____, _____ What is the amount that would appear on Ms. Smith's claim form? _____

d. Based on the patient's summary sheet, what are some value codes that may be listed in box 39 to assist the processing of the claim? _____ and _____

e. How many nights was Ms. Smith in the hospital? Where is this information reflected on the UB-04?

f. Where was Ms. Smith admitted from? _____ Where is this information reflected on the UB-04? _____ What code would be used? _____

g. Where was Ms. Smith discharged to? _____ Where is this information reflected on the UB-04? _____ What code would be used? _____

h. What would be entered in FL74?

i. What information would be entered in FL76? _____

j. What information would be entered in FL 69? _____

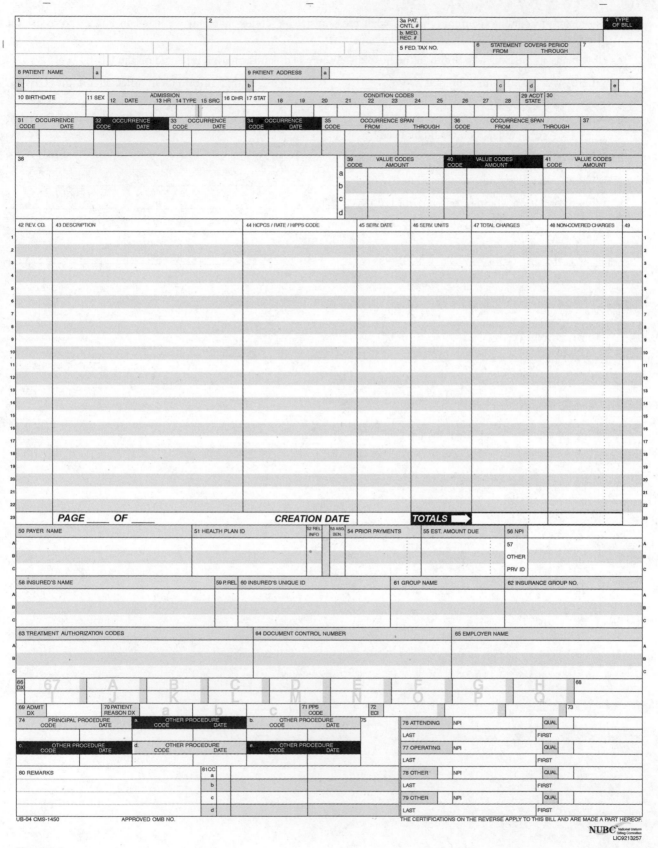

Fig. 19.1

General Hospital		Tax. ID# 12-3456789
123 Main Street		NPI: 1234567890
Anytown, XX 55343		
(888) 123-4567		

PATIENT INFORMATION

Admit: 05/01/20XX 0815	Discharge: 05/04/20XX 1154	Type of admission: Elective	MRN: 25-68-46	Acct#: 987654321	Assignment on file: Yes
Patient Name: Mary Smith	DOB: 01/01/19XX	Address: 629 Mill Rd Anytown, XX 55343	Phone: (869) 555-5555	Condition: pt in SNF, spouse retired	Marital Status: M
Admission source: SNF	Sex: F				Discharge: SNF

INSURANCE INFORMATION

Primary Insurance: Medicare	Insured's Name: Mary Smith	Pt. relationship: self	Identification #: XYZ00533698	Authorization: n/a
Secondary Insurance: ANYPLAN	Insured's Name: Harrold Smith	Pt. relationship: spouse	Identification#: 25568AB8	Authorization: 869580501XX

Attending Physician: Roger Orthostein, MD	Attending Physician NPI: 0987654321
Admitting diagnosis: primary osteoarthritis right knee	Principal diagnosis: primary osteoarthritis right knee, M17.11
Additional diagnoses: HTN	
Principal procedure: 0SRC0JZ right total knee arthroplasty with synthetic prosthesis	Date of principal procedure: 05/01/20XX
Other Procedures:	

CHARGE DETAIL

Revenue Code	Description	HCPCS/Rate	Units	Total Charges	Non-covered Charges
0128	Semiprivate room/board	$3000.00	3	9000.00	
025X	Anesthesia		3	300.00	
0730	EKG/ECG	93000	1	150.00	
0300	Laboratory	85025	1	200.00	
0272	Sterile surgical tray	A4550	1	100.00	
0360	Operating room		2	2500.00	
0250	Pharmacy		10	340.00	
0710	Recovery room		1	200.00	
0278	Synthetic knee prosthesis	JointsRUs	1	4000.00	
0420	Physical Therapy	200.00	4	800.00	
	Medical/surgical		56	10820.00	
TOTAL CHARGE:				$28410.00	

Fig. 19.2

285

20 Seeking a Job and Attaining Professional Advancement

Linda M. Smith

KEY TERMS

Your instructor may wish to select some words pertinent to this chapter for a test. For definitions of the terms, further study, and/or reference, the words, phrases, and abbreviations may be found in the glossary at the end of the textbook. Key terms for this chapter follow.

American Academy of Professional Coders (AAPC)
American Health Information Management
    Association (AHIMA)
application form
auditor
blind mailing
business associate agreement
certification
Certified Coding Specialist
Certified Coding Specialist-Physician
Certified Medical Assistant
Certified Medical Billing Specialist
Certified Professional Coder
Chargemaster Coordinator
chronologic résumé
Clinical Documentation Improvement Specialist
coding specialist

combination résumé
compliance specialist
continuing education
cover letter
employment agencies
functional résumé
interview
mentor
National Certified Insurance and Coding Specialist
networking
portfolio
Registered Medical Assistant
Registered Medical Coder
résumé
Revenue Cycle Manager
self-employment
service contract

KEY ABBREVIATIONS

See how many abbreviations and acronyms you can translate, and then use this as a handy reference list. Definitions for the key abbreviations are located near the back of the textbook in the glossary.

AAPC _____

AHIMA _____

CAP _____

CCAP _____

CCS _____

CCS-P _____

CECP _____

CMA _____

CMBS _____

CMRS _____

CPC _____

CPC-A _____

CPC-H _____

ECP _____

EEOC _____

FCS _____

HRS _____

NCICS _____

PAHCOM _____

RMA _____

RMC _____

USCIS _____

PERFORMANCE OBJECTIVES

The student will be able to:

- Define and spell the key terms and key abbreviations for this chapter, given the information from the *textbook* glossary, within a reasonable time period and with enough accuracy to obtain a satisfactory evaluation.

- After reading the chapter, answer the fill-in-the-blank, multiple choice, and true/false review questions with enough accuracy to obtain a satisfactory evaluation.

- Research information in preparation for creating a résumé, given a worksheet to complete, within a reasonable time period and with enough accuracy to obtain a satisfactory evaluation.

- Create an accurate résumé in a suitable font and print onto plain paper, within a reasonable time period, to obtain a satisfactory evaluation.

- Compose and print on plain paper a letter of introduction to go with the résumé and place it in a typed envelope, using one sheet of plain typing paper and a number 10 envelope, within a reasonable time period, to obtain a satisfactory evaluation.

- Complete an application form for a job, given an application for position form, within a reasonable time period and with enough accuracy to obtain a satisfactory evaluation.

- Compose and print a follow-up thank-you letter onto one sheet of plain paper. Print the address on a number 10 envelope, within a reasonable time period, to obtain a satisfactory evaluation.

- Access the internet and visit websites to research and/or obtain data, within a reasonable time period and with enough accuracy to obtain a satisfactory evaluation.

STUDY OUTLINE

Employment Opportunities
  Insurance Billing Specialist
  Advanced Job Opportunities
Professional Organizations
  Certification
Job Search
  Online Job Search
  Job Fairs
  Application
  Letter of Introduction
  Résumé
  Interview
  Portfolio
  Proof of Citizenship
  Follow-Up Letter
Self-Employment
  Planning your Business
  Professional Mailing Address

Finances to Consider
Business Name and License
Insurance
Business Associate Under the Health Insurance
  Portability and Accountability Act
Service Contract
Pricing Your Services
Security and Equipment
Marketing, Advertising, Promotion, and Public
  Relations
Business Incubator
Reassess and Continue With Success
Attaining Professional Advancement
  Networking
  Find a Mentor

Part I Fill in the Blank

Review the objectives, key terms, glossary definitions of key terms, chapter information, and figures before completing the following review questions.

1. Name three job titles that the insurance billing specialist may find advertised.

   a. _____

   b. _____

   c. _____

2. A _____ specialist works with physicians and other health care professionals to ensure that the documentation in the health record is complete and granular.

3. The process of earning a credential through a professional organization by gaining advanced education and experience is known as _____.

4. You have just completed a 1-year medical insurance billing course at a college. Name some preliminary job search contacts to make on campus.

   a. _____

   b. _____

   c. _____

   d. _____

5. When completing a job application form, the first step should be _____. Why? _____
   _____

6. Name skills that an applicant could list on an application form or in a résumé when they are seeking a position as an insurance billing specialist.

   a. _____

   b. _____

   c. _____

   d. _____

   e. _____

   f. _____

7. A question appears on a job application form about salary. Two ways in which to handle this question are:

   a. _____.

   b. _____.

8. State the chief purpose of a cover letter when a résumé is sent to a prospective employer.
   _____

9. What information may be omitted from a résumé, under the Civil Rights Act of 1964, informed by the EEOC?
   _____

10. A/an _____ is a formal consultation with an employer to evaluate the qualifications of a prospective job applicant.

11. List the items to be compiled in a portfolio.

    a. _____

    b. _____

    c. _____

    d. _____

    e. _____

    f. _____

    g. _____

    h. _____

    i. _____

12. You are being interviewed for a job and the interviewer asks this question: "What is your religious preference?" How would you respond?

    _____

    _____

13. If a short period of time elapses after an interview and the applicant has received no word from the prospective employer, what follow-up steps may be taken?

    a. _____

    b. _____

14. If an individual creates a billing company and coding services are to be part of the offerings, the coding professional should have what type of professional status?

    _____

15. When considering self-employment, remember that the key to a successful business is to begin with a _____
    _____ .

16. Hugh Beason was the owner of XYZ Medical Reimbursement Service. A fire occurred, damaging some of the equipment and part of the office premises requiring him to stop working for a month so that repairs could be made. What type/types of insurance would be helpful for this kind of problem?

    _____

17. A document that outlines the obligations of a billing service and a health care organization stating the responsible party for each specific duty and task is a/an

    _____ .

18. List three methods a self-employed insurance billing specialist may use to price their services.

    a. _____

    b. _____

    c. _____

19. A business _____ is an environment that grows and nurtures small businesses in their early years of existence by offering a wide range of business assistance and shared resources.

20. Gwendolyn Stevens has an insurance billing company and is attending a professional meeting where she has given business cards to a few attendees. Give two reasons for using this business marketing strategy.

    a. _____

    b. _____

21. Give the names of at least two national organizations that certify billers and coders.

    a. _____

    b. _____

Part II Multiple Choice

Choose the best answer.

22. A résumé format that emphasizes work experience dates is known as:
    a. functional.
    b. combination.
    c. business.
    d. chronologic.

23. When an individual plans to start an insurance billing company, he or she should have enough funds to operate the business for a period of:
    a. 6 months or more.
    b. 18 months or more.
    c. 1 year or more.
    d. 2 years.

24. Under Health Insurance Portability and Accountability Act (HIPAA) regulations, if a physician's insurance billing is outsourced to a person, this individual is known as a/an _____ because he or she uses and discloses individuals' identifiable health information.
    a. billing specialist
    b. business associate
    c. outside contractor
    d. outside vendor

25. When insurance billing is outsourced to a company, a document that defines the duties and obligations of each party involved should be created, signed, and notarized by both parties; it is known as a:
    a. contract agreement.
    b. business agreement.
    c. service contract.
    d. legal contract.

26. A guide who offers advice, criticism, and guidance to an inexperienced person to help him or her reach a goal is known as a/an:
    a. mentor.
    b. counselor.
    c. associate.
    d. instructor.

Part III True/False

Write "T" or "F" in the blank to indicate whether you think the statement is true or false.

_____ 27. A résumé format that stresses job skills is known as functional.

_____ 28. When job applicants have similar skills and education, surveys have shown that hiring by employers has been based on bilingual skills.

_____ 29. Enhancing knowledge and keeping up-to-date are responsibilities of an insurance billing specialist.

_____ 30. Professional status of an insurance billing specialist may be obtained by passing a national examination for a Certified Medical Reimbursement Specialist (CMRS).

_____ 31. To earn the status of a claims assistance professionals, this may be obtained by passing a national examination as a certified coding specialist (CCS).

Performance Objective

Task: Read these job advertisements. Then read the interests and abilities of the applicants to decide which job title belongs to each job hunter.

Conditions: Use the job advertisements and a pen or a pencil.

Standards: Time: _____ minutes

                 Accuracy: _____

                 (Note: The time element and accuracy criteria may be given by your instructor.)

Directions: These job openings appeared on various health care websites. Read the ads and then read the interests and abilities of each job applicant. Insert the job title for each applicant.

Job Titles

Insurance Biller	**Insurance Coder**	**Bilingual Collections Manager**
HS grad, computer exp, typing 40 wpm needed for busy output clinic, insurance claims knowledge	Detail-oriented individual, Dx and proc coder. 2 years exp preferred	Self-motivated individual with good communications skills. Bilingual. Enjoys working in health care.

Trudy

Trudy is bilingual in English and Spanish and enjoys working with people. She is especially good with the telephone and likes communications.

Job Title: _____

Walter

Walter wants to work in the health care field. He has taken diagnostic and procedure coding classes and enjoys problem solving.

Job Title: _____

Ilona

Ilona has experience with inputting patient data and transmitting insurance claims. She says she is honest and dependable.

Job Title: _____

           Chapter **20** *Seeking a Job and Attaining Professional Advancement*

Performance Objective

Task: Respond to a job advertisement by completing a worksheet and typing a résumé by abstracting data from your worksheet.

Conditions: Use two sheets of plain typing paper, a newspaper advertisement (Fig. 20.1), and a computer.

Standards: Time: _____ minutes

      Accuracy: _____

      (Note: The time element and accuracy criteria may be given by your instructor.)

Directions: An advertisement appeared on a health care organization's website (see Fig. 20.1). You decide to apply for the position. Complete a worksheet in preparation for typing your résumé. Some of the information requested on the worksheet should not appear on the résumé but should be available if you are asked to provide it. Ask a classmate to review and comment about the information in your worksheet. Extract data that you think are relevant from the worksheet, and type a rough draft of your résumé. Ask the instructor for suggestions to improve the rough draft.

1. Insert title of personal data sheet from worksheet.

2. Insert heading: name, address, telephone number, and so on.

3. Select one of three formats for data.

4. Insert heading and data for education information.

5. Insert heading and data for skill information.

6. Insert heading and data for employment information.

7. Insert reference information.

8. Proofread résumé.

9. Print résumé.

MEDICAL INSURANCE CODING/REIMBURSEMENT SPECIALIST

Mid-Atlantic Clinic, a 20-physician, multi-specialty group practice in Chicago, Illinois, has a need for a coding and reimbursement specialist. Knowledge of medical terminology, CPT and ICD-10-CM coding systems, Medicare regulations, third-party insurance reimbursement, and physician billing procedures required. Proficiency in the interpretation and coding of procedural and diagnostic codes is strongly preferred. Successful candidates must have excellent communication and problem-solving skills. This position offers a competitive salary and superior benefits. Please send resume to:

George B. Pason, Personnel Director
Mid-Atlantic Clinic
1230 South Main Street
Chicago, IL 60611

Fig. 20.1

ASSIGNMENT 20.4 COMPLETE A COVER LETTER

Performance Objective

Task: Compose a cover letter to accompany your résumé.

Conditions: Use one sheet of plain typing paper, a number 10 envelope, computer, printer, thesaurus, and English dictionary.

Standards: Time: _____ minutes

              Accuracy: _____

              (Note: The time element and accuracy criteria may be given by your instructor.)

Directions: Compose a cover letter introducing yourself, and create a rough draft. Consult the instructor for suggestions. Print the cover letter on plain bond paper in a form that can be mailed. Type the name and address of the employer on a number 10 envelope, and insert the letter with the résumé from Assignment 20.3.

ASSIGNMENT 20.5 COMPLETE A JOB APPLICATION FORM

Performance Objective

Task: Complete a job application form by using data from your résumé.

Conditions: Use an application form (Fig. 20.2), your résumé, and a computer.

Standards: Time: _____ minutes

                 Accuracy: _____

                 (Note: The time element and accuracy criteria may be given by your instructor.)

Directions: Assume that the employer asked you to come to his or her place of business to complete an application form and make an appointment for an interview. Using your data and résumé, complete an application form (see Fig. 20.2).

APPLICATION FOR EMPLOYMENT
For Insurance Billing Specialist

Personal Information

Name (Last, First, Middle)	
Area Code/Phone Number	
Present Address (Street)	
Present Address (City, State, Zip)	
Are you a US Citizen? If no, type of Visa, Visa No/ Date of Entry.	

Employment Information

Position you are applying for?	
Full time or part time?	
Date available for employment?	
Wage/salary expectation?	

Professional Licenses and/or Certifications

Organization or State Issued	Date Issued	Number
1.		
2.		
3.		

Education

School	School, Address and Telephone	Dates Attended (To-From)	Did you graduate?	Degree/Major
High School			Yes/No	
College			Yes/No	
Graduate Study			Yes/No	
Other Training			Yes/No	

Fig. 20.2

Special Skills and Abilities

Special Skill/Ability	Yes/No	Explain Experience/Proficiency Level
Claim Form Completion	Yes/No	
Coding - CPT	Yes/No	
Coding – ICD-10	Yes/No	
Collections	Yes/No	
Electronic/Paper Billing	Yes/No	
Payment Posting	Yes/No	
Other:	Yes/No	
Other:	Yes/No	
Other:	Yes/No	

Employment Record (List most recent first)

1.Employer Name Address/Phone Number	A.Position Held B.Supervisor	Dates (From and To)	Reason for Leaving
2.Employer Name Address/Phone Number	Position Held	Dates (From and To)	
3.Employer Name Address/Phone Number	Position Held	Dates (From and To)	
4.Employer Name Address/Phone Number	Position Held	Dates (From and To)	

Personal or Professional References (Other than Relatives

Name Address	Relationship to Applicant and Occupation	Phone Number Email Address
1.		
2.		
3.		

I certify that all answers given by me on this application are true, correct and complete to the best of my knowledge. I acknowledge that the information contained in this application are subject to check.

Signature: _____   Date:_____

Fig. 20.2, cont'd

ASSIGNMENT 20.6 PREPARE A FOLLOW-UP THANK-YOU LETTER

Performance Objective

Task: Prepare a follow-up thank-you letter after the interview, sending it to the interviewer.

Conditions: Use one sheet of plain typing paper, a number 10 envelope, computer, printer, thesaurus, and English dictionary.

Standards: Time: _____ minutes

                Accuracy: _____

                (Note: The time element and accuracy criteria may be given by your instructor.)

Directions: After the interview, you decide to send a follow-up thank-you letter to the person who interviewed you. Compose a letter and address a number 10 envelope

ASSIGNMENT 20.7 VISIT WEBSITES FOR JOB OPPORTUNITIES

Performance Objective

Task: Access the internet and visit several websites.

Conditions: Use a computer with a printer and/or a pen or a pencil to make notes.

Standards: Time: _____ minutes

              Accuracy: _____

              (Note: The time element and accuracy criteria may be given by your instructor.)

Directions: Visit at least five websites by using either a search engine (Yahoo, Google, Bing) or a job-search website. Some suggestions are:

    www.indeed.com
    www.juju.com
    www.linkedin.com
    www.topusajobs.com
    www.monster.com
    www.ziprecruiter.com

Enter a keyword or job title, such as "medical billing specialist" or "medical coder." Enter your city and state to locate listings near you. Click on the search button. If you get some results, print the listings that appeal to you for sharing and discussing in class.

Performance Objective

Task: Write a paragraph describing the benefits of becoming certified in this field.

Conditions: Use a computer with printer and/or a pen or a pencil.

Standards: Time: _____ minutes

               Accuracy: _____

               (Note: The time element and accuracy criteria may be given by your instructor.)

Directions: Write a paragraph or two describing why you would like to become certified in this field, and incorporate a numbered list of benefits. Make sure grammar, punctuation, and spelling are correct.

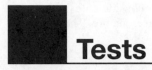

Tests

TEST 1: PROCEDURE (E/M AND MEDICINE SECTIONS) AND DIAGNOSTIC PROCEDURE CODE TEST

Directions: Using a *Current Procedural Terminology* (CPT) codebook insert the correct code numbers and modifiers for each service rendered. Give a brief description for each professional service rendered. An optional exercise is to abstract the pertinent data from each case, then use the *International Classification of Diseases*, Tenth Revision, Clinical Modifications (ICD-10-CM) codebook to insert the diagnosis code.

Insert year of the CPT codebook used:

_____

Insert year of the ICD-10-CM codebook used:

_____

1. Dr. Input sees a new patient, Mrs. Post, in the office for acute abdominal distress. The physician spends approximately 1 hour obtaining a comprehensive history and physical examination with high-complexity decision-making. Several diagnostic studies are ordered, and Mrs. Post is given an appointment to return in 1 week.

Description

_____ CPT # _____
_____ ICD-10-CM # _____

2. Mr. Nakahara, an established patient, sees Dr. Practon in the office on January 11 for a reevaluation of his type 2 diabetic condition. Dr. Practon takes a detailed history and performs a detailed examination. Decision-making is moderately complex.

Description

_____ CPT # _____
_____ ICD-10-CM # _____

3. Dr. Cardi sees Mrs. Franklin for a follow-up office visit for her hypertension. A problem-focused history and examination of her cardiovascular system are obtained and reveal a blood pressure of 140/100. Decision-making is straightforward, with medication being prescribed. The patient is advised to return in 2 weeks to have her blood pressure checked by the nurse. Mrs. Franklin returns 2 weeks later, and the nurse checks her blood pressure.

Description

_____ CPT # _____
_____ ICD-10-CM # _____
_____ CPT # _____
_____ ICD-10-CM # _____

4. Dr. Skeleton receives a call at 7 PM from Mrs. Snyder. Her husband, a patient of Dr. Skeleton's, has been very ill for 2 hours with profuse vomiting. Dr. Skeleton goes to their home to see Mr. Snyder and spends considerable time obtaining a detailed history and examination. The medical decision-making is of a highly complex nature. The physician administers an injection of prochlorperazine (Compazine).

Description

_____ CPT # _____

_____ CPT # _____

_____ ICD-10-CM # _____

5. Dr. Cutis sees an established patient, a registered nurse, for determination of pregnancy. A detailed history and examination are obtained, with moderate-complexity medical decision-making. A Papanicolaou smear is taken, a blood sample is drawn, and the specimens are sent to an independent laboratory for a qualitative human chorionic gonadotropin (hCG) test. The patient also complains of something she has discovered under her armpit. On examination, there is a furuncle of the left axilla, which is incised and drained during this visit. The laboratory requires CPT coding on the laboratory requisition. List how these laboratory procedures would appear on the requisition sheet. The Papanicolaou smear is processed according to the Bethesda System and under physician supervision.

Professional Service Rendered by Dr. Cutis

_____ CPT # _____

_____ CPT # _____

_____ CPT # _____

_____ CPT # _____

_____ ICD-10-CM # _____

_____ ICD-10-CM # _____

Laboratory Service on Requisition Sheet

_____ CPT # _____

_____ CPT # _____

6. Dr. Antrum makes a house call on Betty Mason, an established patient, for a problem-focused history of acute otitis media. A problem-focused examination is performed, with straightforward medical decision-making. While there, Dr. Antrum also sees Betty's younger sister, Sandra, whom she has seen previously in the office, for acute tonsillitis. A problem-focused history and examination are performed with low-complexity decision-making. In addition to the examinations, Dr. Antrum gives both children injections of penicillin.

Professional Service Rendered to Betty

_____ CPT # _____

_____ CPT # _____

_____ ICD-10-CM # _____

Professional Service Rendered to Sandra

_____ CPT # _____

_____ CPT # _____

_____ ICD-10-CM # _____

7. Two weeks later, Dr. Antrum is called to the emergency department at College Hospital at 2 AM on Sunday to see Betty Mason for recurrent chronic otitis media with suppuration. A problem-focused history and examination are performed with straightforward decision-making. Dr. Antrum administers a second injection of penicillin.

Description

_____ CPT # _____
_____ CPT # _____
_____ CPT # _____
_____ ICD-10-CM # _____

8. While at the hospital, Dr. Antrum is asked to see another patient in the emergency department, who is new to her. She performs an intermediate 3.5 cm laceration repair of the scalp. The patient is advised to come to the office in 4 days for a dressing change. Four days later, the patient comes into the office for a dressing change by the nurse.

Description

_____ CPT # _____
_____ ICD-10-CM # _____

9. Dr. Menter, a psychiatrist, sees the following patients in the hospital. Code each procedure.

Ms. Blake: consultation, expanded problem-focused history and
examination and straightforward decision-making; referred by Dr. Practon CPT # _____

Mrs. Clark: group psychotherapy (50 min) CPT # _____

Mrs. Samson: group psychotherapy (50 min) CPT # _____

Mr. Shoemaker: group psychotherapy (50 min) CPT # _____

Miss James: individual psychotherapy (25 min) CPT # _____

10. Dr. Input, a gastroenterologist, sees Mrs. Chan in the hospital at the request of Dr. Practon for an esophageal ulcer. In addition to the detailed history and examination and the low-complexity decision-making, Dr. Input performs a flexible, transoral esophagogastroduodenoscopy with washings. Two days later, he sees Mrs. Chan in a follow-up hospital visit and obtains a problem-focused interval history and examination with low-complexity decision-making.

Description

_____ CPT # _____
_____ CPT # _____
_____ ICD-10-CM # _____

_____
_____ CPT # _____

11. Mrs. Galati, a new patient, goes to Dr. Cardi because of chest pain (moderate to severe), weakness, fatigue, and dizziness. Dr. Cardi takes a comprehensive history and performs a comprehensive examination, followed by a treadmill ECG with interpretation and report. He also performs a vital capacity test and dipstick urinalysis, and draws blood for triiodothyronine () testing and for analysis by sequential multiple analyzer computer (SMAC) (16 panel tests, including complete blood cell count [CBC]), which are sent to and billed by a laboratory. Medical decision-making is of high complexity.

Description

_____ CPT # _____
_____ CPT # _____
_____ CPT # _____
_____ CPT # _____

305

_____ CPT # _____
_____ CPT # _____
_____ ICD-10-CM # _____
_____ ICD-10-CM # _____
_____ ICD-10-CM # _____

12. Jake Wonderhill has not had his eyes examined by Dr. Lenser for about 5 years. He is seen by Dr. Lenser, who performs the following ophthalmologic procedures in addition to a comprehensive eye examination: fluorescein angioscopy and electroretinography (full field). Mr. Wonderhill receives a diagnosis of retinitis pigmentosa.

Description

_____ CPT # _____
_____ CPT # _____
_____ CPT # _____
_____ ICD-10-CM # _____

13. Dr. Practon is making rounds at the College Hospital and answers an urgent call on Third Floor East. He performs cardiopulmonary resuscitation on Mr. Sanchez for cardiac arrest and orders the patient taken to the critical care unit. Chest radiographs, laboratory work, blood gas measurements, and ECG are performed. The physician is detained 2 hours in constant attendance on the patient.

Description

_____ CPT # _____
_____ CPT # _____
_____ CPT # _____
_____ ICD-10-CM # _____

14. Mrs. Powers, a new patient, sees Dr. Skeleton for sciatica with lumbago. Dr. Skeleton takes a detailed history and performs a detailed examination of the patient's lower back and extremities. Medical decision-making is of low complexity. Diathermy (30 minutes) is given. The next day the patient comes in for therapeutic exercises in the Hubbard tank (30 minutes).

Description

_____ CPT # _____
_____ CPT # _____
_____ ICD-10-CM # _____
_____ CPT # _____
_____ ICD-10-CM # _____

15. a. Mrs. Garcia, a new patient, is seen by Dr. Caesar for occasional vaginal bleeding (detailed history/examination and low-complexity decision-making). The doctor determines that the bleeding is coming from the cervix and asks her to return in 3 days for cryocauterization of the cervix. During the initial examination, Mrs. Garcia asks for an evaluation for possible infertility. Dr. Caesar advises her to wait 2 to 3 weeks and make an appointment for two infertility tests.

    b. When the patient returns in 3 days for cryocauterization, the doctor also takes a wet mount for bacteria/fungi, which is sent to and billed by a laboratory.

    c. Three weeks later, an injection procedure for hysterosalpingography and endometrial biopsy are performed.

Description

a. _____ CPT # _____

   _____ ICD-10-CM # _____

b. _____ CPT # _____

   _____ CPT # _____

   _____ ICD-10-CM # _____

c. _____ CPT # _____

   _____ CPT # _____

   _____ ICD-10-CM # _____

Multiple Choice

After reading the boxed codes with descriptions, select the answer/answers that is/are best in each case.

59120	Surgical treatment of ectopic pregnancy; tubal or ovarian, requiring salpingectomy and/or oophorectomy, abdominal or vaginal approach
59121	tubal or ovarian, without salpingectomy and/or oophorectomy
59130	abdominal pregnancy
59135	interstitial, uterine pregnancy requiring total hysterectomy
59136	interstitial, uterine pregnancy with partial resection of uterus
59140	cervical, with evacuation

16. In regard to this section of CPT codes, which of the following statements is true about codes 59120 through 59140? Mark all that apply.
    a. They refer to abdominal hysterotomy.
    b. They involve laparoscopic treatment of ectopic pregnancy.
    c. They refer to treatment of ectopic pregnancy by surgery.
    d. They involve tubal ligation.

17. In regard to this section of CPT codes, for treatment of a tubal ectopic pregnancy, necessitating oophorectomy, the code to select is
    a. 59121.
    b. 59120.
    c. 59135.
    d. 59136.
    e. 59130.

18. In regard to this section of CPT codes, for treatment of an ectopic pregnancy (interstitial, uterine) requiring a total hysterectomy, the code/codes to select is/are
    a. 59135.
    b. 59135 and 59120.
    c. 59120.
    d. 59130 and 59120.
    e. 59121.

Directions: Match the description given in the right column with the procedure code/modifier combination in the left column. Write the letter in the blank.

Procedure With Modifier   **Description**

1. 99214-25 _____   a. Dr. Practon assisted Dr. Caesar with a total abdominal hysterectomy and bilateral salpingo-oophorectomy.

2. 99204-57 _____   b. Dr. Skeleton interprets a thoracolumbar x-ray film that was taken at College Hospital.

3. 58150-80 _____   c. Mrs. Ulwelling saw Dr. Antrum for an office visit as a new patient, and she recommended that the patient undergo a laryngoscopy, with stripping of vocal cords to be done the following day.

4. 32440-55 _____   d. Mrs. Gillenbach walked through a plate glass window and underwent a rhinoplasty, performed by Dr. Graff on February 16, 20xx. On February 26, 20xx, she came to see Dr. Graff for a consultation regarding reconstructive surgery on her right leg.

5. 72080-26 _____   e. An established patient, Mrs. Mercado, is seen in a follow-up exam for type 2 diabetes. The patient asks Dr. Langerhans to look at some skin tags. The doctor examines them and says they need to be removed (11200). The evaluation and management service was detailed and of a moderate complexity.

6. 29425-58 _____   f. Dr. Cutler performed a bilateral orchiopexy (inguinal approach) on baby Kozak.

7. 54640-50 _____   g. Dr. Skeleton applied a short leg-walking cast to Mrs. Belchere's right leg 4 weeks after his initial treatment of her fractured tibia.

8. 99253-24 _____   h. Dr. Cutler went on vacation, and Dr. Coccidioides took care of Mrs. Ash during the postoperative period after her total pneumonectomy.

Directions: Using a CPT codebook, insert the correct code numbers and modifiers for each service rendered. Give a brief description for each professional service rendered.

9. Dr. Input performs a gastrojejunostomy for carcinoma in situ of the duodenum and calls in Dr. Scott to administer the anesthesia and Dr. Cutler to assist. This intraperitoneal surgery takes 2 hours, 30 minutes. The patient is otherwise normal and healthy. List the procedure and diagnostic code numbers with appropriate modifiers for each physician.

Professional Service Rendered by Dr. Input
_____ CPT # _____
_____ ICD-10-CM # _____

Professional Service Rendered by Dr. Scott
_____ CPT # _____
_____ ICD-10-CM # _____

Professional Service Rendered by Dr. Cutler
_____ CPT # _____
_____ ICD-10-CM # _____

10. Dr. Rumsey assists Dr. Cutler with a total colectomy (intraperitoneal procedure) with ileostomy. Dr. Scott is the anesthesiologist. Surgery takes 2 hours, 55 minutes. The patient has a secondary malignant neoplasm of the colon (severe systemic disease). List the procedure code numbers with appropriate modifiers and diagnostic code numbers for each physician.

Professional Service Rendered by Dr. Rumsey

_____ CPT # _____
_____ ICD-10-CM # _____

Professional Service Rendered by Dr. Scott

_____ CPT # _____
_____ ICD-10-CM # _____

Professional Service Rendered by Dr. Cutler

_____ CPT # _____
_____ ICD-10-CM # _____

11. Dr. Cutis removes a malignant tumor from a patient's back (1.5 cm) and does the local anesthesia herself.

Description

_____ CPT # _____
_____ ICD-10-CM # _____

12. Dr. Skeleton sees Mr. Richmond, a new patient worked into the office schedule on an emergency basis after a motor vehicle traffic accident with another car. Mr. Richmond has multiple lacerations of the face, arm, and chest and a fracture of the left tibia. The physician takes a comprehensive history and performs a comprehensive examination. Decision-making is moderately complex. Dr. Skeleton orders bilateral radiographs of the tibia and fibula and two views of the chest and left wrist to be taken in his office. Then he closes the following lacerations: 2.6 cm, simple, face; 2.0 cm, intermediate, face; 7.5 cm, intermediate, right arm; 4.5 cm, intermediate, chest. All radiographs are negative except that of the left tibia. Dr. Skeleton performs a manipulative reduction of the left tibial shaft and applies a cast. Code this case as if you were actually listing the codes on the CMS-1500 claim form.

Description

_____ CPT # _____ and _____
_____ CPT # _____
_____ CPT # _____
_____ CPT # _____
_____ CPT # _____
_____ CPT # _____
_____ CPT # _____
_____ CPT # _____
_____ CPT # _____
_____ CPT # _____
_____ ICD-10-CM # _____
_____ ICD-10-CM # _____
_____ ICD-10-CM # _____
_____ ICD-10-CM # _____
_____ ICD-10-CM # _____

Six weeks later, Dr. Skeleton sees the same patient for an office visit and obtains radiographs (two views) of the left tibia and fibula. Treatment involves application of a cast below the patient's left knee to the toes, including a walking heel.

Description

_____ CPT # _____
_____ CPT # _____
_____ CPT # _____
_____ ICD-10-CM # _____

13. Dr. Cutler performs an incisional biopsy of a patient's breast for a breast lump, which requires 40 minutes of anesthesia. Dr. Scott is the anesthesiologist. The patient is otherwise normal and healthy. List the procedure and diagnostic code numbers for each physician.

Professional Service Rendered by Dr. Cutler

_____ CPT # _____

_____ ICD-10-CM # _____

Professional Service Rendered by Dr. Scott

_____ CPT # _____

_____ ICD-10-CM # _____

14. Mrs. DeBeau is aware that Dr. Input will be out of town for 6 weeks; however, she decides to have him perform the recommended combined anterior-posterior colporrhaphy with enterocele repair for vaginal enterocele. Dr. Practon agrees to perform the follow-up care and assist. Dr. Scott is the anesthesiologist. The anesthesia time is 2 hours, 15 minutes. The patient is normal and healthy. List the procedure and diagnostic code numbers for each physician. Note: Emphasis for this problem should be placed on the choice of CPT modifiers.

Professional Service Rendered by Dr. Input

_____ CPT # _____

_____ ICD-10-CM # _____

Professional Service Rendered by Dr. Practon

_____ CPT # _____

_____ CPT modifier _____

_____ CPT modifier _____

_____ ICD-10-CM # _____

Professional Service Rendered by Dr. Scott

_____ CPT # _____

_____ ICD-10-CM # _____

15. Mr. Wong is seen in the College Hospital. Dr. Coccidioides performs a bronchoscopy with biopsy. Results of the biopsy confirm the diagnosis: malignant neoplasm of upper left lobe of lung. The following day the physician performs a total pneumonectomy. Dr. Cutler assists on the total pneumonectomy (pulmonary resection), and Dr. Scott is the anesthesiologist. Surgery takes 3 hours, 45 minutes. The patient has mild systemic disease. List the procedure and diagnostic code numbers for each physician.

Professional Service Rendered by Dr. Coccidioides

_____ CPT # _____

_____ CPT # _____

_____ ICD-10-CM # _____

Professional Service Rendered by Dr. Cutler

_____ CPT # _____

_____ ICD-10-CM # _____

Professional Service Rendered by Dr. Scott

_____ CPT # _____

_____ ICD-10-CM # _____

When completing the CMS-1500 claim form for Dr. Scott, in which block would you list anesthesia minutes? _____

_____

TEST 3: PROCEDURE (RADIOLOGY AND PATHOLOGY SECTIONS) AND DIAGNOSTIC CODE TEST

Directions: Using a CPT codebook, insert the correct procedure code numbers and modifiers and diagnostic codes for each service rendered. Give a brief description for each professional service rendered.

1. Mrs. Cahn sees Dr. Skeleton because of severe pain in her right shoulder. She is a new patient. Dr. Skeleton takes a detailed history and performs a detailed examination. A complete x-ray study of the right shoulder is done. Decision-making is of low complexity. A diagnosis of bursitis is made, and an injection into the bursa is administered.

Description

_____ CPT # _____
_____ CPT # _____
_____ CPT # _____
_____ ICD-10-CM # _____

2. John Murphy comes into the Broxton Radiologic Group, Inc., for an extended radiation therapy consultation for prostatic cancer. The radiologist takes a detailed history and does a detailed examination. Decision-making is of low complexity. The physician determines a simple treatment plan involving simple simulation-aided field settings. Basic dosimetry calculations are done, and the patient returns the following day and receives radiation therapy to a single treatment area (6-10 MeV).

Description

_____ CPT # _____
_____ CPT # _____
_____ CPT # _____
_____ CPT # _____
_____ CPT # _____

Diagnosis:

_____ ICD-10-CM # _____

3. Dr. Input refers Mrs. Horner to the Nuclear Medicine Department of the Broxton Radiologic Group, Inc., for a bone marrow imaging of the whole body, and imaging of the liver and spleen. List the procedure code numbers after each radiologic procedure to show how the radiology group would bill. Also, list the diagnosis of malignant neoplasm of the bone marrow.

Description

Total body bone marrow, imaging CPT # _____

Radiopharmaceuticals, diagnostic (iodine I-123) HCPCS # _____

Liver and spleen imaging CPT # _____

Radiopharmaceuticals, diagnostic (iodine I-123) HCPCS # _____

Diagnosis:

_____ ICD-10-CM # _____

4. Dr. Input also refers Mrs. Horner to XYZ Laboratory for the following tests. List the procedure code numbers to indicate how the laboratory would bill.

Description

CBC, automated, and automated differential CPT # _____

Urinalysis, automated with microscopy CPT # _____

Urine culture (quantitative, colony count) CPT # _____

Urine antibiotic sensitivity (microtiter) CPT # _____

5. The general laboratory at College Hospital receives a surgical tissue specimen (ovarian biopsy) for gross and microscopic examination from a patient with Stein-Leventhal syndrome. List the procedure and diagnostic code numbers to indicate what the hospital pathology department would bill.

Description

_____ CPT # _____

Diagnosis:

_____ ICD-10-CM # _____

6. Dr. Langerhans refers Jerry Cramer to XYZ Laboratory for a lipid panel. He has a family history of cardiovascular disease. List the procedure and diagnostic code number or numbers to indicate how the laboratory would bill.

Description

_____ CPT # _____

Diagnosis:

_____ ICD-10-CM # _____

7. Dr. Caesar is an OB/GYN specialist who has her own ultrasound machine. Carmen Cardoza, age 45, is referred to Dr. Caesar for an obstetric consultation and an amniocentesis with ultrasonic guidance. The diagnosis is Rh incompatibility. The doctor performs a detailed history and physical examination, and decision-making is of low complexity.

Description

_____ CPT # _____
_____ CPT # _____
_____ CPT # _____

Diagnosis:

_____ ICD-10-CM # _____

8. Mr. Marcos's medical record indicates that a retrograde pyelogram followed by a percutaneous nephrostolithotomy, with basket extraction of a 1 cm stone, was performed by Dr. Ulibarri for nephrolithiasis.

Description

_____ CPT # _____
_____ CPT # _____

Diagnosis:

_____ ICD-10-CM # _____

9. Broxton Radiologic Group, Inc., performs the following procedures on Mrs. Stephens at the request of Dr. Input. List the procedure code numbers after each radiologic procedure. On the laboratory slip, the following congenital diagnoses are listed: diverticulum of the stomach and colon; cystic lung. Locate the corresponding diagnostic codes.

Barium enema CPT # _____

Evaluation of upper gastrointestinal tract with small bowel CPT # _____

Complete chest x-ray CPT # _____

Diagnosis:

_____ ICD-10-CM # _____

Diagnosis:

_____ ICD-10-CM # _____

Diagnosis:

_____ ICD-10-CM # _____

10. Two weeks later, Mrs. Stephens is referred again for further radiologic studies for flank pain. List the procedure and diagnostic code numbers after each radiologic procedure.

Intravenous pyelogram (IVP) with drip infusion CPT # _____

Oral cholecystography CPT # _____

Diagnosis:
_____ ICD-10-CM # _____

Performance Objective

Task: Complete a CMS-1500 claim form for a private case

Conditions: Use the patient's record (Fig. 1) one health insurance claim form; a computer or a pen; procedural and diagnostic codebooks; and Appendix A in this *Workbook*.

Standards: Claim Productivity Management

                     Time: _____ minutes

                     Accuracy: _____

                     (Note: The time element and accuracy criteria may be given by your instructor.)

Directions:

1. Using NUCC guidelines, complete a CMS-1500 claim form and direct it to the private carrier. Refer to Jennifer T. Lacey's patient record for information and Appendix A in this *Workbook* to locate the fees to record on the claim, and post them to the financial statement. Date the claim August 15 of the current year. Dr. Caesar is accepting assignment, and the patient's signatures to release information to the insurance company and to have the payment forwarded directly to the physician are on file.

2. Use your CPT codebook to determine the correct five-digit code numbers and modifiers for each professional service rendered. Use your HCPCS Level II codebook for HCPCS procedure codes and modifiers. Use your ICD-10-CM coding manual to code each active diagnosis.

PATIENT RECORD NO. T-4

Lacey	Jennifer	T.	11-12-55	F	555-549-0098
LAST NAME	FIRST NAME	MIDDLE NAME	BIRTH DATE	SEX	HOME PHONE

451 Roberts Street	Woodland Hills	XY	12345
ADDRESS	CITY	STATE	ZIP CODE

555-443-9899	555-549-0098		lacey@wb.net
CELL PHONE	PAGER NO.	FAX NO.	E-MAIL ADDRESS

430-XX-7709	Y0053498
PATIENT'S SOC. SEC. NO.	DRIVER'S LICENSE

legal secretary	Higgins and Higgins Attorneys at Law
PATIENT'S OCCUPATION	NAME OF COMPANY

430 Second Avenue, Woodland Hills, XY 12345	555-540-6675
ADDRESS OF EMPLOYER	PHONE

SPOUSE OR PARENT	OCCUPATION

EMPLOYER	ADDRESS	PHONE

American Commercial Insurance Company, 5682 Bendix Blvd., Woodland Hills, XY 12345	
NAME OF INSURANCE	INSURED OR SUBSCRIBER

5789022	444
POLICY/CERTIFICATE NO.	GROUP NO.

REFERRED BY: Clarence Cutler, MD

Fig. 1

DATE	PROGRESS NOTES No. T-4
8-1-xx	New pt referred by Dr. Cutler, came into office for consultation and additional opinion.
	CC: Full feeling in stomach and low abdominal region.
	Irregular menstruation. Ultrasonic report showed
	leiomyoma of uterus and rt ovarian mass; however, visualization of mass poor and type
	cannot be identified. Pap smear Class I. No personal or family hx of CA.
	Comprehensive hx and physical examination performed on healthy appearing white female.
	Wt: 136 lbs. BP 128/60. T 98.6 F. Palpated rt adnexal mass and
	enlarged uterus; vulva and cervix appear normal; LMP 7/16/XX.
	Medical decision-making: mod complex
	Tx plan: Adv hospital admit and additional tests to R/O carcinoma.
	Tentatively scheduled abdominal hysterectomy with bilateral salpingo-oophorectomy.
	Moderate medical decision making
	BC/llf *Bertha Caesar, MD*
8-2-xx	Adm to College Hosp. A comprehensive history and exam was performed; moderate medical decision-making.
	Scheduled surgery at 7:00 A.M. tomorrow.
	BC/llf *Bertha Caesar, MD*
8-3-xx	Perf abdominal
	hysterectomy with bilateral salpingo-oophorectomy.
	BC/llf *Bertha Caesar, MD*
8-4-xx	Hospital Visit. An expanded problem-focused history and exam was performed; moderate medical decision
	making. Path report revealed Leiomyoma of uterus and corpus luteum cyst of rt ovary. Pt C/O PO pain,
	otherwise doing well. BC/llf *Bertha Caesar, MD*
8-5-xx	Hospital visit. An expanded problem-focused history and exam was performed; moderate medical decision-
	making. Pt ambulating well, pain decreased. Dressing changed, wound healing well.
	BC/llf *Bertha Caesar, MD*
8-6-xx	Hospital visit; problem-focused history and exam; straight forward medical decision-making. Pain minimal.
	Pt ambulating without assistance. Removed staples, no redness or swelling. Pln DC tomorrow.
	BC/llf *Bertha Caesar, MD*
8-7-xx	Discharged home; pt doing well. RTO next wk. Disability from 8-1 to 8-23-xx.
	BC/llf *Bertha Caesar, MD*

Fig. 1 cont'd

Performance Objective

Task: Complete a CMS-1500 claim form for a private case and post transactions to the patient's financial accounting record.

Conditions: Use the patient's record (Fig. 2) and financial statement (Fig. 3), one health insurance claim form, a computer or a pen, procedural and diagnostic codebooks, and Appendixes A in this *Workbook*.

Standards: Claim Productivity Management

                      Time: _____ minutes

                      Accuracy: _____

                      (Note: The time element and accuracy criteria may be given by your instructor.)

Directions

1. Using NUCC guidelines, complete a CMS-1500 claim form and direct it to the private carrier. Refer to Hortense N. Hope's patient record for information and Appendix A in this *Workbook* to locate the fees to record on the claim, and post them to the financial statement. Date the claim July 31 of the current year. Dr. Practon is accepting assignment, and the patient's signatures to release information to the insurance company and to have the payment forwarded directly to the physician are on file.

2. Use your CPT codebook to determine the correct five-digit code numbers and modifiers for each professional service rendered. Use your HCPCS Level II codebook for HCPCS procedure codes and modifiers. Use your ICD-10-CM coding manual to code each active diagnosis.

3. Record the proper information on the financial record and claim form, and note the date that you billed the insurance company.

PATIENT RECORD NO. T-5

Hope	Hortense	N.	04-12-56	F	555-666-7821
LAST NAME	FIRST NAME	MIDDLE NAME	BIRTH DATE	SEX	HOME PHONE

247 Lantern Pike	Woodland Hills	XY	12345
ADDRESS	CITY	STATE	ZIP CODE

	555-323-1687	555-666-7821	hope@wb.net
CELL PHONE	PAGER NO.	FAX NO.	E-MAIL ADDRESS

321-XX-0009	N0058921
PATIENT'S SOC. SEC. NO.	DRIVER'S LICENSE

Clerk typist	R and S Manufacturing Company
PATIENT'S OCCUPATION	NAME OF COMPANY

2271 West 74 Street, Torres, XY 12349	555-466-5890
ADDRESS OF EMPLOYER	PHONE

Harry J. Hope	carpenter
SPOUSE OR PARENT	OCCUPATION

Jesse Construction Company, 3861 South Orange Street, Torres, XY 12349	555-765-2318
EMPLOYER ADDRESS	PHONE

Ralston Insurance Company, 2611 Hanley Street, Woodland Hills, XY 12345	Hortense N. Hope
NAME OF INSURANCE	INSURED OR SUBSCRIBER

ATC321458809	T8471811A
POLICY/CERTIFICATE NO.	GROUP NO.

REFERRED BY: Harry J. Hope (husband)

DATE	PROGRESS NOTES
7-1-xx	New F pt comes in complaining of lt great toe pain. Incised, drained, and cleaned area
	around nail on lt great toe. Dx: onychia and paronychia. Started on antibiotic and adv to
	retn in 2 days for permanent excision of nail plate. Expanded problem-focused history and exam performed;
	straightforward medical decision making. GP/llf *Gerald Practon, MD*
7-3-xx	Pt returns for nail excision. Injected procaine in lt great toe; removed entire toenail.
	Drs applied. PTR in 5 days for PO check.
	GP/llf *Gerald Practon, MD*
7-7-xx	PO check. Dressing changed, nail bed healing well. Pt to continue on AB until gone.
	Retn PRN Problem-focused history and exam performed. Straightforward medical decision-making.
	GP/llf *Gerald Practon, MD*

Fig. 2

Acct No. T-5

STATEMENT
Financial Account
COLLEGE CLINIC
4567 Broad Avenue
Woodland Hills, XY 12345-0001
Tel. 555-486-9002
Fax No. 555-487-8976

Hortense N. Hope
247 Lantern Pike
Woodland Hills, XY 12345

Phone No. (H) 555-666-7821   (W)   555-466-5890   Birthdate 4/12/56

Primary Insurance Co. Ralston Insurance Company   Policy/Group No. ATC321458809 / T8471811A

Secondary Insurance Co. None   Policy/Group No.

DATE	REFERENCE	DESCRIPTION	CHARGES	CREDITS PYMNTS.	ADJ.	BALANCE	
20xx		BALANCE FORWARD ➔					
7-1-xx		I & D lt great toe					
7-3-xx		Excision lt great toenail					
7-7-xx		PO check					

PLEASE PAY LAST AMOUNT IN BALANCE COLUMN ⬆

THIS IS A COPY OF YOUR FINANCIAL ACCOUNT AS IT APPEARS ON OUR RECORDS

Fig. 3

TEST 6: COMPLETE A CLAIM FORM FOR A MEDICARE CASE

Performance Objective

Task: Complete a CMS-1500 claim form and post transactions to the patient's financial accounting record.

Conditions: Use the patient's record (Fig. 4) and financial statement (Fig. 5), one health insurance claim form, a computer or a pen, procedural and diagnostic codebooks, and Appendix A in this *Workbook*.

Standards: Claim Productivity Management

Time: _____ minutes

Accuracy: _____

(Note: The time element and accuracy criteria may be given by your instructor.)

Directions

1. Using NUCC guidelines, complete a CMS-1500 claim form and direct it to your local Medicare Administrative Contractor. Refer to the CMS website to locate your local Medicare Administrative Contractor's address to mail the claim to. Refer to Frances F. Foote's patient record for information and Appendix A in this *Workbook* to locate the fees to record on the claim, and post them to the financial statement. Date the claim October 31 of the current year. Dr. Practon is a participating provider, and the patient's signatures to release information to the insurance company and to have the payment forwarded directly to the physician are on file.

2. Use your CPT codebook to determine the correct five-digit code numbers and modifiers for each professional service rendered. Use your HCPCS Level II codebook for HCPCS procedure codes and modifiers. Use your ICD-10-CM coding manual to code each active diagnosis.

3. Record the proper information on the patient's financial accounting record and claim form, and note the date that you billed the insurance company.

PATIENT RECORD NO. T-6

Foote	Frances	F.	08-10-32	F	555-678-0943
LAST NAME	FIRST NAME	MIDDLE NAME	BIRTH DATE	SEX	HOME PHONE

984 North A Street	Woodland Hills	XY	12345
ADDRESS	CITY	STATE	ZIP CODE

555-443-9908	555-320-7789	555-678-0943	foote@wb.net
CELL PHONE	PAGER NO.	FAX NO.	E-MAIL ADDRESS

578-XX-8924	B4309811
PATIENT'S SOC. SEC. NO.	DRIVER'S LICENSE

retired legal secretary	
PATIENT'S OCCUPATION	NAME OF COMPANY

ADDRESS OF EMPLOYER	PHONE

Harry L. Foote	roofer
SPOUSE OR PARENT	OCCUPATION

BDO Construction Company, 340 North 6th Street, Woodland Hills, XY 12345	555-478-9083
EMPLOYER ADDRESS	PHONE

Medicare	self
NAME OF INSURANCE	INSURED OR SUBSCRIBER

578-XX-8924A	
POLICY/CERTIFICATE NO.	GROUP NO.

REFERRED BY: G. U. Curette, MD, 4780 Main Street, Ehrlich, XY 12350 Tel: 555-430-8788   NPI #34216600XX

DATE	PROGRESS NOTES
10-11-xx	NP pt referred by Dr. Curette with a CC of foot pain centering around rt great toe and
	sometimes shooting up her leg. Problem-focused history taken. Problem-focused exam revealed severe
	overgrowth of nail into surrounding tissues. AP and lat right foot x-rays taken & interpreted which
	indicate no fractures or arthritis. Pt has had a N workup for gout by Dr. Curette.
	DX: Severe onychocryptosis both margins of rt hallux. Adv to sched. OP surgery at
	College Hospital for wedge resection of skin of nail fold to repair ingrown nail.
	No disability from work (Straight forward medical decision-making).
	NP/llf *Nick Pedro, MD*
10-13-xx	Pt admitted for OP surgery at College Hospital. Complete wedge resection performed for
	repair of rt hallux ingrown nail. Pt will stay off foot over the weekend and retn next wk for
	PO re ch.
	NP/llf *Nick Pedro, MD*
10-20-xx	PO visit. Problem-focused history and exam. Straight forward medical decision-making. Rt hallux healing well.
	RTC as necessary. NP/llf *Nick Pedro, MD*

Fig. 4

Acct No. T-6

STATEMENT
Financial Account
COLLEGE CLINIC
4567 Broad Avenue
Woodland Hills, XY 12345-0001
Tel. 555-486-9002
Fax No. 555-487-8976

Frances F. Foote
984 North A Street
Woodland Hills, XY 12345

Phone No. (H) 555-678-0943   (W) _____   Birthdate 8/10/32

Primary Insurance Co. Medicare   Policy/Group No. 578-XX-8924A

DATE	REFERENCE	DESCRIPTION	CHARGES	CREDITS		BALANCE	
				PYMNTS.	ADJ.		
20xx		BALANCE FORWARD					
10-11-xx		NP OV					
10-11-xx		X-rays					
10-13-xx		Wedge excision/skin of nail fold					
10-20-xx		PO					

PLEASE PAY LAST AMOUNT IN BALANCE COLUMN

THIS IS A COPY OF YOUR FINANCIAL ACCOUNT AS IT APPEARS ON OUR RECORDS

Fig. 5

Performance Objective

Task: Complete two CMS-1500 claim forms for a Medicare/Medigap case and post transactions to the patient's financial accounting record.

Conditions: _____Use patient's record (Fig. 6) and financial statement (Fig. 7), two health insurance claim forms, a computer or a pen, procedural and diagnostic codebooks, and Appendix A in this *Workbook*.

Standards: Claim Productivity Management

                        Time: _____ minutes

                        Accuracy: _____

                        (Note: The time element and accuracy criteria may be given by your instructor.)

Directions

1. Using NUCC guidelines, complete two CMS-1500 claim forms and direct them to your local Medicare Administrative Contractor. Refer to the CMS website to locate your local Medicare Administrative Contractor's address to mail the claim to. Refer to Charles B. Kamb's patient record for information and Appendix A to locate the fees to record on the claim, and post them to the financial statement. Be sure to include the Medigap information on the claim form so that it will be crossed over (sent to the Medigap insurance carrier) automatically. Date the claim June 30 of the current year. Dr. Practon is a participating provider with both Medicare and the Medigap program, and the patient's signatures to release information to the insurance companies and to have the payment forwarded directly to the physician are on file.

2. Use your CPT codebook to determine the correct five-digit code numbers and modifiers for each professional service rendered. Use your HCPCS Level II codebook for HCPCS procedure codes and modifiers. Use your ICD-10-CM coding manual to code each active diagnosis.

3. Record the proper information on the patient's financial accounting record and claim form, and note the date that you billed the insurance company.

PATIENT RECORD NO. T-7

Kamb	Charles	B.	01-26-27	M	555-467-2601
LAST NAME	FIRST NAME	MIDDLE NAME	BIRTH DATE	SEX	HOME PHONE

2600 West Nautilus Street	Woodland Hills	XY	12345	
ADDRESS	CITY	STATE	ZIP CODE	

CELL PHONE	PAGER NO.	FAX NO.	E-MAIL ADDRESS

454-XX-9569	M3200563
PATIENT'S SOC. SEC. NO.	DRIVER'S LICENSE

retired TV actor	Amer. Federation of TV & Radio Artists (AFTRA)
PATIENT'S OCCUPATION	NAME OF COMPANY

30077 Ventura Boulevard, Woodland Hills, XY 12345	555-400-3331
ADDRESS OF EMPLOYER	PHONE

Jane C. Kamb	homemaker
SPOUSE OR PARENT	OCCUPATION

EMPLOYER	ADDRESS	PHONE

Medicare (Primary)	self	National Insurance Company (Medigap)
NAME OF INSURANCE	INSURED OR SUBSCRIBER	

454-XX-9569A	Medigap Policy No. 5789002
POLICY/CERTIFICATE NO.	GROUP NO.

REFERRED BY: Mrs. O. S. Tomy (friend) National PAYRID NAT234567

DATE	PROGRESS NOTES
6-1-xx	New pt comes into ofc to est new PCP in area; recently moved from Ohio. W obese M c/o
	nasal bleeding for two and a half months c̄ headaches and nasal congestion. Pt states he
	has had HBP for 1 yr. Taking med: Serpasil prescribed by dr in Ohio; does not know dosage.
	A comprehensive history and physical were performed which revealed post nasal hemorrhage.
	Moderate medical decision-making which revealed post nasal hemorrhage. Coagulation time (Lee and White)
	and microhematocrit (spun) done in ofc are WNL. BP 180/100. Used nasal cautery and post nasal packs to control
	hemorrhage. Rx prophylactic antibiotic to guard against sinusitis NKA. Adv retn tomorrow, bring hypertensive
	medication. Pt signed authorization to request med records from dr in Ohio. D: Recurrent epistaxis
	due to nonspecific hypertension. No disability from work.
	GP/llf Gerald Practon, MD
6-2-xx	Pt retns and nasal hemorrhage is reevaluated. Postnasal packs
	removed and replaced. BP 182/98. Pt forgot medication for hypertension but states he is
	taking it 2 X d. Adv retn in 1 day, bring medication.
	GP/llf Gerald Practon, MD
6-3-xx	Pt retns and nasal hemorrhage is reevaluated. Postnasal packs removed. BP 178/100. Expanded problem-
	focused history and exam performed to evaluate HTN. Low medical decision-making. Verified
	hypertensive medication. Pt to increase dosage to 4 X d. Pt referred to Dr. Perry Cardi (int) for future care of HTN
	GP/llf Adv retn in 5 days. Gerald Practon, MD
6-8-xx	Pt retns and nasal hemorrhage is reevaluated Pt referred to Dr. Perry Cardi (int) for future care of hypertension.
	Prev medical records arrived and reviewed. BP 190/102.
	GP/llf Gerald Practon, MD

Fig. 6

Acct No. __T-7__

STATEMENT
Financial Account
COLLEGE CLINIC
4567 Broad Avenue
Woodland Hills, XY 12345-0001
Tel. 555-486-9002
Fax No. 555-487-8976

Charles B. Kamb
2600 West Nautilus Street
Woodland Hills, XY 12345

Phone No. (H) ___555-467-2601___ (W) ___None/retired___ Birthdate ___1-26-27___

Primary Insurance Co. ___Medicare___ Policy/Group No. ___454-XX-9569A___

Secondary Insurance Co. ___National Insurance Company (Medigap)___ Policy/Group No. ___5789002___

DATE	REFERENCE	DESCRIPTION	CHARGES	CREDITS PYMNTS.	ADJ.	BALANCE	
20xx		BALANCE FORWARD ⟶					
6-1-xx		NP OV					
6 -xx		Coagulation time					
6-1-xx		Microhematocrit					
6-1-xx		Post nasal pack/cautery					
6-2-xx		Subsequent nasal pack					
6-3-xx		OV					
6-8-xx		OV					

PLEASE PAY LAST AMOUNT IN BALANCE COLUMN ⬆

THIS IS A COPY OF YOUR FINANCIAL ACCOUNT AS IT APPEARS ON OUR RECORDS

Fig. 7

Performance Objective

Task: Complete a CMS-1500 claim form for a Medicaid case and post transactions to the patient's financial accounting record.

Conditions: _____ Use the patient's record (Fig. 8) and financial statement (Fig. 9), one health insurance claim form, a computer or a pen, procedural and diagnostic codebooks, and Appendix A in this *Workbook*.

Standards: _____Claim Productivity Management

Time: _____ minutes

Accuracy: _____

(Note: The time element and accuracy criteria may be given by your instructor.)

Directions

1. Using NUCC guidelines, complete a CMS-1500 claim form and direct it to the Medicaid fiscal intermediary for your state. Refer to Louise K. Herman's patient record for information and Appendix A to locate the fees to record on the claim, and post them to the financial statement. Date the claim May 31 of the current year.

2. Use your CPT codebook to determine the correct five-digit code numbers and modifiers for each professional service rendered. Use your HCPCS Level II codebook for HCPCS procedure codes and modifiers. Use your ICD-10-CM coding manual to code each active diagnosis.

3. Record the proper information on the patient's financial accounting record and claim form and note the date that you billed the insurance company.

4. Post the payment of $350 (voucher number 4300), received from the Medicaid fiscal intermediary 40 days after claim submission, and write off (adjust) the balance of the account.

PATIENT RECORD NO. T-8

Herman	Louise	K.	11-04-60	F	555-266-9085
LAST NAME	FIRST NAME	MIDDLE NAME	BIRTH DATE	SEX	HOME PHONE

13453 Burbank Boulevard	Woodland Hills	XY	12345
ADDRESS	CITY	STATE	ZIP CODE

555-466-7003		555-266-9085	herman@wb.net
CELL PHONE	PAGER NO.	FAX NO.	E-MAIL ADDRESS

519-XX-0018	T0943995
PATIENT'S SOC. SEC. NO.	DRIVER'S LICENSE

unemployed budget analyst	
PATIENT'S OCCUPATION	NAME OF COMPANY

ADDRESS OF EMPLOYER	PHONE

Harold D. Herman	retired salesman
SPOUSE OR PARENT	OCCUPATION

EMPLOYER	ADDRESS	PHONE

Medicaid	self
NAME OF INSURANCE	INSURED OR SUBSCRIBER

0051936001X	
MEDICAID NO.	GROUP NO.

REFERRED BY: Raymond Skeleton, MD

DATE	PROGRESS NOTES
5-6-xx	NP pt referred by Dr. Skeleton. CC: Rectal bleeding. Took a comprehensive history and
	performed a comprehensive physical examination. Diagnostic anoscopy revealed
	bleeding int and ext hemorrhoids and 2 infected rectal polyps. Rx antibiotic. Retn in
	2 days for removal of hemorrhoids and polyps. Moderate medical decision-making.
	RR/llf *Rex Rumsey, MD*
5-8-xx	Pt returned to office for simple internal/external hemorrhoidectomy.
	Continue on AB until gone. Adv. sitz baths daily.
	Retn in 1 wk.
	RR/llf *Rex Rumsey, MD*
5-15-xx	DNS Telephoned pt and rescheduled.
	Mary Bright, CMA
5-17-xx	PO OV Expanded problem-focused history and exam performed. Low complexity medical decision-making.
	Pt progressing well. No pain, discomfort or bleeding. Discharged from care, retn PRN.
	RR/llf *Rex Rumsey, MD*

Fig. 8

Tests

Copyright © 2023 by Elsevier, Inc. All rights reserved.

Acct No. T-8

STATEMENT
Financial Account
COLLEGE CLINIC
4567 Broad Avenue
Woodland Hills, XY 12345-0001
Tel. 555-486-9002
Fax No. 555-487-8976

Louise K. Herman
13453 Burbank Boulevard
Woodland Hills, XY 12345

Phone No. (H)   555-266-9085   (W) _____   Birthdate ____ 11/4/60 _____

Primary Insurance Co.   Medicaid _____   Policy/Group No.   0051936001X _____

Secondary Insurance Co. _____   Policy/Group No. _____

| DATE | REFERENCE | DESCRIPTION | CHARGES | CREDITS | | BALANCE | |
				PYMNTS.	ADJ.		
20xx			BALANCE FORWARD ⟶				
5-6-xx		NP OV					
5-6-xx		Dx anoscopy					
5-8-xx		Int/Ext Hemorrhoidectomy					
5-17-xx		PO OV					

PLEASE PAY LAST AMOUNT IN BALANCE COLUMN ⟰

THIS IS A COPY OF YOUR FINANCIAL ACCOUNT AS IT APPEARS ON OUR RECORDS

Fig. 9

TEST 9: COMPLETE A CLAIM FORM FOR A TRICARE CASE

Performance Objective

Task: Complete a CMS-1500 claim form for a TRICARE case and post transactions to the patient's financial accounting record.

Conditions: _____Use the patient's record (Fig. 10) and financial statement (Fig. 11), one health insurance claim form, a computer or a pen, procedural and diagnostic codebooks, and Appendix A in this *Workbook*.

Standards: _____Claim Productivity Management

Time: _____ minutes

Accuracy: _____

(Note: The time element and accuracy criteria may be given by your instructor.)

Directions

1. Using NUCC guidelines, complete a CMS-1500 claim form and direct it to the TRICARE carrier for your area. Refer to Darlene M. Cash's patient record for information and Appendix A to locate the fees to record on the claim, and post them to the financial statement. Date the claim February 27 of the current year. Dr. Cutler is accepting assignment, and the patient's signatures to release information to the insurance company and to have the payment forwarded directly to the physician are on file.

2. Use your CPT codebook to determine the correct five-digit code numbers and fees for each professional service rendered. Use your HCPCS Level II codebook for HCPCS procedure codes and modifiers. Use your ICD-10-CM coding manual to code each active diagnosis.

3. Record the proper information on the patient's financial accounting record and claim form, and note the date that you billed the insurance company.

PATIENT RECORD NO. T-9

Cash	Darlene	M.	3-15-70	F	555-666-8901
LAST NAME	FIRST NAME	MIDDLE NAME	BIRTH DATE	SEX	HOME PHONE

5729 Redwood Avenue	Woodland Hills	XY	12344
ADDRESS	CITY	STATE	ZIP CODE

555-290-5400		555-666-8901	cash@wb.net
CELL PHONE	PAGER NO.	FAX NO.	E-MAIL ADDRESS

298-XX-6754	J3457789
PATIENT'S SOC. SEC. NO.	DRIVER'S LICENSE

teacher	City Unified School District
PATIENT'S OCCUPATION	NAME OF COMPANY

Century High School, 2031 West Olympic Boulevard, Dorland, XY 12345	555-678-1076
ADDRESS OF EMPLOYER	PHONE

David F. Cash	Navy Petty Officer—Grade 8 (active status)
SPOUSE OR PARENT	OCCUPATION

United States Navy	HHC, 2nd Batt, 26th Infantry, APO New York, NY, 10030	
EMPLOYER	ADDRESS	PHONE

TRICARE Standard	David Cash (DOB 4-22-70)
NAME OF INSURANCE	INSURED OR SUBSCRIBER

767 XX 9080	
POLICY/CERTIFICATE NO.	GROUP NO.

REFERRED BY: Hugh R. Foot, MD, 2010 Main St., Woodland Hills, XY 12345   NPI #61 25099XX

DATE	PROGRESS NOTES
1-4-xx	New pt, referred by Dr. Foot comes in complaining of head pain which began yesterday.
	Performed an expanded problem-focused history and physical exam. Lt parietal area of skull slightly
	tender, some redness of scalp. Pain localized and not consistent with HA syndromes. Rest of
	exam N. Imp: head pain, undetermined nature, possible cyst. Apply hot compresses and
	observe. Take Ibuprofen for pain prn (200 mg up to 2 q. 4 h). Retn in 1 wk, no disability
	from work. Straight forward medical decision-making.
	CC/llf *Clarence Cutler, MD*
1-11-xx	Pt retns and states that the hot compresses have helped but is concerned with some
	swelling in area. On exam noticed slt elevation of skin in lt parietal area of scalp, no
	warmth over area. Slt pain on palpation. Exam otherwise neg. Imp: Subcutaneous nodule.
	Continue with same tx plan: Hot compresses daily and Ibuprofen prn. Retn in 2-3 wks
	if not resolved. Expanded problem-focused history and exam performed. Low complexity medical decision
	making. CC/llf *Clarence Cutler, MD*
2-3-xx	Pt retns for reexamination of parietal skull. Elevation of skin still persisting. It has now
	come to a head, is warm to the touch, and consistent with an inflammatory cystic lesion.
	A decision is made to excise the benign lesion. Scalp cyst, 1.5 cm removed under
	procaine block with knife dissection; closed wound with six #000 black silk sutures.
	Adv to retn 1 wk for removal of sutures
	CC/llf *Clarence Cutler, MD*
2-10-xx	Pt presents for suture removal. Sutures removed and slight oozing occurs in midsection
	of wound. Wound dressed and pt advised to apply antibacterial cream daily. Retn in 4 to
	5 days for final check. Problem-focused history and exam. Straight forward medical decision-making.
	CC/llf *Clarence Cutler, MD*
2-15-xx	Pt presents for PO check of head wound. Parietal area healed well. RTO prn
	Problem-focused history and exam. Straight forward medical decision-making.
	CC/llf *Clarence Cutler, MD*

Fig. 10

329

Acct No. ___T-9___

STATEMENT
Financial Account
COLLEGE CLINIC
4567 Broad Avenue
Woodland Hills, XY 12345-0001
Tel. 555-486-9002
Fax No. 555-487-8976

Darlene M. Cash
5729 Redwood Avenue
Woodland Hills, XY 12345

Phone No. (H) ___555-666-8901___ (W) ___555-678-1076___   Birthdate ___3/15/70___

Primary Insurance Co. _TRICARE Standard_____   Policy/Group No. ___767-XX-9080___

Secondary Insurance Co._____   Policy/Group No._____

DATE	REFERENCE	DESCRIPTION	CHARGES	CREDITS		BALANCE	
				PYMNTS.	ADJ.		
20xx		BALANCE FORWARD ⟶					
1-4-xx		NP OV					
1-11-xx		OV					
2-3-xx		Excision inflammatory cystic scalp lesion					
2-10-xx		OV					
2-15-xx		OV					
		PLEASE PAY LAST AMOUNT IN BALANCE COLUMN ⇧					

THIS IS A COPY OF YOUR FINANCIAL ACCOUNT AS IT APPEARS ON OUR RECORDS

Fig. 11

Performance Objective

Task: Complete two CMS-1500 claim forms for a private case and post transactions to the patient's financial accounting record.

Conditions: Use the patient's record (Fig. 12) and financial statement (Fig. 13), two health insurance claim forms, a computer or a pen, procedural and diagnostic codebooks, and Appendix A in this *Workbook*.

Standards: _____Claim Productivity Management

Time: _____ minutes

Accuracy: _____

(Note: The time element and accuracy criteria may be given by your instructor.)

Directions

1. Using NUCC guidelines, complete two CMS-1500 claim forms and direct them to the private carrier. Refer to Gertrude C. Hamilton's patient record for information and Appendix A in this *Workbook* to locate the fees to record on the claim, and post them to the financial statement. Date the first claim August 15 and the second one October 15. Dr. Cardi is accepting assignment, and the patient's signatures to release information to the insurance company and to have the payment forwarded directly to the physician are on file.

2. Use your CPT codebook to determine the correct five-digit code numbers and modifiers for each professional service rendered. Use your HCPCS Level II codebook for HCPCS procedure codes and modifiers. Use your ICD-10-CM coding manual to code each active diagnosis. Frequently, surgeons wait to receive the pathology report before entering a final diagnosis on the claim form. In this case, the claim was submitted before the pathology report was received.

3. Record the proper information on the financial record and claim form, and note the date that you billed the insurance company.

4. Mrs. Hamilton makes a payment of $200, check number 5362, on her account on October 26. Post the proper entry for this transaction.

PATIENT RECORD NO. T-10

Hamilton	Gertrude	C.	03-06-57	F	555-798-3321
LAST NAME	FIRST NAME	MIDDLE NAME	BIRTH DATE	SEX	HOME PHONE

5320 Phillips Street	Woodland Hills	XY	12345
ADDRESS	CITY	STATE	ZIP CODE

555-399-4990	555-312-6677	555-798-3321	hamilton@wb.net
CELL PHONE	PAGER NO.	FAX NO.	E-MAIL ADDRESS

540-XX-7677   D9043557
PATIENT'S SOC. SEC. NO.   DRIVER'S LICENSE

retired secretary
PATIENT'S OCCUPATION   NAME OF COMPANY

ADDRESS OF EMPLOYER   PHONE

deceased
SPOUSE OR PARENT   OCCUPATION

EMPLOYER   ADDRESS   PHONE

Colonial Health Insurance, 1011 Main Street, Woodland Hills, XY 12345   self
NAME OF INSURANCE   INSURED OR SUBSCRIBER

540XX7677   4566 (through previous employment)
POLICY/CERTIFICATE NO.   GROUP NO.

REFERRED BY: Gerald Practon, MD, 4567 Broad Avenue, Woodland Hills, XY 12345

Fig. 12

DATE	PROGRESS NOTES No. T-10
7-29-xx	Dr. Practon asked me to consult on this 57-year-old pt adm to College Hosp today.
	Duplex carotid ultrasonography indicates bilateral carotid stenosis. Comprehensive history: Suffered CVA lt
	hemisphere 1 yr prior to adm. Marked rt arm & leg weakness c̄ weakness of rt face and
	slurring of speech. Comprehensive exam revealed lt carotid bruit, II/IV, & right carotid bruit, II/IV.
	Performed hand-held Doppler vascular study on bilateral carotids which indicated
	decreased blood flow. Adv brain scan and lt carotid thromboendarterectomy; rt carotid
	thromboendarterectomy at a later date. High complexity medical decision-making.
	PC/llf *Perry Cardi, MD*
7-30-xx	Hospital visit. Expanded problem-focused history and exam. Moderate medical decision-making. Dr. Practon
	asked me to take over pt's care. Pt had a brain scan done today, ECG, and lab work.
	PC/llf *Perry Cardi, MD*
7-31-xx	Hospital visit. Expanded problem-focused history and exam. Moderate medical decision-making. Brain scan
	indicates prior CVA; no new findings. ECG, normal sinus rhythm with occasional premature ventricular
	contractions. Lab work WNL. Discussed test results with Mrs. Hamilton.
	PC/llf *Perry Cardi, MD*
8-1-xx	Hospital visit. Problem-focused history and exam. Low complexity medical decision-making. Decision made
	for surgery, to be scheduled tomorrow. PC/llf *Perry Cardi, MD*
8-2-xx	Pt taken to the operative suite. Performed lt carotid thromboendarterectomy by neck
	incision (see op report). The Surgery went as planned, pt in recovery.
	PC/llf *Perry Cardi, MD*
8-3-xx	Hospital visit. Problem-focused history and exam. Straightforward medical decision-making. The operative site
	appears normal. Pt resting comfortably. PC/llf *Perry Cardi, MD*
8-4-xx	DC from hosp. Pt to be seen in ofc in 1 week.
	PC/llf *Perry Cardi, MD*
8-12-xx	PO Office visit. Detailed history and exam. Moderate complexity medical decision making. Discussed the outcome
	of surgery. Pt making satisfactory progress. Adv rt carotid thromboendarterectomy. Pt would like it done as soon
	as possible; next month if there is an operative time. Scheduled surgery for September 16, 20XX at
	College Hospital.
	PC/llf *Perry Cardi, MD*
9-16-xx	Adm to College Hospital. Performed a detailed history, detailed physical examination, and straightforward
	medical decision-making. Rt carotid thromboendarterectomy performed by neck incision.
	DX: Rt carotid stenosis.
	PC/llf *Perry Cardi, MD*
-17-xx	Hospital visit. Problem-focused history and exam. Straightfoward medical decision-making. Pt stable and doing
	well. Operative site looks good. Plan for discharge tomorrow.
	PC/llf *Perry Cardi, MD*
9-8-xx	DC from hosp to home. RTC 1 wk.
	PC/llf *Perry Cardi, MD*
9-2-xx	PO visits Office visit. Problem-focused history and exam. Straightforward medical decision-making. Pt making
	a satisfactory recovery. Her neighbor will monitor BP daily. Retn 1 month.
	PC/llf *Perry Cardi, MD*

Fig. 12 cont'd

STATEMENT

COLLEGE CLINIC
4567 Broad Avenue
Woodland Hills, XY 12345-0001
Tel. 555-486-9002
Fax No. 555-487-8976

Acct No. T-10

Gertrude C. Hamilton
5320 Phillips Street
Woodland Hills, XY 12345

Phone No. (H) ____(555) 798-3321____ (W) _____ Birthdate ____03-06-57____

Insurance Co ____Colonial Health Insurance_____ Policy/Group No. 540Xx7677 4566

20xx	REFERENCE	DESCRIPTION	CHARGES	CREDITS PYMNTS.	ADJ.	BALANCE
20xx		BALANCE FORWARD →				
7-29-xx		Inpatient consult				
7-30-xx		HV				
7-31-xx		HV				
8-1-xx		HV				
8-2-xx		L carotid thromboendarterectomy				
8-3-xx		HV				
8-4-xx		Discharge				
8-12-xx		PO OV				
9-16-xx		Admit				
9-16-xx		R carotid thromboendarterectomy				
9-17-xx		HV				
9-18-xx		Discharge				
9-25-xx		PO OV				

PLEASE PAY LAST AMOUNT IN BALANCE COLUMN ⬆

THIS IS A COPY OF YOUR FINANCIAL ACCOUNT AS IT APPEARS ON OUR RECORDS

Fig. 13

Tests

College Clinic Office Policies and Mock Fee Schedule

College Clinic

In this simulation, you are employed as an insurance billing specialist for a group of medical doctors, other allied health specialists, and podiatrists. Each clinic is configured in its own way. The College Clinic has staff physicians who are employed, receive monthly paychecks, and are given Wage and Tax Statements (Form W-2) at the end of the tax year. These doctors are on the staff of a nearby hospital, College Hospital.

Medical practices can have different configurations. For example, individuals or groups can be incorporated. Physicians can be independent contractors, running their own practices outside of the clinic; receive payment by the job and not a salary; and receive a Form 1099 at the end of the tax year.

Reference information to complete insurance claim forms for each assignment follows. Claim forms are to be submitted for the group unless a case involves a physician working as an independent contractor.

Office address:
College Clinic
4567 Broad Avenue
Woodland Hills, XY 12345-0001
Telephone: 555-486-9002

FAX: 555-487-8976
Clinic e-mail: cclinic@cmail.net
Staff e-mail: insert physician's last name followed by a period (.) then cclinic@cmail.net
(example: Pedro Atrics, MD, would have an e-mail address of atrics.cclinic@cmail.net
Group practice, National Provider Identifier (NPI): 3664021CC
Medicare durable medical equipment (DME) supplier number: 3400760001
Group Federal tax ID #: XX12210XX

Hospital address:
College Hospital
4500 Broad Avenue
Woodland Hills, XY 12345-0001
Telephone: 555-487-6789
FAX: 555-486-8900
Hospital NPI: X950731067

College Clinic Staff

Patient records in this *Workbook* include the doctors' names, specialties, subspecialties, and physicians' identification numbers of the College Clinic staff. They are shown in Table 1.

Table 1. College Clinic Staff.

Name	Specialty (Abbreviation)	Social Security No.[a]	State License No.	EIN No. or Federal Tax Identification No.	Medicare CMS-Assigned National Provider Identifier (NPI)[b]
Concha Antrum, MD	Otolaryngologist (OTO) or Ear, Nose, and Throat Specialist (ENT)	082–XX–1707	C 01602X	74–10640XX	12458977XX
Pedro Atrics, MD	Pediatrician (PD)	134–XX–7600	D 06012X	71–32061XX	37640017XX
Bertha Caesar, MD	Obstetrician and Gynecologist (OBG)	230–XX–6700	A 01817X	72–57130XX	43056757XX
Perry Cardi, MD	Internist (I) Subspecialty: Cardiovascular Disease (CD)	557–XX–9980	C 02140X	70–64217XX	67805027XX
Brady Coccidioides, MD	Internist (I) Subspecialty: Pulmonary Disease (PUD)	670–XX–0874	C 04821X	75–67321XX	64211067XX
Vera Cutis, MD	Dermatologist (D)	409–XX–8620	C 06002X	71–80561XX	70568717XX
Clarence Cutler, MD	General Surgeon (GS)	410–XX–5630	B 07600X	71–57372XX	43050047XX
Max Glutens, RPT	Physical Therapist (PT)	507–XX–4300	87610X	79–36500XX	65132277XX
Cosmo Graff, MD	Plastic Surgeon (PS)	452–XX–9899	C 08104X	74–60789XX	50307117XX
Malvern Grumose, MD	Pathologist (Path)	470–XX–2301	A 01602X	72–73651XX	
Gaston Input, MD	Internist (I) Subspecialty: Gastroenterologist (GE)	211–XX–6734	C 08001X	75–67210XX	32783127XX
Adam Langerhans, MD	Endocrinologist	447–XX–6720	C 06051X	60–57831XX	47680657XX
Cornell Lenser, MD	Ophthalmologist (OPH)	322–XX–8963	C 06046X	61–78941XX	54037217XX
Michael Menter, MD	Psychiatrist (P)	210–XX–5302	C 07140X	73–66577XX	67301237XX
Astro Parkinson, MD	Neurosurgeon (NS)	210–XX–8533	C 02600X	75–44530XX	46789377XX
Nick Pedro, DPM	Podiatrist	233–XX–4300	E 08340X	62–74109XX	54022287XX
Gerald Practon, MD	General Practitioner (GP) or Family Practitioner (FP)	123–XX–6789	C 01402X	70–34597XX	46278897XX
Walter Radon, MD	Radiologist (R)	344–XX–6540	C 05001X	95–46137XX	40037227XX
Rex Rumsey, MD	Proctologist (Proct)	337–XX–9743	C 03042X	95–32601XX	01999047XX
Sensitive E. Scott, MD	Anesthesiologist (Anes)	220–XX–5655	C 02041X	72–54203XX	99999267XX
Raymond Skeleton, MD	Orthopedist (ORS, Orthop)	432–XX–4589	C 04561X	74–65412XX	12678547XX
Gene Ulibarri, MD	Urologist (U)	990–XX–3245	C 06430X	77–86531XX	25678831XX

[a]Social Security numbers are shown in the table because each individual is issued one and this is a realistic picture because they would be on file.

[b]Providers began using the NPI on May 23, 2007, except for small health plans, whose compliance date was May 23, 2008.

Abbreviations and Symbols

Abbreviations and symbols may appear on patient records, prescriptions, hospital charts, and patient ledger cards. Abbreviation styles differ, but the current trend is to omit periods in capital letter abbreviations except for doctors' academic degrees. Following is a list of abbreviations and symbols used in this *Workbook* and their meanings.

Abbreviations

A	allergy
AB	antibiotics
Abdom	abdomen
abt	about
a.c.	before meals
Adj[a]	adjustment
adm	admit; admission; admitted
adv	advise(d)
aet	at the age of
agit	shake or stir
AgNO$_3$	silver nitrate
ALL	allergy
AM, a.m.	ante meridiem (time—before noon)
ant	anterior
ante	before
AP	anterior-posterior; anteroposterior
approx	approximate
appt	appointment
apt	apartment
ASA	acetylsalicylic acid (aspirin)
ASAP	as soon as possible
ASCVD	arteriosclerotic cardiovascular disease
ASHD	arteriosclerotic heart disease
asst	assistant
auto	automated, automobile
AV	atrioventricular
Ba	barium (enema)
Bal/fwd[a]	balance forward
BE	barium enema
B/F[a]	balance forward; brought forward
b.i.d.	two times daily
BM	bowel movement
BMR	basal metabolic rate
BP	blood pressure
Brev	Brevital sodium
BX, bx	biopsy
C	cervical (vertebrae); comprehensive (history/examination)
Ca, CA	cancer, carcinoma
c/a[a]	cash on account
CABG	coronary artery bypass graft
CAT	computed axial tomography
cau	Caucasian
CBC	complete blood count
CBS	chronic brain syndrome
cc	cubic centimeter
CC	chief complaint
chr	chronic
ck[a]	check
cm	centimeter
CO, c/o	complains of; care of
compl, comp	complete; comprehensive
Con, CON, Cons	consultation
Cont	continue
CPX	complete physical examination
C&R	compromise and release
Cr[a]	credit
C&S	culture and sensitivity
cs, CS[a]	cash on account
C-section	cesarean section
CT	computed or computerized tomography
CVA	cardiovascular accident; cerebrovascular accident
CXR	chest radiograph
cysto	cystoscopy
D, d	diagnosis; detailed (history/examination); day(s)
D&C	dilatation and curettage
dc	discontinue
DC	discharge
DDS	Doctor of Dental Surgery
def[a]	charge deferred
Del	delivery; obstetrics and gynecology
Dg	diagnosis
dia	diameter
diag	diagnosis; diagnostic
dil	dilate (stretch, expand)
Disch	discharge
DM	diabetes mellitus
DNA	does not apply
DNS	did not show
DPM	Doctor of Podiatric Medicine
DPT	diphtheria, pertussis, and tetanus
Dr	Doctor
Dr[a]	debit
DRG	diagnosis-related group
Drs	dressing
DUB	dysfunctional uterine bleeding
Dx	diagnosis
E	emergency
EC[a]	error corrected
ECG, EKG	electrocardiogram; electrocardiograph
echo	echocardiogram; echocardiography
ED	emergency department
EDC	estimated date of confinement
EEG	electroencephalograph
EENT	eye, ear, nose, and throat

[a]Bookkeeping abbreviation.

EGD	esophagogastroduodenoscopy		I&D	incision and drainage
EKG, ECG	electrocardiogram; electrocardiograph		I/f[a]	in full
E/M	Evaluation and Management (*Current Procedural Terminology* code)		IM	intramuscular (injection)
			imp, imp.	impression (diagnosis)
			incl.	include; including
EMG	electromyogram		inflam	inflammation
EPF	expanded problem-focused (history/examination)		init	initial (office visit)
			inj, INJ	injection
epith	epithelial		ins, INS[a]	insurance
ER	emergency room		int	internal
Er, ER[a]	error corrected		intermed	intermediate (office visit)
ESR	erythrocyte sedimentation rate		interpret	interpretation
est	established (patient); estimated		IUD	intrauterine device
Ex, exam	examination		IV	intravenous (injection)
exc	excision		IVP	intravenous pyelogram
Ex MO[a]	express money order		K 35	Kolman (an instrument used in urology)
ext	external		KUB	kidneys, ureters, and bladder
24F, 28F	French (size of catheter)		L	left; laboratory
F	female		lab, LAB	laboratory
FBS	fasting blood sugar		lat	lateral; pertaining to the side
FH	family history		lbs	pounds
ft	foot, feet		LC	low-complexity (decision making)
FU	follow-up (examination)		LMP	last menstrual period
fwd[a]	forward		LS	lumbosacral
Fx	fracture		lt	left
gb, GB	gallbladder		ltd	limited (office visit)
GGE	generalized glandular enlargement		L & W	living and well
GI	gastrointestinal		M	medication; married
Grav, grav	gravida, a pregnant woman; used with Roman numerals (I, II, III) to indicate the number of pregnancies		MC	moderate-complexity (decision making)
			MDM	medical decision making
			med	medicine
GU	genitourinary		mg	milligram(s)
H	hospital call		mg/dL	milligrams per deciliter
HA	headache		MI	myocardial infarction
HBP	high blood pressure		micro	microscopy
HC	hospital call or consultation; high-complexity (decision making)		mL, ml	milliliter
			mo	month(s)
HCD	house call (day)		MO[a]	money order
HCN	house call (night)		N	negative
Hct	hematocrit		NA	not applicable
HCVD	hypertensive cardiovascular disease		NAD	no appreciable disease
Hgb	hemoglobin		NC, N/C[a]	no charge
hist	history		NEC	not elsewhere classifiable
hosp	hospital		neg	negative
H&P	history and physical (examination)		NKA	no known allergies
hr, hrs	hour, hours		NOS	not otherwise specified
h.s.	before bedtime		NP	new patient
HS	hospital surgery		NYD	not yet diagnosed
Ht	height		OB, Ob-Gyn	obstetrics and gynecology
HV	hospital visit		OC	office call
HX, hx	history		occ	occasional
HX PX	history and physical examination		OD	right eye
I	injection		ofc	office
IC	initial consultation			

[a]Bookkeeping abbreviation.

OP	outpatient	rec	recommend
Op, op	operation	rec'd	received
OR	operating room	re ch	recheck
orig	original	re-exam	reexamination
OS	office surgery; left eye	Reg	regular
OV	office visit	ret, retn, rtn	return
oz	ounce	rev	review
PA	posterior-anterior; posteroanterior	RHD	rheumatic heart disease
Pap	Papanicolaou (smear, stain, test)	RN	registered nurse
Para I	woman having borne one child	R/O	rule out
PC	present complaint	ROA[a]	received on account
p.c.	after meals	RPT	registered physical therapist
PCP	primary care physician	rt	right
PD	permanent disability	RTC	return to clinic
Pd, PD[a]	professional discount	RTO	return to office
PE	physical examination	RTW	return to work
perf	performed	RX, Rx, Rx	prescribe; prescription; any medication or treatment ordered
PF	problem-focused (history/examination)		
PFT	pulmonary function test	S	surgery
PH	past history	SC	subcutaneous
Ph ex	physical examination	sched.	scheduled
phys	physical	SD	state disability
PID	pelvic inflammatory disease	SE	special examination
PM, p.m.	post meridiem (time—afternoon)	SF	straightforward (decision making)
PND	postnasal drip	Sig	directions on prescription
PO, P Op	postoperative	SLR	straight leg raising
p.o.	by mouth (per os)	slt	slight
post	posterior	Smr	smear
postop	postoperative	SOB	shortness of breath
PPD	purified protein derivative (such as in tuberculin test)	Sp gr	specific gravity
		SQ	subcutaneous (injection)
preop	preoperative	STAT	immediately
prep	prepared	strep	*Streptococcus*
PRN, p.r.n.	as necessary (pro re nata)	surg	surgery
Proc	procedure	Sx	symptom(s)
Prog	prognosis	T	temperature
P & S	permanent and stationary	T&A	tonsillectomy and adenoidectomy
PSA	prostate-specific antigen (blood test to determine cancer in the prostate gland)	Tb, tb	tuberculosis
		TD	temporary disability
		tech	technician
Pt, pt	patient	temp	temperature
PT	physical therapy	tet. tox.	tetanus toxoid
PTR	patient to return	t.i.d.	three times daily
PVC	premature ventricular contraction	TPR	temperature, pulse, and respiration
PVT ck[a]	private check received	Tr, trt	treatment
PX	physical examination	TURB	transurethral resection of bladder
q	every	TURP	transurethral resection of prostate
qd	one time daily, every day	TX	treatment
qh	every hour	u	units
q.i.d.	four times daily	UA, ua	urinalysis
QNS	quantity not sufficient	UCHD	usual childhood diseases
qod	every other day	UCR	usual, customary, and reasonable (fees)
R	right; residence call; report	UGI	upper gastrointestinal
RBC, rbc	red blood cell (count)	UPJ	ureteropelvic junction or joint

[a]Bookkeeping abbreviation.

UR	urinalysis
URI	upper respiratory infection
Urn	urinalysis
UTI	urinary tract infection
W	work; white
WBC, wbc	white blood cell (count); well baby care
WC	workers' compensation
wk	week; work
wks	weeks
WNL	within normal limits
Wr	Wassermann reaction (test for syphilis)
Wt, wt	weight
X	xray, x-ray(s), times (e.g., 3X means three times)
XR	xray, x-ray(s)
yr(s)	year(s)

Symbols

+	positive
#	pound(s)
$\bar{c}$, /c	with
$\bar{s}$, /s	without
$\bar{cc}$, $\bar{c}$/c	with correction (eye glasses)
$\bar{sc}$, $\bar{s}$/c	without correction (eye glasses)
-	negative
$\bar{0}$	negative
!, +	positive
(L)	left
(R)	right
♂	male
♀	female
$-^a$	charge already made
$\ominus^a$	no balance due
$\surd^a$	posted
($0.00)^a	credit

Laboratory Abbreviations

ABG	arterial blood gas(es)
AcG	factor V (AcG or proaccelerin); a factor in coagulation that converts prothrombin to thrombin
ACTH	adrenocorticotropic hormone
A/C ratio	albumin-coagulin ratio
AFB	acid-fast bacilli
AHB	alpha-hydroxybutyric (dehydrogenase)
AHG	antihemophilic globulin; antihemolytic globulin (factor)
ALA	aminolevulinic acid
ALT	alanine aminotransferase (*see* SGPT)
AMP	adenosine monophosphate
APT test	aluminum-precipitated toxoid test
AST	aspartate aminotransferase (*see* SGOT)
ATP	adenosine triphosphate
BSP	bromosulfophthalein (bromsulphalein; sodium sulfobromophthalein) (test)
BUN	blood urea nitrogen
CBC	complete blood count
CNS	central nervous system
CO	carbon monoxide
CPB	competitive protein binding: plasma
CPK	creatine phosphokinase
CSF	cerebrospinal fluid
D hemoglobin	hemoglobin fractionation by electrophoresis for hemoglobin D
DAP	direct agglutination pregnancy (Gravindex and DAP)
DEAE	diethylaminoethanol
DHT	dihydrotestosterone

---

^aBookkeeping abbreviation.

340

diff	differential
DNA	deoxyribonucleic acid
DRT	test for syphilis
EACA	epsilon-aminocaproic acid (a fibrinolysin)
EMIT	enzyme-multiplied immunoassay technique (for drugs)
ENA	extractable nuclear antigen
esr, ESR	erythrocyte sedimentation (sed) rate
FDP	fibrin degradation products
FIGLU	formiminoglutamic acid
FRAT	free radical assay technique (for drugs)
FSH	follicle-stimulating hormone
FSP	fibrinogen split products
FTA	fluorescent-absorbed treponema antibodies
Gc, Gm, Inv	immunoglobulin typing
GG, gamma G, A, D, G, M	gamma-globulin (immunoglobulin fractionation by electrophoresis)
GG, gamma G E, RIA	immunization E fractionation by radioimmunoassay
GGT	gamma-glutamyl transpeptidase
GLC	gas liquid chromatography
GMP	guanosine monophosphate
GTT	glucose tolerance test
G6PD	glucose-6-phosphate dehydrogenase
HAA	hepatitis-associated agent (antigen)
HBD, HBDH	hydroxybutyrate dehydrogenase
HCT	hematocrit
hemoglobin, electrophoresis	letters of the alphabet used for different types or factors of hemoglobins (includes A_2, S, C, etc.)
Hgb	hemoglobin, qualitative
HGH	human growth hormone
HI	hemagglutination inhibition
HIA	hemagglutination inhibition antibody
HIAA	hydroxyindoleacetic acid (urine), 24-hour specimen
HIV	human immunodeficiency virus
HLA	human leukocyte antigen (tissue typing)
HPL	human placental lactogen
HTLV-III	antibody detection; confirmatory test
HVA	homovanillic acid
ICSH	interstitial cell-stimulating hormone
IFA	intrinsic factor, antibody (fluorescent screen)
IgA, IgE, IgG, IgM	immunoglobulins: quantitative by gel diffusion
INH	isonicotinic hydrazide, isoniazid
LAP	leucine aminopeptidase
LATS	long-acting thyroid-stimulating (hormone)
LDH	lactic dehydrogenase
LE Prep	lupus erythematosus cell preparation
L.E. factor	antinuclear antibody
LH	luteinizing hormone
LSD	lysergic acid diethylamide

L/S ratio	lecithin-sphingomyelin ratio
MC (*Streptococcus*)	antibody titer
MIC	minimum inhibitory concentration
NBT	nitro-blue tetrazolium (test)
OCT	ornithine carbamoyltransferase
PAH	para-aminohippuric acid
PBI	protein-bound iodine
pCO$_2$	arterial carbon dioxide pressure (or tension)
PCP	phencyclidine piperidine
pcv	packed cell volume
pH	symbol for expression of concentration of hydrogen ions (degree of acidity)
PHA	phenylalanine
PIT	prothrombin inhibition test
PKU	phenylketonuria—a metabolic disease affecting mental development
PO$_2$	oxygen pressure
P&P	prothrombin-proconvertin
PSP	phenolsulfonphthalein
PT	prothrombin time
PTA	plasma thromboplastin antecedent
PTC	plasma thromboplastin component; phenylthiocarbamide
PTT	prothrombin time; partial thromboplastin time (plasma or whole blood)
RBC, rbc	red blood cells (count)
RIA	radioimmunoassay
RISA	radioiodinated human serum albumin
RIST	radioimmunosorbent test
RPR	rapid plasma reagin (test)
RT$_3$U	resin triiodothyronine uptake
S-D	strength-duration (curve)
SGOT	serum glutamic oxaloacetic transaminase (*see* AST)
SGPT	serum glutamic pyruvic transaminase (*see* ALT)
STS	serologic test for syphilis
T$_3$	triiodothyronine (uptake)
TB	tubercle bacillus, tuberculosis
TBG	thyroxine-binding globulin
T&B differentiation, lymphocytes	thymus-dependent lymphs and bursa-dependent lymphs
THC	tetrahydrocannabinol (marijuana)
TIBC	total iron-binding capacity, chemical
TLC screen	thin-layer chromatography screen
TRP	tubular reabsorption of phosphates
UA	urinalysis
VDRL	Venereal Disease Research Laboratory (agglutination test for syphilis)
VMA	vanillylmandelic acid
WBC, wbc	white blood cells (count)

Mock Fee Schedule

Refer to the Mock Fee Schedule (Table 2) to complete the financial accounting statements (ledgers) and claim forms in this *Workbook*. The fees listed are hypothetical and are intended only for use in completing the questions. For completion of CMS-1500 claim forms, use the amounts in the column labeled Mock Fees, unless instructed otherwise.

When completing the insurance claim forms, use the latest edition of *Current Procedural Terminology* (CPT), the professional code book published by the American Medical Association, to find the correct code numbers and modifiers for the services rendered. The Mock Fee Schedule (Table 2) is arranged in the same sequence as the six CPT code book sections (i.e., Evaluation and Management; Anesthesia; Surgery; Radiology, Nuclear Medicine, and Diagnostic Ultrasound; Pathology and Laboratory; and Medicine).

Note: # indicates that the code is not in numerical sequence.

Table 2. Mock Fee Schedule

Code No.	Description	Mock Fees	Medicare[a] Participating	Nonpartici-pating	Limiting Charge	Follow-Up Days
EVALUATION AND MANAGEMENT						
Office						
New Patient						
99202	Level 2	90.00	74.23	70.52	81.10	
99203	Level 3	120.00	105.25	99.99	114.99	
99204	Level 4	180.00	161.07	153.02	175.97	
99205	Level 5	230.00	203.66	193.48	222.50	
Established Patient						
99211	Level 1	30.00	22.54	21.41	24.62	
99212	Level 2	50.00	44.31	42.09	48.40	
99213	Level 3	90.00	73.37	69.70	80.16	
99214	Level 4	120.00	106.62	101.29	116.48	
99215	Level 5	160.00	143.35	136.18	156.61	
Hospital						
Hospital Observation						
99217	Observation Discharge	80.00	71.74	68.15	78.37	
99219	Level 2	150.00	134.28	127....		
99220	Level 3	200.00	182.89	173.75	199.81	
Subsequent Observation						
#99224	Level 1	50.00	39.19	37.23	42.81	
#99225	Level 2	80.00	71.93	68.33	78.58	
#99226	Level 3	120.00	103.51	98.33	113.08	

[a]Some services and procedures may not be considered a benefit under the Medicare program and when listed on a claim form, no reimbursement may be received. However, it is important to include these codes when billing because Medicare policies may change without an individual knowing of a new benefit. For this reason, some of the services shown in this Mock Fee Schedule do not have any amounts listed under the three Medicare columns.

Continued

Table 2. Mock Fee Schedule—cont'd

Code No.	Description	Mock Fees	Medicare[a] Participating	Nonpartici- pating	Limiting Charge	Follow-Up Days
Initial Inpatient						
99221	Level 1	110.00	100.36	95.34	109.64	
99222	Level 2	150.00	135.96	129.16	148.53	
99223	Level 3	220.00	200.02	190.05	218.56	
Subsequent Hospital						
99231	Level 1	50.00	38.85	36.91	42.45	
99232	Level 2	80.00	71.59	68.01	78.21	
233	Level 3	120.00	103.17	98.01	112.71	
99238	Discharge <30 min	80.00	72.09	68.49	78.76	
99239	Discharge >30 min	120.00	105.84	100.55	115.63	
Consultations						
Office Consultation						
99241	Level 1	60.00				
99242	Level 2	90.00				
99243	Level 3	110.00				
99244	Level 4	150.00				
99245	Level 5	200.00				
Inpatient Consultation						
99251	Level 1	80.00				
99252	Level 2	110.00				
99253	Level 3	130.00				
99254	Level 4	170.00				
99255	Level 5	220.00				
Emergency Department						
99281	Level 1	30.00	22.32	21.20	24.38	
99282	Level 2	50.00	42.96	40.81	46.93	
99283	Level 3	80.00	64.37	61.15	70.23	
99284	Level 4	130.00	117.91	112.01	128.81	
99285	Level 5	190.00	171.25	162.69	187.09	
Critical Care Services						
99291	First 30–74 minutes	310.00	274.85	261.11	300.28	
99292	Each addl. 30 min	140.00	121.69	115.61	132.95	
Neonatal Intensive Care						
#99468	Initial	1000.00	912.70	867.07	997.13	
#99469	Subsequent	440.00	395.23	375.47	431.79	
Initial Nursing Facility						
99304	Level 1	100.00	89.34	84.87	97.60	
99305	Level 2	150.00	128.17	121.76	140.02	
99306	Level 3	190.00	165.21	156.95	180.49	

[a]Some services and procedures may not be considered a benefit under the Medicare program and when listed on a claim form, no reimbursement may be received. However, it is important to include these codes when billing because Medicare policies may change without an individual knowing of a new benefit. For this reason, some of the services shown in this Mock Fee Schedule do not have any amounts listed under the three Medicare columns.

Table 2. Mock Fee Schedule—cont'd

Code No.	Description	Mock Fees	Medicare[a] Participating	Medicare[a] Nonpartici-pating	Medicare[a] Limiting Charge	Medicare[a] Follow-Up Days
Subsequent Nursing Facility Care						
99307	Level 1	50.00	43.42	41.25	47.44	
99308	Level 2	80.00	68.20	64.79	74.51	
99309	Level 3	100.00	90.08	85.58	98.42	
99310	Level 4	150.00	132.98	126.33	145.28	
99315	Discharge, =or <30 minutes	80.00	72.43	68.81	79.13	
99316	Discharge; >30 minutes	120.00	104.22	99.01	113.86	
Domiciliary, Rest Home, Custodial Care						
New Patient						
99324	Level 1	60.00	54.16	51.45	59.17	
99325	Level 2	90.00	78.79	74.85	86.08	
99326	Level 3	130.00	137.24	130.38	149.94	
99335	Level 2	110.00	94.49	89.77	103.24	
99336	Level 3	150.00	133.51	126.83	145.85	
99337	Level 4	220.00	192.26	182.65	210.05	
Home Services						
New Patient						
99341	Level 1	60.00	54.16	51.45	59.17	
99342	Level 2	90.00	77.76	73.87	84.95	
99343	Level 3	140.00	127.79	121.40	139.61	
99344	Level 4	200.00	180.58	171.55	197.28	
99345	Level 5	250.00	219.69	208.71	240.02	
Established Patient						
99347	Level 1	60.00	54.14	51.43	59.14	
99348	Level 2	100.00	83.22	79.06	90.92	
99349	Level 3	140.00	127.44	121.07	139.23	
99350	Level 4	200.00	177.31	168.44	193.71	
Prolonged Services With Direct (Face-to-Face) Patient Contact (Report in Addition to the Prolonged Services With Direct Contact						
Outpatient						
99354	First hour	150.00	128.27	121.86	140.14	
99355	Each addl. 30 min	110.00	97.47	92.60	106.49	
Inpatient						
99356	First hour	100.00	91.53	86.95	99.99	
99357	Each addl. 30 min	110.00	92.21	87.60	100.74	

[a]Some services and procedures may not be considered a benefit under the Medicare program and when listed on a claim form, no reimbursement may be received. However, it is important to include these codes when billing because Medicare policies may change without an individual knowing of a new benefit. For this reason, some of the services shown in this Mock Fee Schedule do not have any amounts listed under the three Medicare columns.

Continued

345

Table 2. Mock Fee Schedule—cont'd

Code No.	Description	Mock Fees	Medicare[a]			
			Participating	Nonparticipating	Limiting Charge	Follow-Up Days
Prolonged Services Without Direct Contact						
99358	First hour	130.00	110.55	105.02	120.77	
99359	Each addl. 30 min	60.00	53.84	51.15	58.82	
Physician Standby Service						
99360	Each 30 min	100.00				
Case Management Services						
Team Conferences						
99366		90.00				
99367–99368		110.00				
Telephone Calls						
99441	5–10 min	30.00				
99442	11–20 min	40.00				
99443	21–30 min	60.00				
Care Plan Oversight Services						
99374	15–29 minutes	100.00				
99375	30 min or more/month	100.00				
Preventive Medicine						
New Patient						
99381	Infant younger than 1 year	120.00				
99382	1–4 years	120.00				
99383	5–11 years	120.00				
99384	12–17 years	120.00				
99385	18–39 years	120.00				
99386	40–64 years	120.00				
99387	65 years and older	120.00				
Established Patient						
99391	Infant younger than year	100.00				
99392	1–4 years	100.00				
99393	5–11 years	100.00				
99394	12–17 years	100.00				
99395	18–39 years	100.00				
99396	40–64 years	100.00				
99397	65 years and older	100.00				
Counseling (new/est pt)						
Individual						
99401	15 min	50.00				
99402	30 min	70.00				
99403	45 min	90.00				
99404	60 min	100.00				

[a]Some services and procedures may not be considered a benefit under the Medicare program and when listed on a claim form, no reimbursement may be received. However, it is important to include these codes when billing because Medicare policies may change without an individual knowing of a new benefit. For this reason, some of the services shown in this Mock Fee Schedule do not have any amounts listed under the three Medicare columns.

Table 2. Mock Fee Schedule—cont'd

Code No.	Description	Mock Fees	Medicare[a] Participating	Medicare[a] Nonpartici-pating	Medicare[a] Limiting Charge	Medicare[a] Follow-Up Days
Group						
99411	30 min	70.00				
99412	60 min	100.00				
Other Preventive Medicine Services						
99420	Health hazard appraisal	80.00				
99429	Unlisted preventive med service	Variable				
Newborn Care						
99460	Birthing room delivery	110.00	94.88	90.14	103.66	
99461	Other than birthing room	100.00	89.57	85.09	97.85	
99462	Subsequent hospital care	50.00	41.74	39.65	45.60	
99465	Newborn resuscitation	160.00	145.0	137.81	158.48	
Anesthesiology						

Anesthesiology fees are presented here for CPT codes. However, each case would require a fee for time, e.g., every 15 minutes would be worth $55. This fee is determined according to the relative value system, calculated, and added into the anesthesia (CPT) fee. Some anesthetists may list a surgical code using an anesthesia modifier on a subsequent line for carriers that do not acknowledge anesthesia codes.

Code No.	Description	Mock Fees	Medicare[a] Participating	Medicare[a] Nonpartici-pating	Medicare[a] Limiting Charge	Medicare[a] Follow-Up Days
99100	Anes complicated by age	60.00				
99116	Anes complicated use total hypothermia	280.00				
99135	Anes complicated use hypotension	280.00				
99140	Anes complicated emer cond	110.00				
Physician Status Modifier Codes						
P-1	Normal healthy patient	00.00				
P-2	Patient with mild systemic disease	00.00				
P-3	Patient with severe systemic disease	60.00				
P-4	Patient with severe systemic disease that is a constant threat to life	110.0				
P-5	Moribund pt not expected to survive without operation	170				
P-6	Declared brain-dead pt, organs being removed for donor	.00				
Head						
00160	Anes nose/sinus (NEC)	280.00				
00172	Anes repair cleft palate	170.00				
Thorax						
00400	Anes for proc ant integumentary system of chest, incl SC tissue	170.00				
00402	Anes breast reconstruction	280.00				

[a]Some services and procedures may not be considered a benefit under the Medicare program and when listed on a claim form, no reimbursement may be received. However, it is important to include these codes when billing because Medicare policies may change without an individual knowing of a new benefit. For this reason, some of the services shown in this Mock Fee Schedule do not have any amounts listed under the three Medicare columns.

Continued

Appendix **College Clinic Office Policies and Mock Fee Schedule**

Table 2. Mock Fee Schedule—cont'd

Code No.	Description	Mock Fees	Medicare[a]			
			Participating	Nonpartici-pating	Limiting Charge	Follow-Up Days
00546	Anes pulmonary resection with thoracoplasty	280.00				
00600	Anes cervical spine and cord	560.00				
Lower Abdomen						
00800	Anes for proc lower ant abdominal wall	170.00				
00840	Anes intraperitoneal proc lower abdomen: NOS	330.00				
00842	Amniocentesis	220.00				
00914	Anes TURP	280.00				
00942	Anes colporrhaphy, colpotomy, colpectomy	220.00				
Upper Leg						
01210	Anes open proc hip joint; NOS	330.00				
01214	Total hip replacement	440.00				
Upper Arm and Elbow						
01740	Anes open proc humerus/elbow; NOS	220.00				
01758	Exc cyst/tumor humerus	280.00				
Radiologic Procedures						
01922	Anes CAT scan	390.00				
Miscellaneous Procedure(s)						
01999	Unlisted anes proc	Variable				
10060	I & D furuncle, onychia, paronychia; single	130.00	118.99	113.04	130.00	10
11042	Débridement; skin, partial thickness	140.00	123.20	117.04	134.60	10
11043	Debridement; muscle/fascia	250.00	228.58	217.15	249.72	10
11044	Débridement; skin, subcu. muscle, bone	340.00	308.50	293.08	337.04	10
11102	Tangential biopsy; single lesion	110.00	97.91	93.01	106.96	10
11103	Tangential biopsy; each additional	60.00	52.03	49.43	56.84	10
11104	Punch biopsy; single lesion	140.00	123.19	117.03	134.58	10
11105	Punch biopsy; each additional	70.00	59.37	56.40	64.86	10
11106	Incisional biopsy; single lesion	170.00	149.27	141.81	163.08	10
11107	Incisional biopsy; each additional	80.00	70.52	66.99	77.04	10
11200	Exc, skin tags; up to 15	100.00	87.09	82.74	95.15	10
11401	Exc, benign lesion, 0.6–1.0 cm trunk, arms, legs	170.00	150.16	142.65	164.05	10
11402	1.1–2.0 cm	190.00	166.54	158.21	181.94	10
11403	2.1–3.0 cm	210.00	192.08	182.48	209.85	10
11420	Exc, benign lesion, 0.5 cm or less scalp, neck, hands, feet, genitalia	140.00	124.36	118.14	135.86	10

[a]Some services and procedures may not be considered a benefit under the Medicare program and when listed on a claim form, no reimbursement may be received. However, it is important to include these codes when billing because Medicare policies may change without an individual knowing of a new benefit. For this reason, some of the services shown in this Mock Fee Schedule do not have any amounts listed under the three Medicare columns.

Table 2. Mock Fee Schedule—cont'd

Code No.	Description	Mock Fees	Medicare[a] Participating	Medicare[a] Nonparticipating	Medicare[a] Limiting Charge	Follow-Up Days
11421	Exc, benign lesion, 0.6–1.0 cm scalp, neck, hands, feet, genitalia	180.00	156.72	148.88	171.21	10
11422	Exc, benign lesion scalp, neck, hands, feet, or genitalia; 1.1–2.0 cm	200.00	176.16	167.35	192.45	10
11441	Exc, benign lesion face, ears, eyelids, nose, lips, or mucous membrane	190.00	168.40	159.98	183.98	10
11602	Exc, malignant lesion, trunk, arms, or legs; 1.1–2.0 cm dia	270.00	242.60	230.47	265.04	10
11719	Trimming of nondystrophic nails, any number	20.00	13.94	13.24	15.23	0
11720	Débridement of nails, any method, 1–5	40.00	32.2	30.59	35.18	0
11721	6 or more	50.00	44.	42.51	48.89	0
11730	Avulsion nail plate, partial or complete, simple repair; single	120.00	108	103.35	118.85	0
11750	Exc, nail or nail matrix, partial or complete	170.00	1 2	146.70	168.71	10
11765	Wedge excision of nail fold	190.00	.12	157.81	181.48	10
12001	Simple repair (scalp, neck, axillae, ext genitalia, trunk, or extremities incl. hands & feet); 2.5 cm or less	100.00	8.59	84.16	96.78	10
12011	Simple repair (face, ears, eyelids, nose, lips, or mucous membranes); 2.5 cm or less	120.00	107.96	102.56	117.94	10
12013	2.6 5.0 cm	130.00	112.73	107.09	123.15	10
12032	Repair, scalp, axillae, trunk (intermediate)	330.00	296.78	281.94	324.23	10
12034	Repair, intermediate, wounds (scalp, axillae, trunk, or extremities) excl hands or feet, 7.6–12.5 cm	350	318.48	302.56	347.94	10
12051	Repair, intermediate, layer closure of wounds (face, ears, eyelids, nose, lips, or mucous membranes); 2.5 cm or less	.00	266.80	253.46	291.48	10
17000	Cauterization, 1 lesion	70.00	64.01	60.81	69.93	10
17003	Second through 14 lesions, each	10.00	5.91	5.61	6.45	10
17004	Destruction (laser surgery), 15 or more lesions	170.00	155.09	147.34	169.44	10
19020	Mastotomy, drainage/exploration dee abscess	510.00	463.17	440.01	506.01	90
19100	Biopsy, breast, needle	170.00	150.35	142.83	164.25	0
19101	Biopsy, breast, incisional	360.00	328.66	312.23	359.06	10
20610	Arthrocentesis, aspiration or inje on major joint (shoulder, hip, k , or bursa)	70.00	60.97	57.92	66.61	0

[a]Some services and procedures may not be c sidered a benefit under the Medicare program and when listed on a claim form, no reimbursement may be received. Howev it is important to include these codes when billing because Medicare policies may change without an individual knowing of a w benefit. For this reason, some of the services shown in this Mock Fee Schedule do not have any amounts listed under the thre Medicare columns.

Continued

Table 2. Mock Fee Schedule—cont'd

Code No.	Description	Mock Fees	Medicare[a]			
			Participating	Nonpartici- pating	Limiting Charge	Follow-Up Days
21330	Nasal fracture, open treatment complicated	610.00	551.33	523.76	602.32	90
24066	Biopsy, deep, soft tissue, upper arm, elbow	670.00	611.61	581.03	668.18	90
27455	Osteotomy, proximal tibia	1030.00	941.29	894.23	1028.36	90
27500	Treatment closed femoral shaft fracture without manipulation	570.00	513.79	488.10	561.32	90
27530	Treatment closed tibial fracture, proximal, without manipulation	330.00	298.36	283.44	325.96	90
27750	Treatment closed tibial shaft fracture, without manipulation	380.00	339.98	322.98	371.43	90
27752	With manipulation	580.00	528.17	501.76	577.02	90
29280	Strapping of hand or finger	40.00	30.41	28.89	33.22	0
29345	Appl long leg cast (thigh to toes)	150.00	131.98	125.38	144.19	0
29355	Walker or ambulatory type	160.00	138.29	131.38	151.09	0
30110	Excision, simple nasal polyp	260.00	234.81	223.07	256.53	10
30520	Septoplasty	700.00	636.03	604.23	694.86	90
30903	Control nasal hemorrhage; unilateral	250.00	222.93	211.78	243.55	0
30905	Control nasal hemorrhage, posterior with posterior nasal packs and/or cautery; initial	370.00	331.19	314.63	361.82	0
30906	Subsequent	380.00	345.47	328.20	377.43	0
31540	Laryngoscopy with excision of tumor and/or stripping of vocal cords	270.00	238.22	226.31	260.26	0
31541	With operating microscope	290.00	259.95	246.95	283.99	0
31575	Laryngoscopy, flexible fiberoptic; diagnostic	140.00	120.33	114.31	131.46	0
31625	Bronchoscopy with biopsy	380.00	339.37	322.40	370.76	0
32310	Pleurectomy	1000.00	896.70	851.87	979.65	90
32440	Pneumonectomy, total	1690.00	1539.60	1462.62	1682.04	90
33020	Pericardiotomy	890.00	812.76	772.12	887.94	90
33206	Insertion of pacemaker; atrial	500.00	449.29	426.83	490.85	90
33208	Atrial and ventricular	570.00	515.55	489.77	563.24	90
35301	Thromboendarterectomy, with or without patch graft; carotid, vertebral, subclavian, by neck incision	1220.00	1115.96	1060.16	1219.18	90
36005	Intravenous injection for contrast venography	320.00	290.31	275.79	317.16	0
36248	Catheter placement (selective) arterial system, 2nd, 3rd order and beyond	150.00	135.32	128.55	147.83	0
36415	Routine venipuncture for collection of specimen(s)	10.00				0

[a]Some services and procedures may not be considered a benefit under the Medicare program and when listed on a claim form, no reimbursement may be received. However, it is important to include these codes when billing because Medicare policies may change without an individual knowing of a new benefit. For this reason, some of the services shown in this Mock Fee Schedule do not have any amounts listed under the three Medicare columns.

Table 2. Mock Fee Schedule—cont'd

Code No.	Description	Mock Fees	Medicare[a] Participating	Nonpartici- pating	Limiting Charge	Follow-Up Days
38101	Splenectomy, partial	1260.00	1152.91	1095.26	1259.55	90
38220	Bone marrow; aspiration only	180.00	164.15	155.94	179.33	0
38221	Biopsy, needle or trocar	170.00	154.89	147.15	169.22	0
38510	Biopsy/excision deep cervical node/s	570.00	517.88	491.99	565.7?	10
39540	Hernia repair	950.00	861.19	818.13	940.8?	90
42820	T&A under age 12 years	320.00	285.36	271.09	311.7?	90
42821	T&A over age 12 years	330.00	297.67	282.79	325.21	90
43200	Upper GI endoscopy, simple primary exam	260.00	237.07	225.22	259.00	0
43235	Upper GI endoscopy incl. esophagus, stomach, duodenum, or jejunum; complex	310.00	275.17	261.41	300.62	0
43239	Esophagogastro-duodenoscopy, with biopsy, single or multiple	410.00	366.54	348.21	400.44	0
43255	With control of bleeding, any method	710.00	644.38	612.16	703.98	0
43453	Dilation esophagus	950.00	862.17	819.06	941.92	0
43754	Gastric intubation	200.00	177.84	168.95	194.29	0
43820	Gastrojejunostomy	1460.00	1331.48	1264.91	1454.65	90
44150	Colectomy, total, abdominal	2020.00	1847.72	1755.33	2018.63	90
44320	Colostomy or skin level cecostomy	1310.00	1190.30	1130.79	1300.41	90
44950	Appendectomy	700.00	636.90	605.06	695.82	90
45308	Proctosigmoidoscopy; removal of polyp	200.00	179.41	170.44	196.01	0
45315	Multiple polyps	230.00	202.45	192.33	221.18	0
45330	Sigmoidoscopy (flexible), diagnostic (with or without biopsy or collection of specimen by brushing or washing)	190.00	171.45	162.88	187.31	0
45333	Sigmoidoscopy (flexible) with removal of polyps	340.00	306.94	291.59	335.33	0
45380	Colonoscopy with biopsy	460.00	418.79	397.85	457.53	
46255	Hemorrhoidectomy int & ext, simple	560.00	510.46	484.94	557.68	
46258	Hemorrhoidectomy with fistulectomy	510.00	466.78	443.44	509.96	?
46600	Anoscopy; diagnostic	120.00	101.03	96.01	110.41	
46614	With control of hemorrhage	160.00	144.87	137.63	158.27	?
46700	Anoplasty, for stricture, adult	720.00	653.04	620.39	713.45	90
47562	Cholecystectomy; laparoscopic	720.00	652.28	619.67	712.62	90
47600	Cholecystectomy; abdominal excision	1160.00	1059.61	1006.63	1157.62	90
49505	Inguinal hernia repair, age 5 or over	570.00	515.96	490.16	563.68	90
49520	Repair, inguinal hernia, any age; reducible	690.00	625.62	594.34	683.49	90
50080	Nephrostolithotomy, percutaneous	1000.00	871.17	827.61	951.75	90
50780	Ureteroneocystostomy	1210.00	1107.41	1052.04	1209.85	90

[a]Some services and procedures may not be considered a benefit under the Medicare program and when listed on a claim form, no reimbursement may be received. However, it is important to include these codes when billing because Medicare policies may change without an individual knowing of a new benefit. For this reason, some of the services shown in this Mock Fee Schedule do not have any amounts listed under the three Medicare columns.

Continued

Appendix **College Clinic Office Policies and Mock Fee Schedule**

Table 2. Mock Fee Schedule—cont'd

Code No.	Description	Mock Fees	Medicare[a]			
			Participating	Nonpartici-pating	Limiting Charge	Follow-Up Days
51900	Closure of vesicovaginal fistula, abdominal approach	910.00	826.13	784.82	902.54	90
52000	Cystourethroscopy	230.00	206.64	196.31	225.76	0
52601	Transurethral resection of prostate	800.00	730.91	694.36	798.51	90
53040	Drainage of deep periurethral abscess	430.00	392.62	372.99	428.94	90
53060	Drainage of Skene's gland	210.00	185.16	175.90	202.29	10
53230	Excision, female diverticulum (urethral)	670.00	609.20	578.74	665.55	90
53240	Marsupialization of urethral diverticulum, M or F	470.00	424.16	402.95	463.39	90
53270	Excision of Skene's gland(s)	230.00	207.37	197.00	226.55	10
53620	Dilation, urethra, male	160.00	145.98	138.68	159.48	0
53660	Dilation urethra, female	80.00	69.73	66.24	76.18	0
54150	Circumcision	170.00	151.95	144.35	166.00	10
54520	Orchiectomy, simple	360.00	325.59	309.31	355.71	90
55700	Biopsy of prostate, needle or punch	270.00	245.10	232.85	267.78	0
55801	Prostatectomy, perineal subtotal	1200.00	1097.82	1042.93	1199.37	90
57265	Colporrhaphy AP with enterocele repair	950.00	867.74	824.35	948.00	90
57452	Colposcopy	130.00	118.71	112.77	129.69	0
57510	Cauterization of cervix, electro or thermal	170.00	149.04	141.59	162.83	10
57520	Conization of cervix with or without D&C, with or without repair	370.00	330.26	313.75	360.81	90
58100	Endometrial biopsy	110.00	96.38	91.56	105.29	0
58120	D&C, diagnostic and/or therapeutic (non-OB)	310.00	278.19	264.28	303.92	10
58150	TAH w/without salpingo-oophorectomy	1110.00	1007.35	956.98	1100.53	90
58200	Total hysterectomy, extended, corpus	1470.00	1344.53	1277.30	1468.90	90
58210	Radical abdominal hysterectomy with bilateral total pelvic lymphadenectomy	1980.00	1803.30	1713.14	1970.11	90
58300	Insertion of intrauterine device	100.00				0
58340	Hysterosalpingography, inj proc for	210.00	190.31	180.79	207.91	0
58720	Salpingo-oophorectomy, complete or partial, unilateral or bilateral surgical treatment of ectopic pregnancy	820.00	742.01	704.91	810.65	90
59120	Ectopic pregnancy requiring salpingectomy and/or oophorectomy	870.00	793.86	754.17	867.30	90
59121	Without salpingectomy and/or oophorectomy	870.00	794.81	755.07	868.33	90
59130	Abdominal pregnancy	1020.00	924.94	878.69	1010.49	90
59135	Total hysterectomy, interstitial, uterine pregnancy	1000.00	914.31	868.59	998.88	90

[a]Some services and procedures may not be considered a benefit under the Medicare program and when listed on a claim form, no reimbursement may be received. However, it is important to include these codes when billing because Medicare policies may change without an individual knowing of a new benefit. For this reason, some of the services shown in this Mock Fee Schedule do not have any amounts listed under the three Medicare columns.

Table 2. Mock Fee Schedule—cont'd

Code No.	Description	Mock Fees	Medicare[a] Participating	Medicare[a] Nonpartici- pating	Medicare[a] Limiting Charge	Follow-Up Days
59136	Partial uterine resection, interstitial uterine pregnancy	960.00	876.93	833.08	958.04	90
59140	Cervical, with evacuation	450.00	403.66	383.48	441.00	90
59160	Curettage postpartum hemorrhage (separate proc)	260.00	235.08	223.33	256.83	10
59400	OB care—routine, incl. antepartum/ postpartum care	2290.00	2087.85	1983.46	2280.98	0
59510	C-section including antepartum and postpartum care	2630.00	2308.21	2192.80	2521.72	0
59515	C-section, postpartum care only	1370.00	1245.83	1183.54	1361.07	0
59812	Treatment of incompl. abortion, any trimester	370.00	335.20	318.44	366.21	90
61314	Craniotomy infratentorial	1930.00	1762.20	1674.09	1925.20	90
62270	Spinal puncture, lumbar; diagnostic	150.00	136.90	130.06	149.57	0
65091	Evisceration of eye, without implant	750.00	677.79	643.90	740.49	90
65205	Removal of foreign body, ext eye	50.00	37.07	35.22	40.50	0
65222	Removal of foreign body, corneal, with slit lamp	80.00	67.26	63.90	73.49	0
69420	Myringotomy	130.00	116.95	111.10	127.77	10
RADIOLOGY, NUCLEAR MEDICINE, AND DIAGNOSTIC ULTRASOUND						
70120	X-ray mastoids, less than 3 views per side	40.00	35.50	33.73	38.79	
70130	Complete, min., 3 views per side	70.00	58.01	55.11	63.38	
71045	Chest x-ray, single view	30.00	24.85	23.61	27.15	
71046	Chest x-ray, 2 views	40.00	31.79	30.20	34.73	
71048	Chest x-ray, 4 or more views	50.00	43.63	41.45	47.67	
72100	X-ray spine, LS; 2 or 3 views	50.00	36.94	35.09	40.35	
72114	Complete, incl. bending views	70.00	57.69	54.81	63.03	
73100	X-ray wrist, 2 views	40.00	31.68	30.10	34.62	
73501	Hip x-ray, unilateral 1 view	40.00	30.69	29.16	33.53	
73502	Hip x-ray, unilateral 2–3 views	50.00	43.81	41.62	47.86	
73590	X-ray tibia & fibula, 2 views	40.00	29.62	28.14	32.36	
73620	Radiologic exam, foot; 2 views	30.00	26.87	25.53	29.36	
73650	X-ray calcaneus, 2 views	30.00	27.22	25.86	29.74	
74248	X-ray, Small bowel	90.00	80.62	76.59	88.08	
74270	X-ray, colon	170.00	150.31	142.79	164.21	
74290	Cholecystography, oral contrast	90.00	79.72	75.73	87.09	
74400	Urography (pyelography), intravenous, with or without KUB	140.00	124.23	118.02	135.72	
74410	Urography, infusion	140.00	126.29	119.98	137.98	

[a]Some services and procedures may not be considered a benefit under the Medicare program and when listed on a claim form, no reimbursement may be received. However, it is important to include these codes when billing because Medicare policies may change without an individual knowing of a new benefit. For this reason, some of the services shown in this Mock Fee Schedule do not have any amounts listed under the three Medicare columns.

Continued

Appendix **College Clinic Office Policies and Mock Fee Schedule**

Table 2. Mock Fee Schedule—cont'd

Code No.	Description	Mock Fees	Medicare[a] Participating	Medicare[a] Nonpartici-pating	Medicare[a] Limiting Charge	Medicare[a] Follow-Up Days
74420	Urography, retrograde	80.00	72.06	68.46	78.73	
76805	Ultrasound, pregnant uterus, or real time; complete, first gestation	150.00	136.82	129.98	149.48	
76810	Ultrasound, pregnant uterus, complete: each additional gestation, after first trimester	100.00	90.08	85.58	98.42	
76946	Ultrasonic guidance for amniocentesis	40.00	31.72	30.13	34.65	
77065	Diagnostic mammography; unilateral	150.00	130.67	124.14	142.76	
77066	Diagnostic mammography; bilateral	180.00	164.67	156.44	179.91	
77300	Radiation dosimetry	80.00	65.36	62.09	71.40	
77307	Teletherapy, isodose plan, complex	320.00	285.14	270.88	311.51	
78104	Bone marrow imaging, whole body	270.00	245.89	233.60	268.64	
78215	Liver and spleen imaging	210.00	192.20	182.59	209.98	
78800	Tumor localization, limited area	280.00	254.55	241.82	278.09	

PATHOLOGY AND LABORATORY[1]
ORGAN OR DISEASE-ORIENTED PANELS

Code No.	Description	Mock Fees	Medicare[a] Participating	Medicare[a] Nonpartici-pating	Medicare[a] Limiting Charge	Medicare[a] Follow-Up Days
80048	Basic metabolic panel	10.00	8.46			
80050	General health panel	20.00				
80051	Electrolyte panel	10.00	7.01			
80053	Comprehensive metabolic panel	20.00	10.56			
80055	Obstetric panel	50.00	47.81			
80061	Lipid panel	20.00	13.39			
80074	Acute hepatitis panel	50.00	47.63			
80076	Hepatic function panel	10.00	8.17			
81000	Urinalysis, nonautomated, with microscopy	10.00	4.02			
81001	Urinalysis, automated, with microscopy	10.00	3.17			
81002	Urinalysis, nonautomated without microscopy	10.00	3.48			
81015	Urinalysis, microscopy only	10.00	3.05			
82270	Blood, occult; feces screening 1–3	10.00	4.38			
82565	Creatinine; blood	10.00	5.12			
82947	Glucose; quantitative	10.00	3.93			
82951	Glucose tolerance test, 3 spec	20.00	12.87			
82952	Each add spec beyond 3	10.00	3.92			
83020	Hemoglobin, electrophoresis	20.00	12.87			
83700	Lipoprotein, blood; electrophoretic separation	20.00	11.26			
84478	Triglycerides, blood	10.00	5.74			
84480	Triiodothyronine (T-3)	20.00	14.18			

[a]Some services and procedures may not be considered a benefit under the Medicare program and when listed on a claim form, no reimbursement may be received. However, it is important to include these codes when billing because Medicare policies may change without an individual knowing of a new benefit. For this reason, some of the services shown in this Mock Fee Schedule do not have any amounts listed under the three Medicare columns.

Table 2. Mock Fee Schedule—cont'd

Code No.	Description	Mock Fees	Medicare[a] Participating	Nonpartici- pating	Limiting Charge	Follow-Up Days
84520	Urea nitrogen, blood (BUN); quantitative	10.00	3.95			
84550	Uric acid, blood chemical	10.00	4.52			
84702	Gonadotropin, chorionic; quantitative	20.00	15.05			
84703	Gonadotropin, chorionic; qualitative	10.00	7.52			
85013	Microhematocrit (spun)	10.00	7.00			
85025	Complete blood count (hemogram), platelet count, automated, differential WBC count	10.00	7.77			
85032	Manual cell count (erythrocyte, leukocyte, or platelet) each	10.00	4.31			
85345	Coagulation time; Lee & White	10.00	4.69			
86038	Antinuclear antibodies	20.00	12.09			
86580	Skin test, TD, intradermal	10.00	7.74			
87081	Culture, bacterial, screening for single organisms	10.00	6.63			
87181	Sensitivity studies, antibiotic; per antibiotic	10.00	4.75			
87184	Disk method, per plate (12 disks or less)	10.00	7.48			
87210	Smear, primary source, wet mount with simple stain, for bacteria, fungi, ova, and/or parasites	10.00	5.82			
88150	Papanicolaou, cytopath	20.00	15.12			
88302	Surgical pathology, gross & micro exam (skin, fingers, nerve, testis)	30.00	29.61	28.41	32.67	
88305	Bone marrow, interpret	70.00	69.13	65.67	75.52	

MEDICINE PROCEDURES

Immunization Injections

Code No.	Description	Mock Fees	Participating	Nonpartici- pating	Limiting Charge	Follow-Up Days
90700	Diphtheria, tetanus, pertussis	34.00				

Therapeutic Injections

96372	Therapeutic prophylactic or Dx injection; IM or SC	20.00	13.94	13.24	15.23	
96374	Intravenous push, single or initial substance/drug	40.00	38.25	36.34	41.79	
96379	Intravenous therapeutic prophylactic, or diagnostic	30.00				

Psychiatry

90832	Individual psychotherapy 20–30 min	70.00	69.68	66.20	76.13	
90853	Group therapy	30.00	27.62	26.24	30.18	

Hemodialysis

90935	Single phys evaluation	80.00	73.12	69.46	79.88	
90937	Repeat evaluation	110.00	104.49	99.27	114.16	

[a]Some services and procedures may not be considered a benefit under the Medicare program and when listed on a claim form, no reimbursement may be received. However, it is important to include these codes when billing because Medicare policies may change without an individual knowing of a new benefit. For this reason, some of the services shown in this Mock Fee Schedule do not have any amounts listed under the three Medicare columns.

Continued

Appendix **College Clinic Office Policies and Mock Fee Schedule**

Table 2. Mock Fee Schedule—cont'd

Code No.	Description	Mock Fees	Medicare[a] Participating	Nonpartici- pating	Limiting Charge	Follow-Up Days
Gastroenterology						
91010	Esophageal incubation	200.00	197.25	187.39	215.50	
Ophthalmologic Services						
92004	Comprehensive eye exam	150.00	147.98	140.58	161.67	
92100	Tonometry	90.00	80.91	76.86	88.39	
92230	Fluorescein angioscopy	80.00	75.64	71.86	82.64	
92273	Electroretinography, full field	130.00	127.33	120.96	139.10	
92531	Spontaneous nystagmus	30.00				
Audiologic Function Tests						
92557	Comprehensive audiometry	40.00	37.84	35.95	41.34	
92596	Ear measurements	70.00	63.12	59.96	68.95	
Cardiovascular Therapeutic Services						
93000	Electrocardiogram (ECG)	20.00	16.58	15.75	18.11	
93015	Treadmill ECG	70.00	69.61	66.13	76.05	
93040	Rhythm ECG, 1–3 leads	20.00	12.43	11.81	13.58	
93306	Doppler echocardiography	210.00	203.23	193.07	222.03	
93307	Echocardiography without Doppler	140.00	138.18	131.27	150.96	
Pulmonary						
94010	Spirometry	40.00	34.45	32.73	37.64	
94060	Spirometry before and after bronchodilator	60.00	57.54	54.66	62.86	
94150	Vital capacity, total	20.00				
Allergy and Clinical Immunology						
95024	Intradermal tests; immediate reaction	10.00	7.82	7.43	8.54	
95028	Intradermal tests; delayed reaction	20.00	12.27	11.66	13.41	
95044	Patch tests	10.00	5.05	4.80	5.52	
95115	Treatment for allergy, single inj.	10.00	8.83	8.39	9.65	
95117	2 or more inj.	20.00	10.21	9.70	11.16	
95165	Allergen immunotherapy, single or multiple antigens, multiple-dose vials (professional svcs for preparation supervision)	20.00	14.09	13.39	15.40	
Neurology						
95819	Electroencephalogram—awake and	430.00	421.05	400.00	460.00	
95860	Electromyography, 1 extremity	120.00	117.87	111.98	128.78	
Physical Medicine						
97024	Diathermy	10.00	6.87	6.53	7.51	
97036	Hubbard tank, each 15 min	40.00	34.74	33.00	37.95	
97110	Physical therapy, initial 30 min	40.00	30.47	28.95	33.29	

[a]Some services and procedures may not be considered a benefit under the Medicare program and when listed on a claim form, no reimbursement may be received. However, it is important to include these codes when billing because Medicare policies may change without an individual knowing of a new benefit. For this reason, some of the services shown in this Mock Fee Schedule do not have any amounts listed under the three Medicare columns.

Table 2. Mock Fee Schedule—cont'd

| Code No. | Description | Mock Fees | Medicare[a] | | | |
			Participating	Nonpartici-pating	Limiting Charge	Follow-Up Days
97140	Manual therapy (manipulation, traction), one or more regions, each 15 min	30.00	28.03	26.63	30.62	
Chiropractic Manipulative Treatment						
98940	Chiropractic manipulative treatment; spinal 1–2 regions	30.00	28.18	26.77	30.79	
Special Services and Reports						
99000	Handling of specimen (transfer from Dr.'s office to lab)	10.00				
99050	Services provided after office hours, or on Sundays and holidays in addition to basic service in the office	30.00				
99053	Services between 10 PM and 8 AM in addition to basic service	40.00				
99056	Services normally provided in office requested by pt in location other than office	20.00				
99058	Office services provided on an emergency basis	30.00				
99070	Supplies and materials (itemize drugs and materials provided)	30.00				
99080	Special reports:					
	Insurance forms	10.00				
	WC extensive review report	200.00				

[a]Some services and procedures may not be considered a benefit under the Medicare program and when listed on a claim form, no reimbursement may be received. However, it is important to include these codes when billing because Medicare policies may change without an individual knowing of a new benefit. For this reason, some of the services shown in this Mock Fee Schedule do not have any amounts listed under the three Medicare columns.